Biomechanics and Functional Tissue Engineering

Edited by Ziyad S. Haidar, Ibrokhim Y. Abdurakhmonov and Abdelwahed Barkaoui

Published in London, United Kingdom

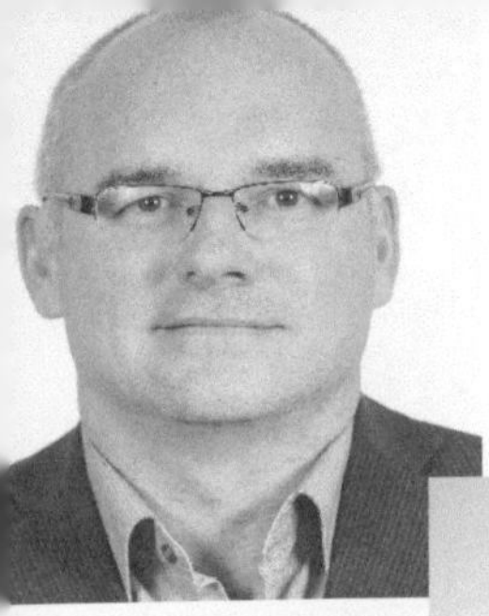
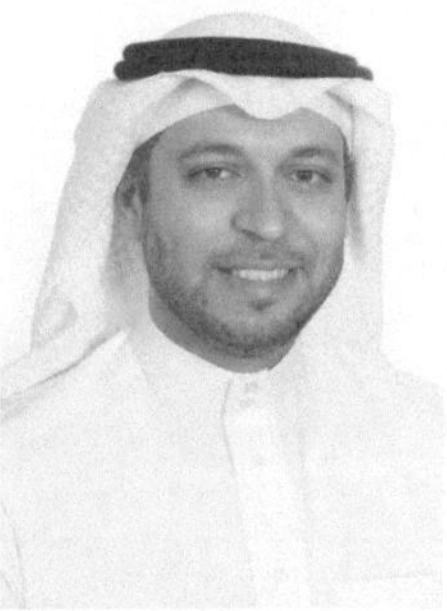
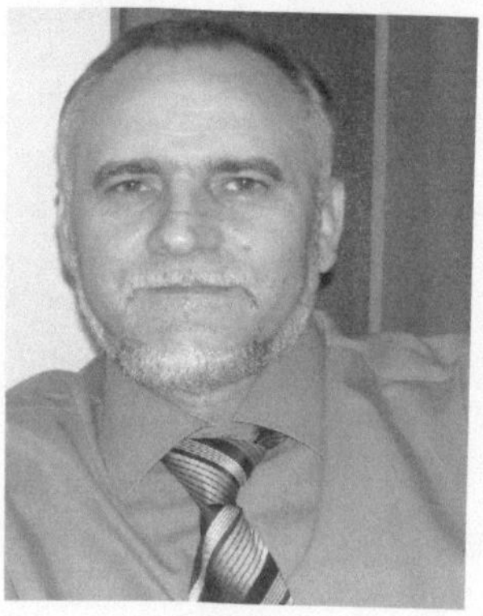
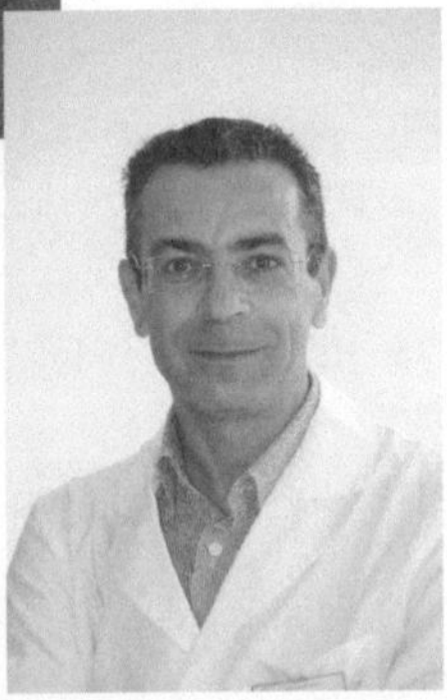
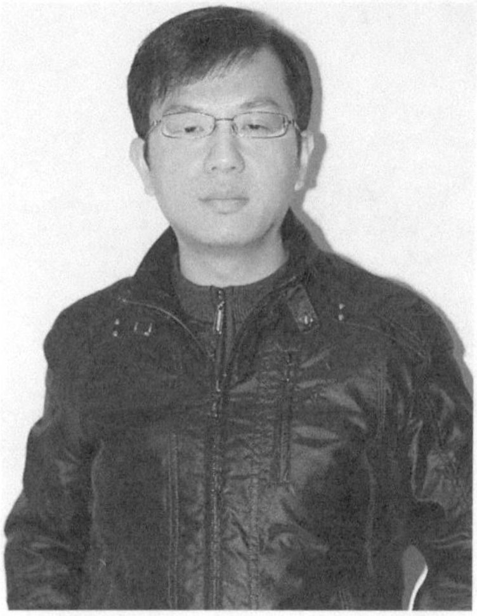
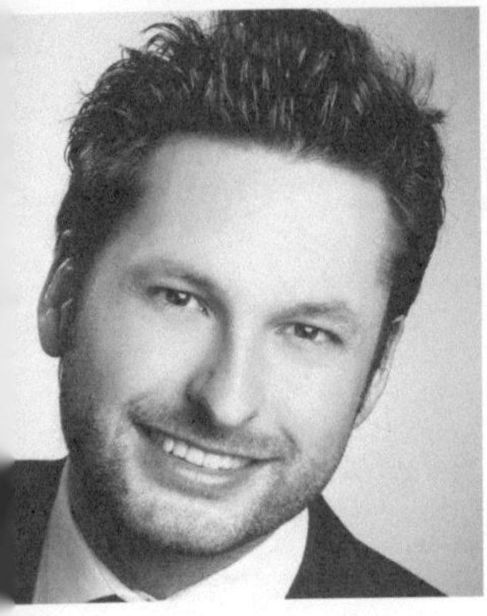
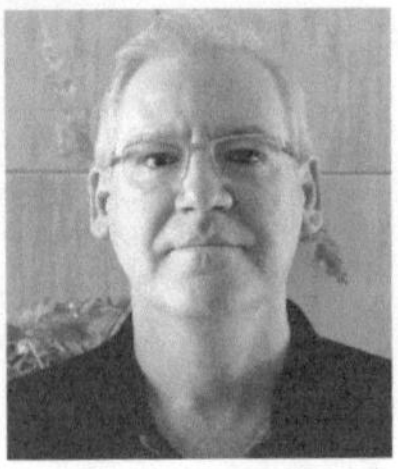

IntechOpen

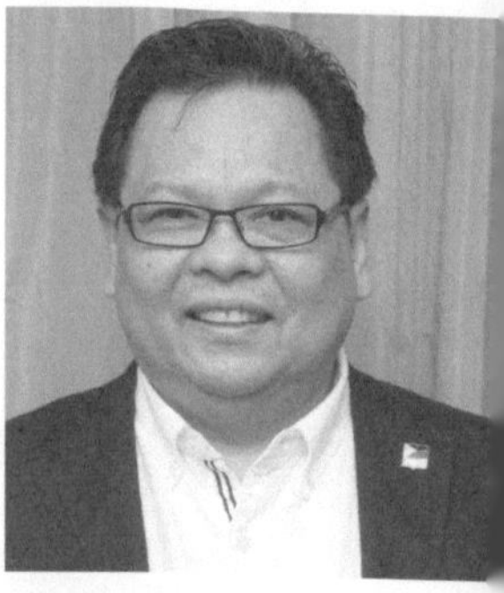
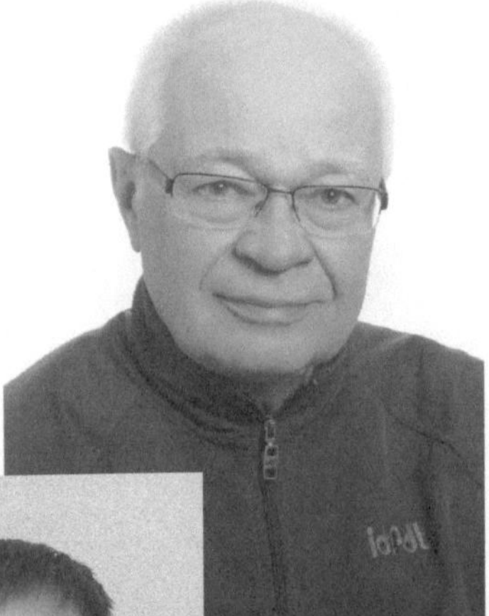
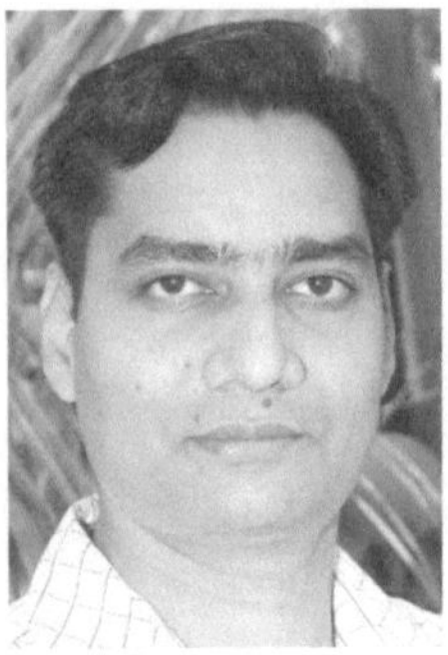
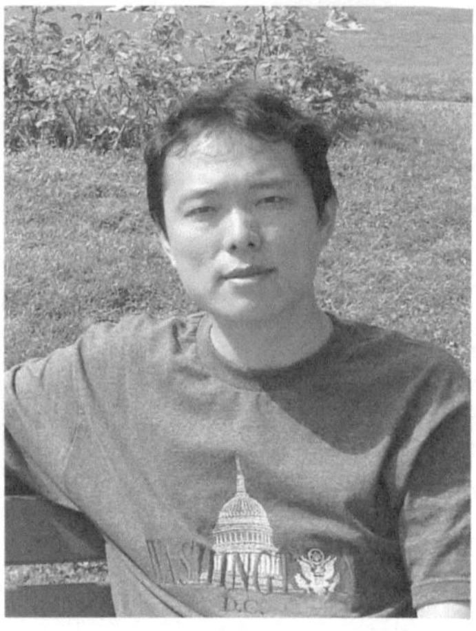
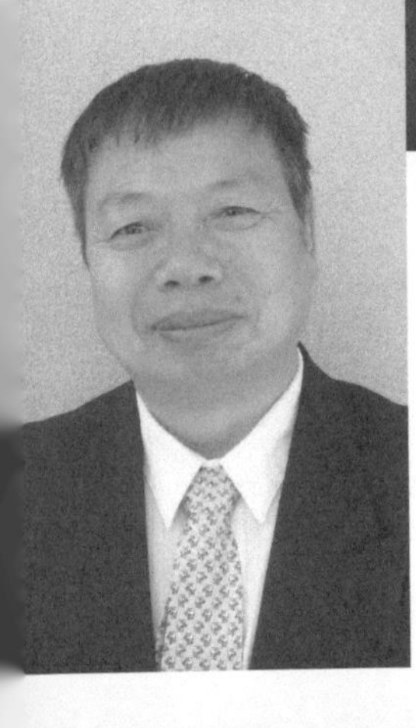
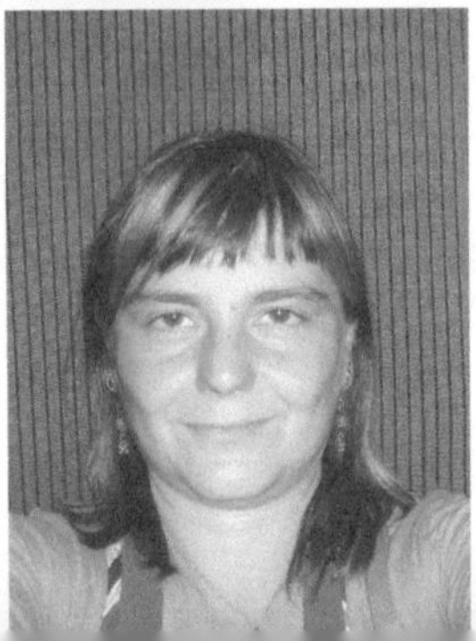

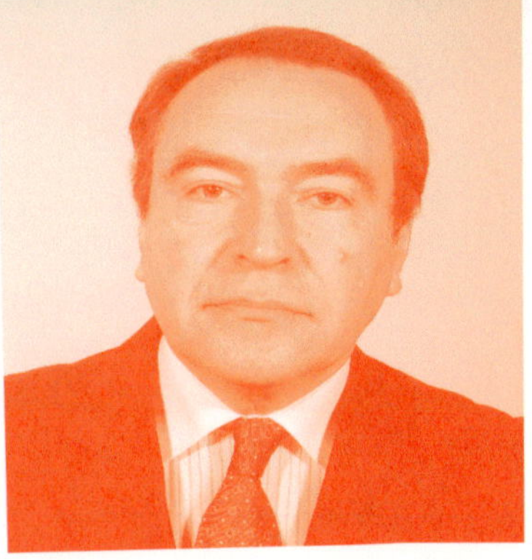

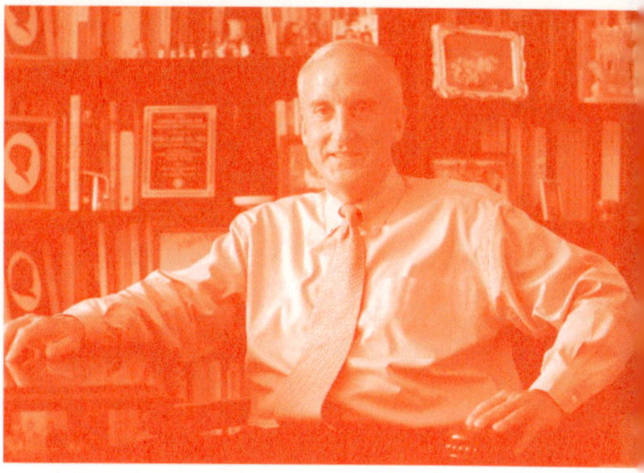

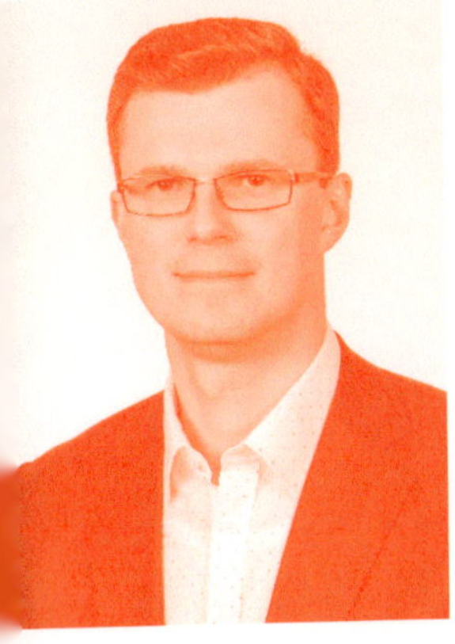

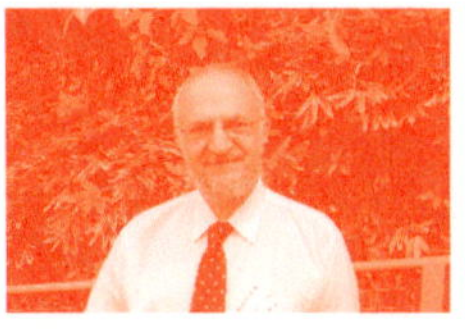

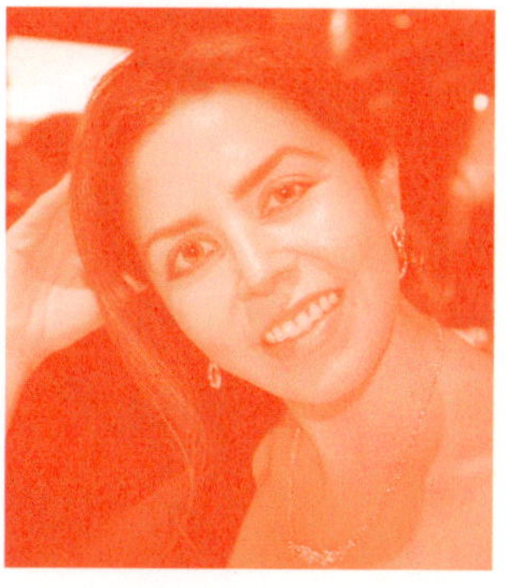

Supporting open minds since 2005

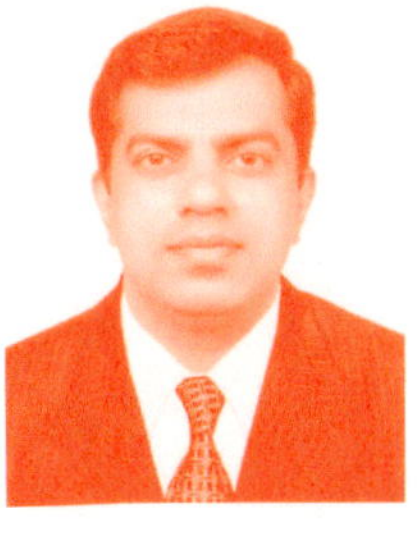

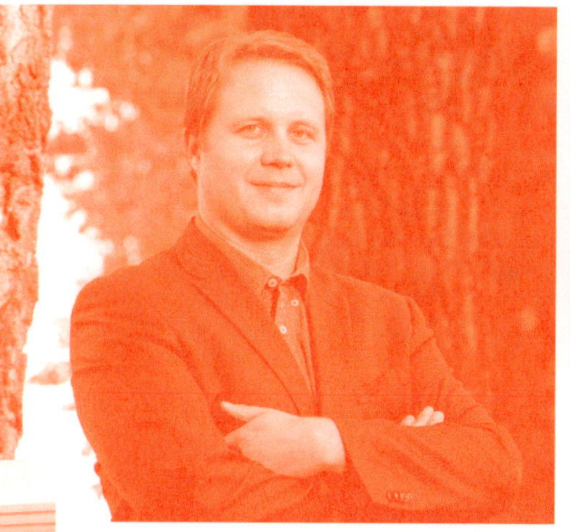

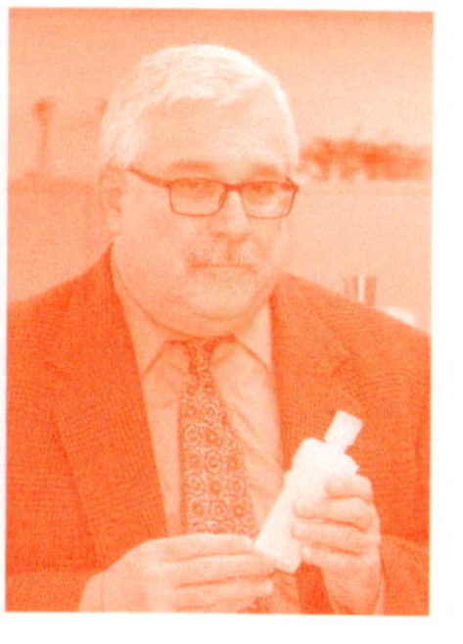

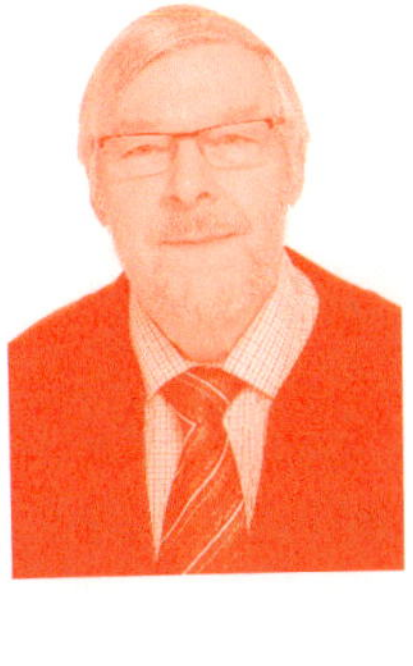

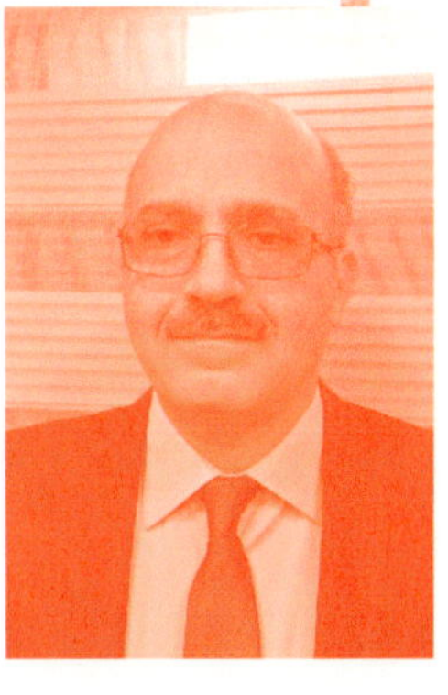

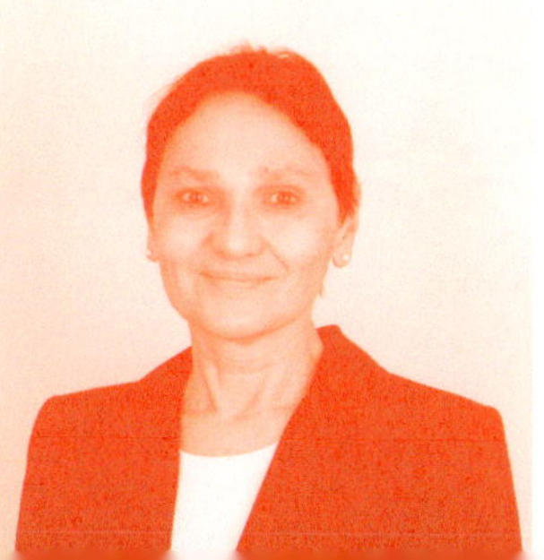

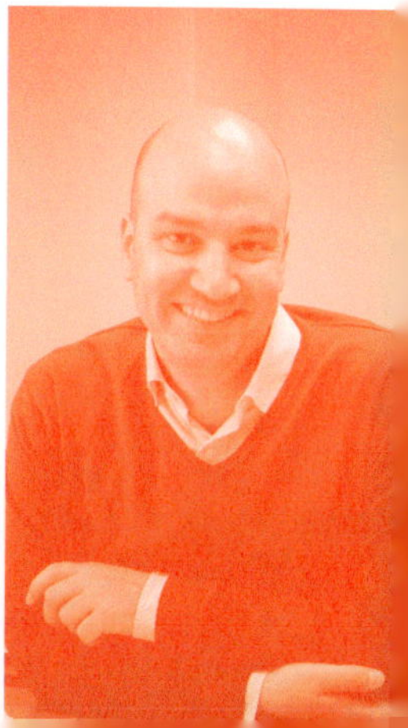

Biomechanics and Functional Tissue Engineering
http://dx.doi.org/10.5772/intechopen.91487
Edited by Ziyad S. Haidar, Ibrokhim Y. Abdurakhmonov and Abdelwahed Barkaoui

Contributors
Abdelwahed Barkaoui, Rabeb Ben Kahla, Fatma Zohra Ben Salah, Moez Chafra, Mohamed Boumaiza, Samia Rourou, Paolo Arosio, Mohamed Nejib Marzouki, Tanmoy Rath, Nilkamal Pramanik, Geetanjali B. Tomar, Nandika Bhattacharya, Sharvari Naik, Shravani Kulkarni, Suraj Math, Jay Dave, Sayali Chandekar, Kaushik Desai, Neha Sapkal, Gangaraju Gedda, Arun Bhupathi, V.L.N. Balaji Gupta Tiruveedhi, Brahim Tlili, H. Guizani, K. Aouadi, M. Nasser, Clotilde Castaldo, Immacolata Belviso, Veronica Romano, Franca Di Meglio, Daria Nurzynska, Imane Ait Oumghar, Patrick Chabrand, Ziyad S. Haidar, Sebastián E. Pérez, Stephen J. J. Fey, Krzysztof Wrzesinski, Søren Alnøe, Peter Willems-Alnøe, Julie S. Vistisen, Torsten D. Bryld, Karoline Mikkelsen, Hans H. Jochumsen

First published in London, United Kingdom, 2021 by IntechOpen
IntechOpen is the global imprint of INTECHOPEN LIMITED, registered in England and Wales, registration number: 11086078, 5 Princes Gate Court, London, SW7 2QJ, United Kingdom
Printed in Croatia

British Library Cataloguing-in-Publication Data
A catalogue record for this book is available from the British Library

Additional hard and PDF copies can be obtained from orders@intechopen.com

Biomechanics and Functional Tissue Engineering
Edited by Ziyad S. Haidar, Ibrokhim Y. Abdurakhmonov and Abdelwahed Barkaoui
p. cm.
Print ISBN 978-1-83880-285-1
Online ISBN 978-1-83880-286-8
eBook (PDF) ISBN 978-1-83880-417-6

Meet the editors

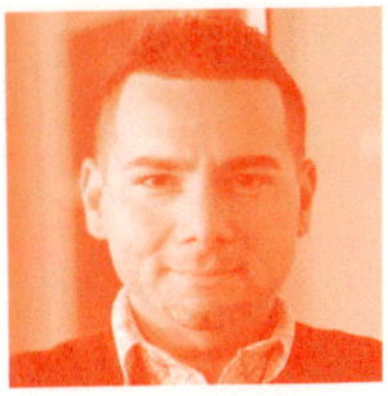

Ziyad S. Haidar, DDS, Cert Implantol, MSC, FRCSc, MBA, Ph.D., is a Full Professor of Biomaterials and Tissue Engineering and the scientific director of the Facultad de Odontología (Faculty of Dentistry), Universidad de los Andes (UAndes), Santiago, Chile. He is also the founder and head of the Biomaterials, Pharmaceutical Delivery, and Cranio-Maxillo-Facial Tissue Engineering Laboratory (BioMAT'X R&D&I Chile – HAIDAR Lab). In addition, he serves as the head of innovation at the Centro de Investigación e Innovación Biomédica (CiiB), a faculty/theses member in the bioMedicine Doctoral (Ph.D. bioMedicina) Program at UAndes, and a visiting clinical and surgical professor at the MaxilloFacial Division of the Universidad de la Frontera and the Department of Head and Neck Surgery, Lautaru Hospital, both in Temuco, Chile. Dr. Haidar is a trained dentist, implantologist, and an oral and maxillofacial surgeon with a Ph.D. in Nanobiomaterials, Pharmaceuticals, and Tissue Engineering from McGill University, Montréal, Canada. He completed a post-doctoral training residency in orthopedics at the Montréal Shriners Hospital, McGill University Health Center, Montréal, Canada. Before moving to Chile, he served as Associate Professor of Bioceramics and the Chair of Excellence in BioEngineering at the Université de Limoges, Limoges, France and was an assistant professor in the Department of Pharmaceutics and Pharmaceutical Chemistry (cross-appointment with the Department of BioEngineering), University of Utah, Salt Lake City, UT, USA. Between 2010 and 2012 Dr. Haidar served as an adjunct professor of Head and Neck Surgery and the scientific director of the joint Utah–Inha R&D Center, Inha University Hospital, Incheon, Seoul, South Korea. He has won several prestigious awards from the International Bone and Mineral Society, Society for Biomaterials, Canadian Biomaterial Society, and the Canadian and Lebanese Societies of Plastic Surgeons, to name a few. His R&D&I focus on patient-oriented development and evaluation of bionanotechnology, biopolymers, bioceramics, and drug delivery systems for the repair, restoration, reconstruction, and regeneration of challenging craniofacial and orthopedic defects. Dr. Haidar is an international speaker with more than 125 publications, conference proceedings, textbooks, and patents to his credit. He is also an editorial board member of several national and international scientific journals and periodicals.

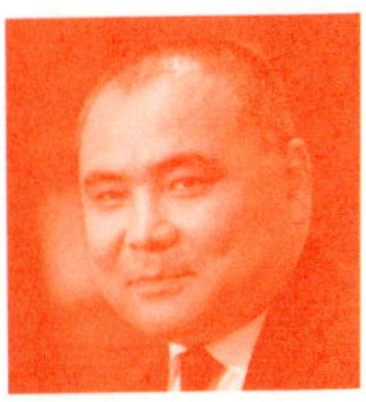

Ibrokhim Y. Abdurakhmonov received his B.S. (1997) *in biotechnology* from the National University, M.S. *in plant breeding* (2001) from Texas A&M University of USA, Ph.D. (2002) *in molecular genetics*, Doctor of Science (2009) *in genetics*, and full professorship (2011) *in molecular genetics and molecular biotechnology* from Academy of Sciences of Uzbekistan. He founded (2012) the Center of Genomics and Bioinformatics of Uzbekistan. He received the 2010 TWAS prize, and "ICAC Cotton Researcher of the Year 2013" for his outstanding contribution to cotton genomics and biotechnology. He was elected as The World Academy of Sciences (TWAS) Fellow (2014) and as a member (2017) of the Academy of Sciences of Uzbekistan. He was appointed (2017) as a Minister of Innovative Development of Uzbekistan.

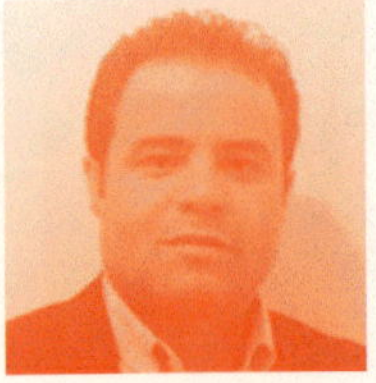

Abdelwahed Barkaoui is an Associate Professor of Mechanical Engineering at the International University of Rabat. He obtained his University habilitation from the University of Tunis El Manar-Tunisia in 2017 and his Ph.D. from the University of Orleans-France in 2012. he has a master's degree in mechanics obtained from the INSA of Lyon-France and a diploma of an engineer in electromechanical from ENI-Sfax Tunisia. Currently, assistant director of LERMA laboratory and coordinator of Modelling & Simulation in Biomechanics & Biomaterials (MS2B) team. He is responsible for mechanical discipline and coordinator of the ABET accreditation project at the Higher School of Energy Engineering. his research mainly concerns problems in biomechanics, mechanobiology, and biomedical engineering. He was a member of the editorial board of several international scientific journals: Frontiers in Bioengineering and Biotechnology "biomechanics" (IF=3,66), Series on Biomechanics, and reviewer for several international journals known in the field of biomechanics and mechanical engineering. Besides, he is the author of more than 60 publications in international journals, books, and conferences.

Contents

Preface

Craniofacial and orodental health are essential components of good overall health and wellbeing. The goal of the medical and dental professions with all their interdisciplinary and multidisciplinary subspecialties is to help the population achieve a stable and healthy head and neck and cranio-maxillofacial complex. Hence, identifying challenges and opportunities is integral, especially considering the increasing ageing population and demand for orodental health care, products, services, and alternative solutions. It is noteworthy that this agrees with and supports the global 2020 vision of the Fédération Dentaire Internationale (FDI) World Dental Federation, the world's leading dental professional organization on oral and dental health. The FDI proposes and urges expansion of the role of existing oral and dental healthcare professionals and fosters fundamental research and translational technologies to better mitigate the impacts of socioeconomic dynamics. In this context, this book focuses on the role of biomechanics and functional tissue engineering.

In brief, innovative engineering solutions that incorporate advanced biomaterials, nanobiotechnology, three-dimensional printing, computer assistance, and robotic systems offer huge potential for augmenting and improving the functional and esthetic cranio-maxillofacial and orodental health profile of patients. A good example, perhaps, is nanodentistry and salivary gland radioprotection in patients with head and neck cancer. Nanodentistry is clearly multidisciplinary and interdisciplinary, building on existing knowledge and accruing expertise in different scientific and technological fields, seeking persistent refinement of traditional approaches, via the development and/or incorporation of advanced biomaterials, new bio-functional tools, and pharmacological formulations to improve overall orodental practice and care. While slowly evolving, such advances are expected to provide dentists and surgeons with more precision-made and tailored functional materials, drugs, and equipment, by which safety, esthetics, biomechanics, function/efficacy, and patient compliance are enhanced. Due to the complex nature of such "outside-the-box" (or even "no-box") healthcare-related bio-engineering problem–solution technologies, they have attracted experts from physics, chemistry, biology, materials science, pharmaceutics, robotics, and bioengineering. The goal is to improve overall healthcare and wellbeing with a positive impact on socioeconomics and quality of life.

This book is a collection of original and state-of-the-art works in orodental and cranio-maxillofacial healthcare and related topics. It presents the latest ideas, concepts, findings, achievements, and future projections as well as promotes awareness of the rapidly evolving and enabling multidisciplinary technology, thereby encouraging a fruitful dialogue to bridge the gap between engineering, medicine, and dentistry (including cell biology and biomechanics subspecialties, extending to the head and neck) for research and innovation collaboration across the fields to address critical and urgent biodental/biomedical concerns. The volume contains eleven original contributions presenting recent advances in biomechanical properties of stem cells, periodontal and bone tissues, and polymer/metal-based biomaterials as pharmaceutical delivery systems and bioimaging agents, as well as stimulating mathematical modeling methods as fundamental and expedited analytical tools, for clinical use. Different areas of engineering solutions, once more, clearly support the previously mentioned growing need and we hope to bridge the disciplinary communication and collaboration gap through this contribution. Finally, while we believe that this book will be useful and inspiring for scientists, researchers, engineers, and clinical practitioners involved in healthcare engineering solutions, it is recommended to pay special attention to the potentially impactful role of applied and functional bio-dental tissue engineering, drug/gene delivery (controlled and metered systems) and cell therapy, bioscaffolds, image-guided and -assisted surgery, nanodentistry and biomechanics towards developing better solutions for problems/conditions of the orodental and cranio-maxillofacial complex.

Ziyad S. Haidar, DDS, Cert Implantol, MSc OMFS, FRCS(c), MBA, Ph.D.
Professor,
Investigador Principal y Director BioMAT'X,
Facultad de Odontología-Facultad de Medicina,
Universidad de los Andes,
Santiago de Chile, Chile

Ibrokhim Y. Abdurakhmonov
Center of Genomics and Bioinformatics,
Academy of Sciences of Uzbekistan,
Tashkent, Uzbekistan

Abdelwahed Barkaoui
International University of Rabat,
Morocco

Acknowledgments

Dr. Haidar would like to express gratitude to all the contributing authors, co-editors, and anonymous reviewers for their driven, careful, and insightful reading, appraisal, commentaries, and suggestions. Dr. Haidar is particularly thankful to Author Service Manager Ms. Marijana Francetic at IntechOpen, the BioMAT'X R&D&I Team (Haidar Laboratory), Faculty of Dentistry, Faculty of Medicine, the Centro de Investigación e Innovación Biomédica (CiiB) and the Department of Innovation at the Universidad de los Andes for their operational and technical support. Acknowledged funding to the Haidar Lab: FAI-UANDESINV-IN-2015-101, FAIN-201905 (Oco ZFAIN2019005) 2021, CONCIYT-FONDEF ID16|10366, CORFO 18COTE-89695 and NAM 2021 (The U.S. National Academy of Medicine - Healthy Longevity Global Grand Challenge Competition).

Section 1

Biomechanics

Chapter 1

Multi-Scale Modeling of Mechanobiological Behavior of Bone

Brahim Tlili, H. Guizani, K. Aouadi and M. Nasser

Abstract

The simulation and theoretical or numerical predictive modeling of the development and growth of biological tissues mainly in the case of bone is a complicated task. As a result, many and various knowledge tools required (experimental, theoretical and numerical) are not yet mastered and even discovered. We will cite here some techniques and methods as well as results specific to the multi-scale numerical modeling methodology, and multiphysics using finite element coupling with neural network computation of biological tissues applied to the predictive behavior of cortical bone based of the microstructure of their local constituents and their reconstruction according to local mechanobiology. It follows that additional work is necessary to give more precision on the different models, the considered approaches show their potential utility to understand this behavior in terms of biological evolutions as well as the subsequent use in medical applications.

Keywords: multiscale, mechanobiology, numerical modeling, coupling, bone

1. Introduction

The human skeleton is made up of 204 articulated bones that perform several essential functions. These bones are the body's backbone, to which muscles and other structures can attach. They also provide a protective function for certain organs, such as those located in the rib cage (heart, lungs, etc.) and facilitate movement. Bones are also involved in the formation of blood cells, the metabolism of calcium and the storage of minerals. The objective of this work is to provide an overview of the bibliography relating to human bone tissue: its structure and composition, its histology and its mechanical behavior at different scales.

2. Bone structure

2.1 Functions

Bone tissue is one of the strongest tissues in the body. It is also a dynamic fabric, constantly remodeled, capable of adapting its density to the stress to minimize stress in the most stressed areas. In addition to this mechanical function of supporting the body and protecting the organs, the skeleton has two other main functions.

- A function of controlling the phosphocalcic metabolism: under the effect of mechanical pressures, the constant remodeling of bone tissue causes the release or storage of mineral salts: it thus ensures (jointly with the intestine and the kidneys) the control of the metabolism phosphocalcic.

- A hematopoietic function: the bones contain the hematopoietic marrow in their medullary spaces. At the level of this marrow are created the various blood cells.

  - Red blood cells or red blood cells are responsible for transporting oxygen from the lungs to cells throughout the body and thus allow them to function.

  - White blood cells or leucocytes are of different types (polynuclear cells, lymphocytes, plasma cells, etc.) and are responsible for the body's defense against infections.

  - Platelets are small elements that have the essential role of initiating blood clotting in the event of a wound.

2.2 Anatomical varieties

Several anatomical varieties of bones are distinguished (**Figure 1**). Each bone has a particular shape that meets a specific need.

- Long bones. This name reflects their morphology and not their size. They include a central body and two ends. The radius, the humerus, the tibia, the femur... belong to this anatomical variety.

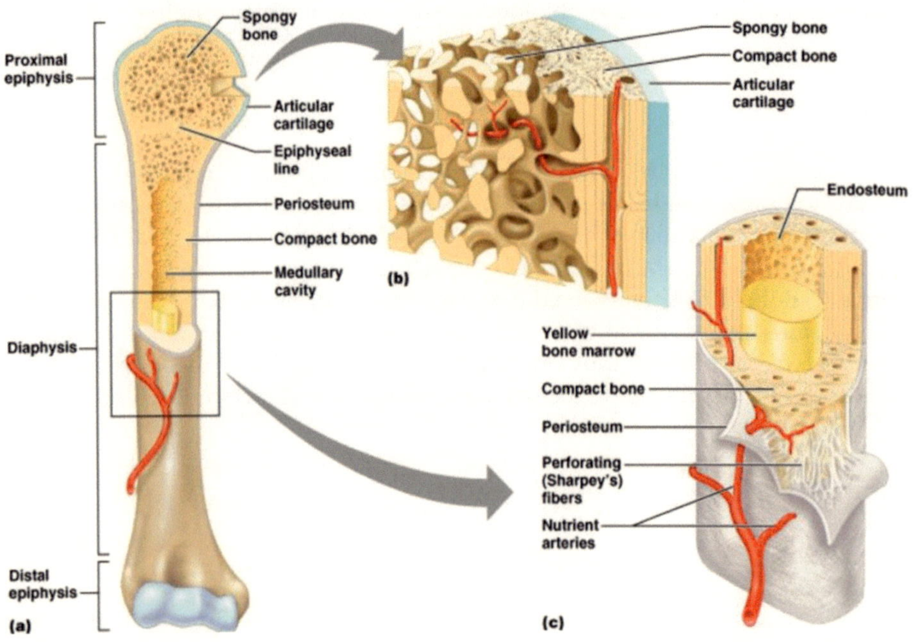

Figure 1.
Structure of a long bone [1].

- Short bones are more or less cubic and mainly contain cancellous bone, the compact bone forms only a thin layer on their surface. This is the case with the bones of the wrist, ankle, phalanges.

- Sesamoid bones are a special type of short bone embedded in a tendon, this is the peculiarity of the kneecap.

- Flat bones are thin and often slightly curved. They have two sides of compact bone more or less parallel, separated by a layer of cancellous bone. The breastbone, ribs, shoulder blades and most of the bones of the skull fall into this category.

- Irregular bones do not belong to any of the above categories. They are complex in shape and consist mostly of cancellous bone covered with thin layers of compact bone. This is the case with certain bones of the skull, vertebrae and iliac bones.

2.3 Constitution

2.3.1 Macroscopic anatomical structure of bones

2.3.1.1 The structure of long bones

Long bones all have the same structure.

- The diaphysis is the body of the bone, its longitudinal part. It's a cylinder of bone relatively thick compact that contains a central medullary canal. In adults, this duct (also called the medullary cavity) contains the yellow marrow, which is mainly from lipids.

- The epiphyses are the ends of the bone, often thicker than the diaphysis. The inside of the epiphyses is made up of cancellous bone, the outside of a thin layer of bone compact. The stressed part of the joint is covered with a thin layer joint cartilage (hyaline cartilage). This dampens the pressure on the end of the bone when moving the joint.

Apart from the articular surfaces where the articular cartilages are located, the bones are surrounded by an outer layer, the periosteum. The central cavity of the long bones is bordered by an internal layer, the endosteum.

- The periosteum is the double membrane, bright white, on the outer surface of the shaft. It mainly contains osteoblasts (cells that produce bone matter) and osteoclasts (cells that destroy bone material), cells described paragraph 1 below. The points of insertion and anchorage of tendons and ligaments are located on this periosteum. Sharpey fibers (collagen fibers which attach the periosteum to the underlying bone) are extremely dense at these points.

- The endosteum is the thin membrane of connective tissue on the internal surfaces of bone. he covers the spans of cancellous bone in the medullary cavities and lines the canals that cut through compact bone. Like the periosteum, the endosteum contains both osteoblasts and osteoclasts.

2.3.2 Cells and extracellular matrix

Bones are mainly made of bone tissue but also contain blood vessels, nerves. Bone tissue is specialized connective tissue called skeletal tissue. It is characterized by the nature of the Extra Cellular Matrix (ECM) which has the property of calcifying and solidifying.

2.3.2.1 Cells

Four types of cells make up bone tissue [1, 2]: on the one hand, bone-forming cells, which include osteoblasts, osteocytes and lining cells, and on the other, bone-resorbent cells, osteoclasts.

- Osteoblasts are bone forming cells located on the outer and inner surface of growing bone tissue. The osteoblasts develop the organic constituents of the Extra Cellular Matrix. They are transformed into osteocytes, or are put to rest in the form of bordering cells.

- Osteocytes are differentiated osteoblasts incapable of dividing and are entirely surrounded by the mineralized Extra Cellular Matrix. Osteocytes sit in cells, osteoclasts, and participate in the maintenance of the bone matrix.

- The bordering cells are osteoblasts at rest which coat the bone surfaces and are liable, if they are called upon, to become active osteoblasts again.

- Osteoclasts, very large cells 20 to 100 μm in diameter, are the seat of the bone resorption process. They are very mobile and able to move on the surface of the bone trabeculae from one resorption site to another.

Osteoclasts, osteoblasts, and bone-lining cells are found on the surface of bone tissue, while osteocytes are located inside the extracellular matrix of bone tissue.

2.3.2.2 The extra cellular matrix

The Extra Cellular Matrix of bone is calcified and has an organic part and a mineral phase.

- The organic matrix is composed of collagen microfibrils, and various elements involved in the mineralization phase of the Extra Cellular Bone Matrix.

- The mineral phase consists of calcium phosphate crystals (apatite) located between the collagen fibers and/or inside them, in the form of small hexagonal needles.

2.3.3 Bone tissue

Most bones are made up of an outer layer that appears smooth and dense to the naked eye, compact bone tissue, and an internal area of trabecular (or cancellous) bone tissue. Bone marrow, red or yellow, is contained in the cavities between the spans of this structure. In the case of long bones, **Figure 1**, the cancellous bone is located at the extremities (epiphyses), the central part of the bone contains the bone marrow.

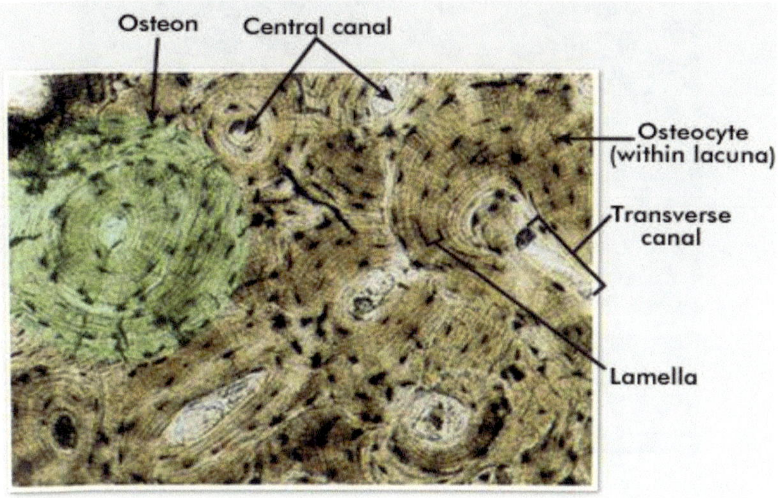

Figure 2.
Compact, cortical bone element [3].

2.3.3.1 Compact bone

The osteon, or Havers' system, is the structural unit of compact bone. Each osteon is of elongated cylindrical shape, parallel to the longitudinal axis of the bone, **Figure 2**. The osteon is made up of a set of hollow cylinders (6 to 15 per osteon) made up of bone matrix and arranged concentrically around its central canal, or Havers' canal, which contains blood capillaries and nerve fibers. These canals are interconnected with the medullary cavity and with the surface of the bone by transverse or oblique canals, the Volkmann canals. Each matrix cylinder is a lamella of the osteon: the compact bone is often called the lamellar bone. In a given lamella, the collagen fibers are all parallel but the fibers of two adjacent lamellae are always oriented in different directions. This alternation strengthens the adjacent lamellae, which provides remarkable resistance to the torsional forces to which the bones are subjected. The osteocytes are found in small empty spaces at the junction of the lamellae, called lacunae. These gaps are connected to each other and to the central osteon canal by the canaliculi, very fine canals, which allow nutrients and waste to easily pass from one osteocyte to another. Thus, the osteocytes are well nourished even though the bone matrix is hard and impermeable to nutrients. The arrangement of the osteons, with the axis oriented in the direction of the mechanical stresses, gives the compact bone maximum strength. If we consider the compressive strength in relation to the density, bone is a reference structure in the field of cellular materials [1, 3].

2.3.3.2 Cancellous bone

Spongy (trabecular) bone tissue is mainly present in short bones and flat bones (sternum, iliac wings) as well as in epiphyses of long bones. It is formed by a three-dimensional network of trabeculae (walls) of bone tissue, branched, delimiting a labyrinth of interconnected spaces reserved by the bone marrow and vessels, **Figure 3**. The shape and density of the alveolar cells depend on the intensity and direction of the stress that the bone must withstand. Cells tend to line up in the direction of greatest stress, and their density increases with the intensity of loading. Cancellous bone has no osteons, but its spans form irregular lamellae and osteocytes connected by canaliculi.

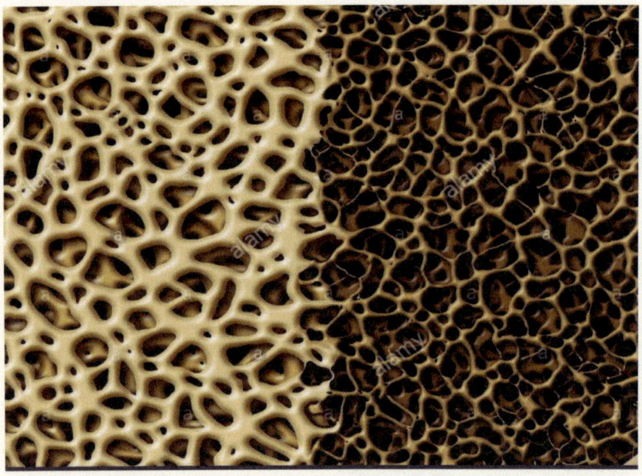

Figure 3.
spongy bone tissue. Side of the cube: 5 mm. Photo UMR 791 INSERM [3].

The nutrients leave the medullary spaces between the spans and arrive at the osteocytes of the cancellous bone by diffusion through the canaliculi.

There are three phases in the life of the bone.

- The growth phase, during which bone is synthesized. Peak bone mass is reached three years after puberty.
- Adulthood in which the phenomenon of bone remodeling maintains an approximately constant mass. Bone is a tissue that is constantly renewed during its existence. It is resorbed by osteoclasts and then reconstructed by osteoblasts. The sustainability of the bone matrix depends on the balance of this cycle. With this process, the bone can adapt to loads and rebuild itself in the event of a fracture.
- With advancing age of the individual, degradation and synthesis are unbalanced, bone mass decreases.

3. Bone development

Osteogenesis and ossification refers to the process of bone formation that leads to the formation of the bone skeleton in the embryo (**Figure 4**). Bone growth is another form of ossification that continues into adulthood as long as the subject continues to grow. In adults, ossification is mainly used for rearrangement and to bone consolidation. The embryo's skeleton is made up entirely of fibrous membranes and hyaline (joint) cartilage until the 6th week of gestation. Then most of these structures are gradually replaced by bone tissue. Two bone formation processes then exist: intramembranous ossification and endochondral ossification.

3.1 Inside the membrane ossification

Intramembranous bone is formed from a fibrous membrane. The bones produced are flat bones. The ground substance of the bone matrix is deposited between the collagen fibers, inside the fibrous membrane, to form cancellous

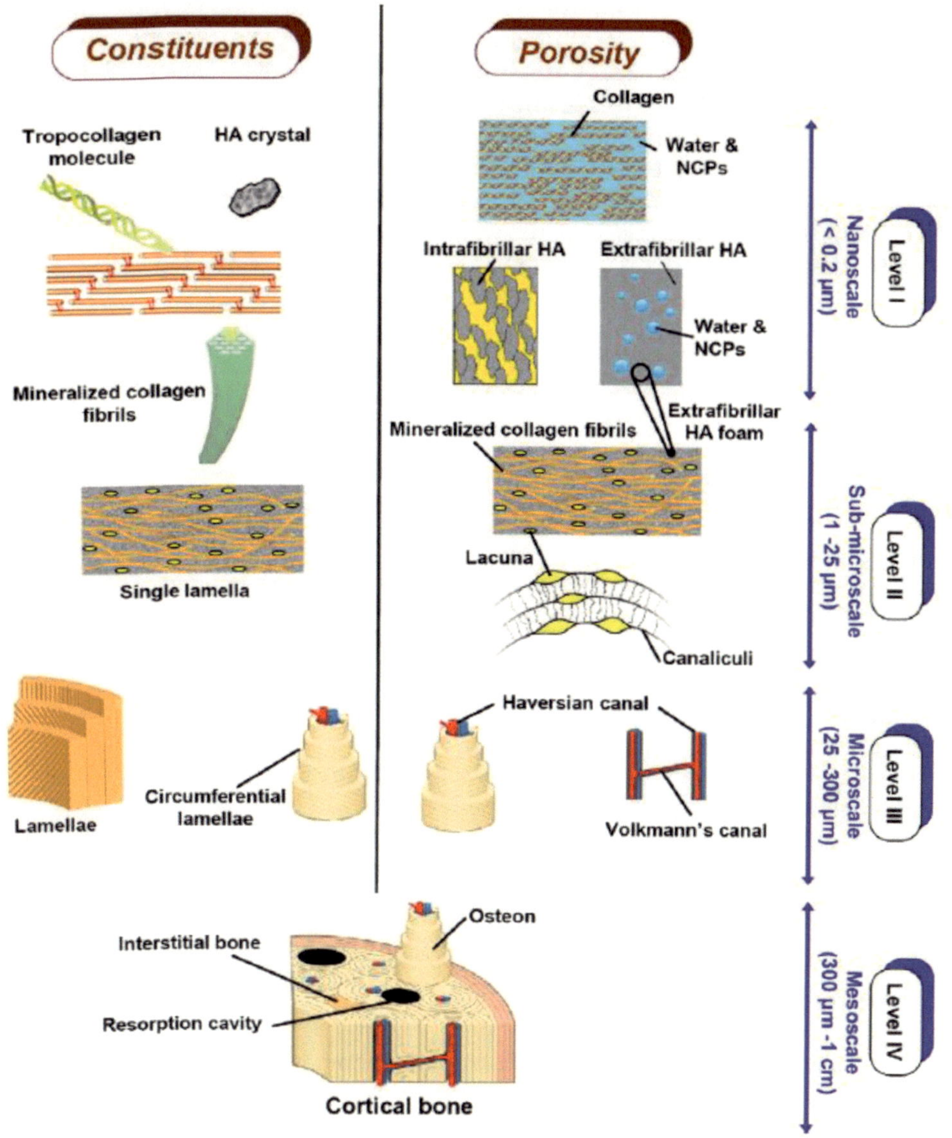

Figure 4.
Hierarchical structure of cortical bone constituents and associated porosity. HA = hydroxyapatite, NCP = non-collagenous proteins [4].

bone. Plates of compact bone eventually enclose the diploe. The successive stages of ossification are:

- the formation of an ossification point in the fibrous membrane;
- the formation of a bone matrix inside the fibrous membrane;
- the formation of fibrous bone and periosteum;
- the formation of compact bone plates and red marrow.
- Endochondral ossification.

Ossification starts from hyaline cartilage and leads to endochondral bone or cartilaginous bone. This process is more complex than the previous one because the cartilage must be disintegrated as the ossification progresses. The majority of the bones of the skeleton are formed by this ossification. The osteoblasts that lie below the periosteum secrete a bone matrix modeled on hyaline cartilage, thus forming a bone sheath. The deterioration of the cartilaginous matrix forms cavities, which allows the entry of a bud which is at the origin of the point of primary ossification: it contains an artery and a nourishing vein, lymphatic vessels, neurofibers, red marrow elements, osteoblasts and osteoclasts. Bone matrix is deposited around the remains of cartilage.

3.2 Bone growth

Bone growth takes place mainly during childhood and adolescence. Most bones stop growing in early adulthood.

3.2.1 Growth in length of bones

Long bones elongate as a result of the interstitial growth of epiphyseal cartilages and the replacement of cartilage with bone material. Growth in length is accompanied by an almost continuous rearrangement of the extremities (epiphyses), in order to maintain the correct proportions between the diaphysis and the epiphyses.

3.2.2 Growth in thickness or diameter of bones

The bones thicken with the efficient activity of the periosteum. Osteoblasts, located below the periosteum, secrete a bone matrix on the outer surface of the bone; osteoclasts, located on the endostate of the diaphysis, destroy the bone surrounding the medullary cavity. The resorption is generally less important than the formation of bone material, the bone thickens and its diameter increases.

4. Bone remodeling

In compact bone as well as in trabecular bone, bone tissue is constantly renewing [1, 4, 5]. This bone remodeling occurs by successive resorption and formation of bone tissue, a process in which osteoclasts and osteoblasts are closely associated. Bone tissue is renewed about every four months in adults. The renewal mechanism consists of several phases.

- Activation phase: under the effect of osteoresorbent factors the lining cells, which normally cover the bone surface, allow osteoclasts (bone resorption cells) to pass. At the same time, osteoblasts differentiate into osteoclasts.

- Bone tissue resorption phase: each osteoclast that becomes active binds to the Extra Cellular Matrix. The resorption phase begins with the dissolution of the mineral phase (acidification) and continues with the degradation of the organic matrix under the action of enzymes.

- Inversion phase: once the osteoclasts have created a gap in the bone tissue, they die. Macrophages then come to replace them, to smooth the bottom of the gap.

- Bone tissue formation phase: this phase, also made up of two stages, is the longest. Once the resorption is complete, the cells at the bottom of the gap differentiate into osteoblasts which synthesize a new Extra Cellular Matrix which is progressively mineralized thereafter. In young, healthy adults, total bone mass remains constant because overall the rates of bone deposition and resorption are equal. The redesign process is not always uniform or balanced:

- bone deposition may occur in an area where the bone has sustained an injury;
- the formation of bone tissue is less rapid than the resorption as the individual advances in age, which is what leads to osteoporosis.

5. Mechanical properties of bone

5.1 Compact bone

The behavior of fresh compact bone, loaded in the longitudinal direction, is elastic up to a strain of 0.7% in tension or in compression [1, 3], failure occurs at 3% strain (**Figure 5**). In the transverse direction, in tension, the bone is less rigid and the rupture occurs at a strain of 0.6%. These values correspond to fresh bones. If they are dry, the Young's modulus increases and the tensile strength decreases. Dry bone is also more fragile. The Young's modulus of fresh compact bone is about 17 GPa longitudinally and 11.5 GPa transversely. The maximum compressive stress is 193 MPa in the longitudinal direction and 133 MPa in the transverse direction. In traction, the maximum stresses are 148 MPa in the longitudinal direction and 49 MPa in the transverse direction.

The elastic mechanical properties of bone ultrastructure scale levels depends on several geometrical and mechanical parameters such as Young's modulus bone elementary com- pounds (mineral, collagen) [6, 7], the nature of collagen (dry, wet) [6], size of the mineral crystal and the number of cross- links [8]. In order to clarify, the averaged elastic constants have been presented in **Table 1** to compare

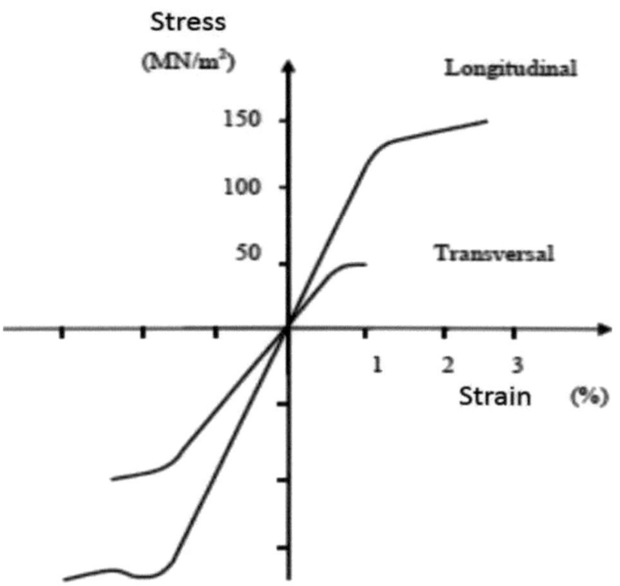

Figure 5.
Tensile-compression test of compact bone [5].

	Young's modulus (GPa)	Poisson's ratio
MCM	0.755	0.264
MCF	40.8	0.271

Table 1.
The average elestic mechanical properties of the bone ultrastructure scales [8].

our results with experi- mental and numerical results of further works performed on the same components. There are few works focused on the mechanical properties characterization of MCFR (mineralized collagen fibers (MCFRs)), for this reason, the comparison of the results is limited on MCM (Mineralized Collagen Microfibrils) and MCF (Mineralized Collagen Fibrils) scale levels.

MCFRs are formed by the assembly of MCFs surrounded by a matrix of mineral and are offset from each other with an apparent pe- riodicity noted D. Then, MCFs are made the same way by MCMs related to each other by cross-links. Finally, MCMs, a particu- lar assembly of five helical TC molecules, longitudinally offset them with the same apparent periodicity D.

5.2 Bone remodeling or renewal

Bone is constantly being renewed. It is a continuous cycle of bone formation and destruction, which is living tissue. This phenomenon is called "bone remodeling". Two types of cell are involved: osteoclasts which will first destroy the bone that has been formed in the past, and osteoblasts which will rebuild new bone.

At first, the osteoclasts arrive and dig real "holes" called gaps: this is the resorption phase.

Then, the osteoblasts arrive in the gaps dug previously. These cells will then fill in with bone tissue without calcium (called osteoid tissue), this is the formation phase. Finally, on this young osteoid bone tissue, the calcium will be fixed: this is the phase of the mineralization.

Bone tissue is a dynamic tissue which is constantly renewed by synthesis and resorption. This mechanism is induced by the action of hormones and local factors (parathyroid hormone, vitamin D3, prostaglandin E2) or mechanical constraints (stresses, alterations in bone tissue). Permanent remodeling makes it possible to renew bone tissue to compensate for the aging of osteocytes, to modify the architecture of bone tissue according to mechanical constraints and finally to control phosphocalcic homeostasis by recirculating calcium and phosphorus during the resorption phase.

There are 5 main phases in the bone remodeling process: the activation phase, the resorption phase, the inversion phase, the formation phase and the quiescence phase. Bone remodeling is a cellular cooperation between osteoblasts and osteoclasts. The phenomenon of bone remodeling takes place within a multicellular temporary remodeling unit called the BMU "Bone Multicellular Unit".

5.2.1 The activation phase

The activation phase is initiated by the osteocytes. These cells are anchored in the bone matrix and have numerous cytoplasmic extensions. They are able to communicate with other cell types, but also to detect mechanical signals (stresses, alterations in bone tissue such as microfractures) or hormonal signals. Faced with these signals, the osteocytes die by apoptosis and induce, through this programmed cell death, the retraction of the bordering cells to expose the bone surface which must be remodeled. Stromal cells, mesenchymal stem cells, which are found in the environment on the surface of bone tissue, differentiate into pre-osteoblasts. These express on their surfaces RANKL, a cytokine-type ligand whose role is the recruitment of pre-osteoclastic cells, coming from the medullary environment, and the differentiation of these into mature cells by the RANK bond (expressed at the surface of pre-osteoclasts) and RANKL. Mature osteoclasts thus formed adhere to the bone surface.

5.2.2 The resorption phase

Mature osteoclasts on the surface of the bone will secrete acids which will decalcify the bone and then enzymes which will digest the collagen in the bone. In about 12 days [9], mature osteoclasts will create a resorption gap of about 40 μm [10]. By digesting bone, osteoclasts release growth factors. The osteoclasts then die by apoptosis.

5.2.3 The reversal phase

After the resorption phase, the osteoclasts are replaced by mononuclear cells of the macrophage type.

5.2.4 The training phase

Osteoblast precursors, derived from pluripotent mesenchymal stem cells in the bone marrow, are rapidly attracted to growth factors released during resorption, proliferate and differentiate into mature osteoblasts. Osteoblasts release a protein,

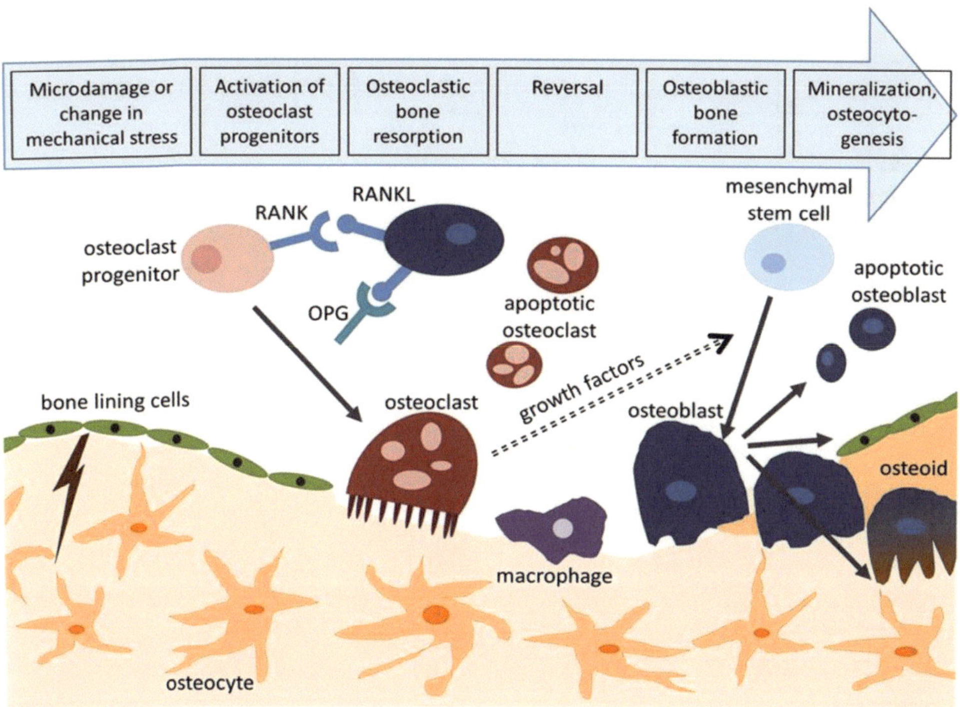

Figure 6.
Bone remodeling according to [11].

osteoprotegerin, which binds to RANKL preventing RANK-RANKL binding and therefore the activation of osteoclastic differentiation [10].

Mature osteoblasts migrate to the bottom of the resorption gap and release type I collagen microfibrils, thus creating new osteoid matrix and alkaline phosphatase, an enzyme involved in bone matrix mineralization [10]. The bone formation phase lasts about 3 months [9]. During the formation phase, certain osteoblasts (approximately 1/40) attach themselves to the bone matrix and differentiate into osteocytes.

5.2.5 The quiescence phase

The remaining osteoblast cells differentiate into bordering cells and the newly formed osteocytes rebuild their connecting network (**Figure 6**) [10].

6. Finite ellement modeling of bone mechanobiological behavior

This section presents the hybrid multiscale modeling ap-proach (Finite Element EF/Neural Network NN) of bone ultrastructure (**Figure 7**).

This approach, which is summarized in **Figure 8**, is composed of four steps: (i) development and simulation of geometric FE models for each level scale separately (microfi- bril, fibril and fiber), (ii) use of the results obtained from FE simulation in each scale level for the neural network program training phase, (iii) generalization of the results in neural network prediction phase, (iv) transition between the different scales using the same NN program.

The forth step is constituted from three NN blocks as Sembled in series (NN block for each scale level) so each NN (i + 1) Block uses as inputs the Nni block outputs (being i = 1,2). Finally, NN3 outputs allow obtaining MCFR elastic properties.

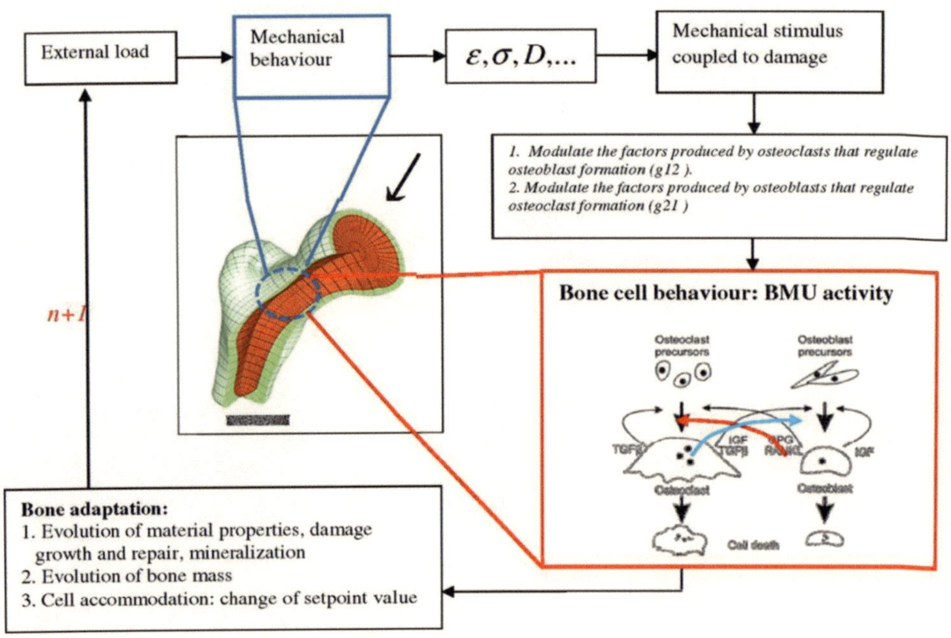

Figure 7.
Schematic representation of bone remodeling based on BMU activity coupled to mechanical stimulus: at the remodeling cycle (n), the applied load generates mechanical stress, strain, and fatigue damage states at every FE of the mesh.

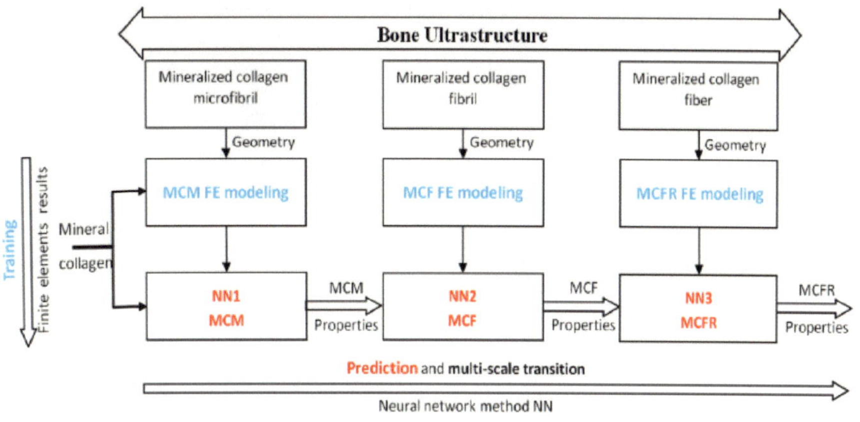

Figure 8.
Hybrid (FE/NN) multiscale modeling of bone ultrastructure [7, 12].

6.1 Results and discussions

In this study, the main results are focused on the new multi-scale hybrid modeling developed during the numerical simulation. By showing the synthetic results obtained with the NN method according to three levels of scale MCM, MCF and MCFR (**Figure 9**). By showing the variation of the generalized Young's modulus MCM as a function of the Young's modulus of the two essential bone constituents according to this scale (mineral and collagen) (**Figure 9a**). In the light of various investigations, these results found under the NN1 analysis are integrated in **Figure 9a** to construct the generalized Young's modulus MCF, obviously by integrating the elastic properties of the mineral. By analogy, the results of NN2 are likewise used to evaluate the Young MCFR's modulus (**Figure 9c**). It must be taken into account that the quantity of the mineral NN degrades in the matrix depending on the level of the scale. Our studies are flexible to have flexibility on the variation of the Young's modulus of the mineral under the effect of a significant difference between the subject amorphous structure [13]. **Figure 9a** shows that the Young's modulus of mineral has a very significant effect compared to the effect of TC modulus of Young's molecules for the MCM level scale. On the other hand, the synthesis in **Figure 9b** shows us that the elastic properties of the mineral are also slightly influential, compare to the Young's modulus of MCMs for the different scale levels of MCF. These results found, are comparable with other studies in literature [12, 14]. On the other hand, the curve of **Figure 9c** shows that the Young's modulus MCFs has a remarkable effect on the equivalent Young's modulus of the MCFR compared to the Young's modulus of the mineral.

Generally, rehological properties of the scale levels of the bone ultrastructure are related to several geometric and mechanical parameters such as the elementary bone compounds of Young's modulus (mineral, collagen), the nature of collagen (dry, wet), the size of the mineral crystal and the number of crossed links. Therefore, the estimated elastic constants have been shown in **Table 2** to compare our results with the experimental and numerical results of other studies in the literature. The literature study dealing with the characterization of the mechanical properties of MCFR are very little and even are not sufficiently developed, for this reason, the comparison of the results is limited to the MCM and MCF scale levels (see **Figures 10** and **11**, respectively).

Figure 10, configures a good correlation between predicted NN (our numerical study) and the experimental study for the small strain margin based on X-ray

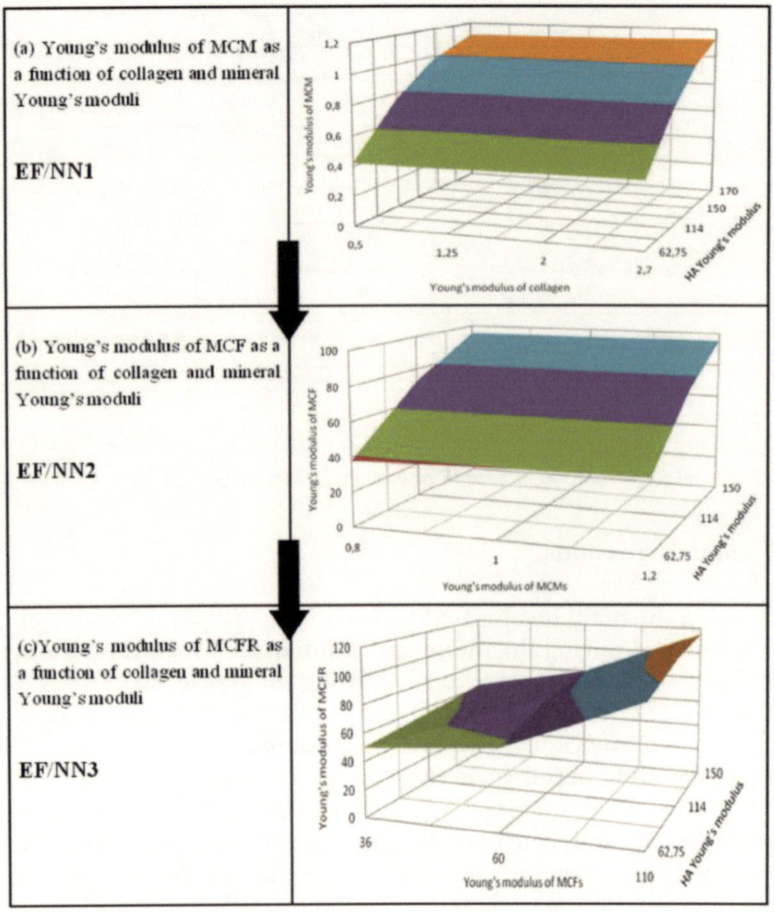

Figure 9.
Evolution of elastic moduli (GPa) of MCM and MCF as function of the mineral Young's modulus and passage between the MCM and MCF [7].

diffraction, atomic force microscopy (AFM) and the calculation of molecular dynamics. (MD).

Also, **Figure 11** records a good agreement between our study predicted NN for the MCF and the numerical and experimental results: analysis by DRX, calculation of molecular dynamics (MD) and calculation by the finite element method. However, there is a slight uncertainty which can be introduced by different sources: the different methods used, the size and nature (hydrated or dehydrated) of the MCM and MCF tested and the hypotheses considered by each. As an indication during this work, consider the mineral as a homogeneous matrix without taking into account the presence of water (PCNs are negligible). These assumptions may explain the differences mentioned above. However, due to the living nature of the materials studied (bone), the Young's modulus of MCM can be on average about 1 ± 0.2 GPa and 40 ± 2 GPa for the Young's modulus of MCF.

Moreover, the comparative study of NN predicted the average Young's modulus of MCF and also comparable to the study carried out in the literature.

The elastic properties are closely linked to several material and structural parameters at the level of our study scale. This translates into a great sensitivity in terms of mechanical properties and service life. Indeed, if the boundary conditions are specified, we can assign to each scale level a unique value of the elastic properties of the bone. As a result, carrying out experimental tests or numerical

Parameters	Notation	Trabecular bone	Cortical bone
GENERAL PARAMETERS			
Initial elastic modulus	E_0 (MPa)	2000	17,000
Poisson ratio	ν	0.3	0.3
Initial density	ρ (g/cm^3)	0.764	1.4
Density coefficient	C (g/cm^3)	4000	80,003
Density exponent	P	3	3
Ash exponent	Q	2.74	2.74
DAMAGE LAW PARAMETERS			
Fatigue parameter	γ	0.2	0.2
Fatigue exponent	β	0.4	0.4
MINERALIZATION PARAMETERS			
Initial ash fraction	α_0	0.6	0.6
Maximum physiological value	α_{max}	0.7	0.7
Velocity of the mineralization	k (days^{-1})	0.0003387	0.0003387
STIMULUS PARAMETERS			
Mechanosensitivity of the osteocyte	μ_k (nmol mm J^{-1} h^{-1})	0.5	0.5
Osteocytes density	N_{oc} (mm^{-3})	10,625	10,625
Spatial influence factor	d_0 (μm)	0.1	0.1
Accommodation velocity parameter	λ (days^{-1})	0.002	0.002
Initial setpoint value	S_k^0 (J m^{-3})	0.0025	0.0025

Parameters		Notation	Trabecular bone	Cortical bone	
BMU PARAMETERS					
Osteoclasts				**Osteoblasts**	
Notation	**Trabecular**	**Cortical**	**Notation**	**Trabecular**	**Cortical**
α_1 (osteoclasts/day)	3	3	α_2 (osteoblasts/day)	4	4
β_1 (osteoclasts/day)	0.2	0.2	β_2 (osteoblasts/day)	0.0017	0.0017
k_1 (osteoclasts/day)	0.24	0.024	k_2 (osteoblasts/day)	0.02	0.002
A_1	1.6	1.6	A_1	−1.6	−1.6
B_1	−0.49	−0.49	B_2	0.6	0.6
γ_1 (g/J)	16.67	16.67	γ_2 (g/J)	33.37	33.37
x_C (t = 0) (osteoclasts)	15	15	x_B (t = 0) (osteoblasts)	1	1

Table 2.
Material properties for bone used for the remodeling simulation [15–17].

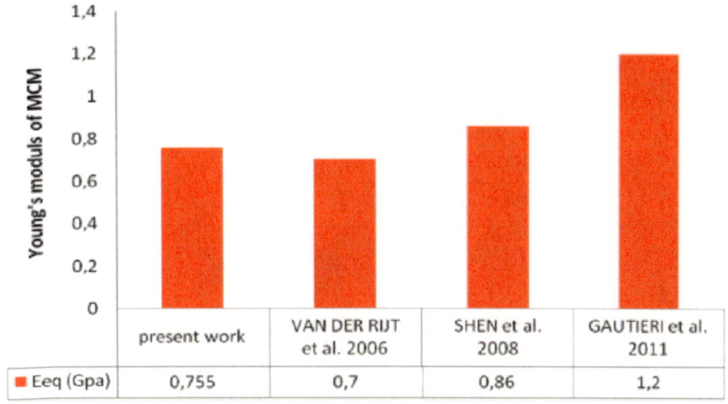

Figure 10.
Comparison between NN predicted average Young's modulus of MCM and literature results [7].

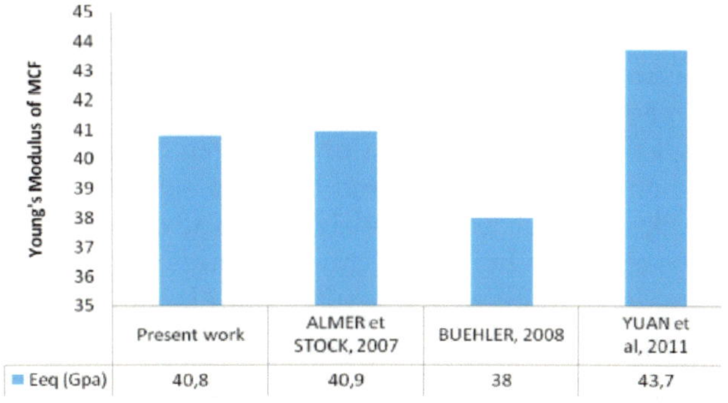

Figure 11.
Comparison between NN predicted average Young's modulus of MCF and literature results [7].

simulations on a case-by-case basis can waste time and become more expensive, hence the growing interest in the use of intelligent digital methods, such as the artificial neural networks method. This method offers a good balance between cost/quality/performance. In this study, the combinations of artificial neural network method and finite element analysis were implemented and used to determine the elastic mechanical properties at different scale levels of the bone tissue nanostructure. Second step, an approach multi-scale using neural networks has been developed. This approach uses the results of finite element analysis for the learning phase. It makes it possible to generalize the results obtained by finite elements and to make the transition between the different scale levels. The results were compared and validated by other studies in the literature and good agreement was observed. This hybrid multi-scale approach makes it possible to quickly determine (a few seconds) the equivalent mechanical properties according to the parameters entered. Here, the method was only used to determine elastic properties but can be approved to identify equivalent mechanical properties related to fracture behavior.

6.2 Relationship between the mechanics and the activities of bone cells in the process of bone remodeling

On the other hand, the complement of this work aims to develop an FE model to show the methodology of bone remodeling, by considering the activities of osteoclasts and osteoblasts (**Figure 12**). The mechanical properties of bone are demonstrated by carefully considering the accumulation and mineralization of

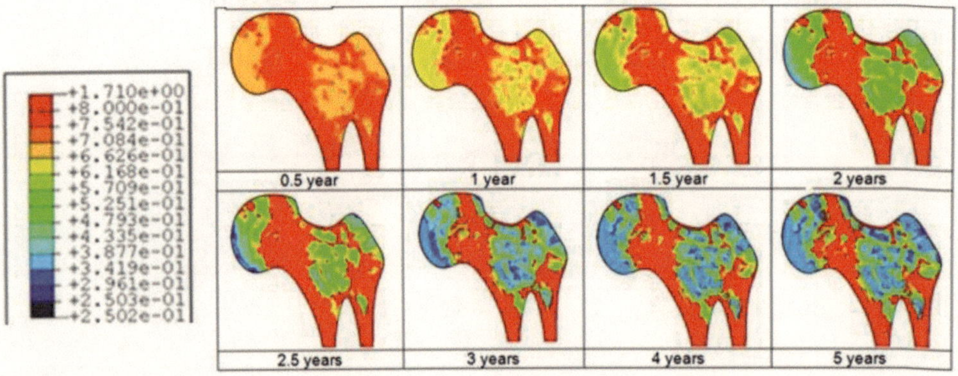

Figure 12.
Predicted bone adaptation sequences in the form of apparent bone density variation in gram per cubic centimeter [18].

failures under the effect of fatigue of the bone material. The strain-damage coupled stimulation phase is shown, which monitors the level of autocrine and paracrine factors. Cell phones and their behavior are based on the dynamic equation of, who describes autocrine and paracrine interactions between osteoblasts and osteoclasts and calculates cell population dynamics and bone mass changes at a discrete site of bone remodeling (**Figure 13**). The FE model developed was implemented in the FE Abaqus code. An example of a human proximal femur is studied using the developed model. The model was able to predict the final adaptation of the human proximal femur similar to models seen in a human proximal femur. The results obtained reveal a complex spatio-temporal bone adaptation [18]. The proposed FEM model provides insight into how bone cells adapt their architecture to the mechanical and biological environment.

The loads on the hip joint sacrificed in the current work constitute the majority of load located on the mediolateral plane of a femur and its margin is clearly greater than the other loads. Therefore, the 2D femur was a reasonable representation of the 3D remodeling behavior. Furthermore, the simulations employed the fixed model parameters given in **Table 2**. The recorded values may be subject to change due to several factors (disease, age, drugs, sex, bone sites, etc.). Finally, the analysis considers only one factor for a single parameter value of the model has been modified of all data, unlike the other parameters, which were fixed. This hypothesis showed in particular that the levels of bone cells play an important role in the process of bone adaptation, which can be modulated by specific bone drugs. Nevertheless, for a future general analysis of AS, it is necessary to consider the full variation of the factor parameters simultaneously for different geometries of femurs.

6.3 Examples of multiscale and multiphysics numerical modeling of biological tissues

The theoretical-numerical simulation and predictive modeling of the behavior and growth of biological tissues is a strange and new technique. As a result, different and multiple knowledge.

tools necessary, it is an overlap between experimentation, digital and also the theoretical, which are not yet well studied or even understood. George D. et al. [19] presented some specific multiscale multiphysics techniques and analyzes for biological tissues applied to the predictive behavior of cortical veins as a function of microstrural properties, taking into account bone remodeling and growth as a

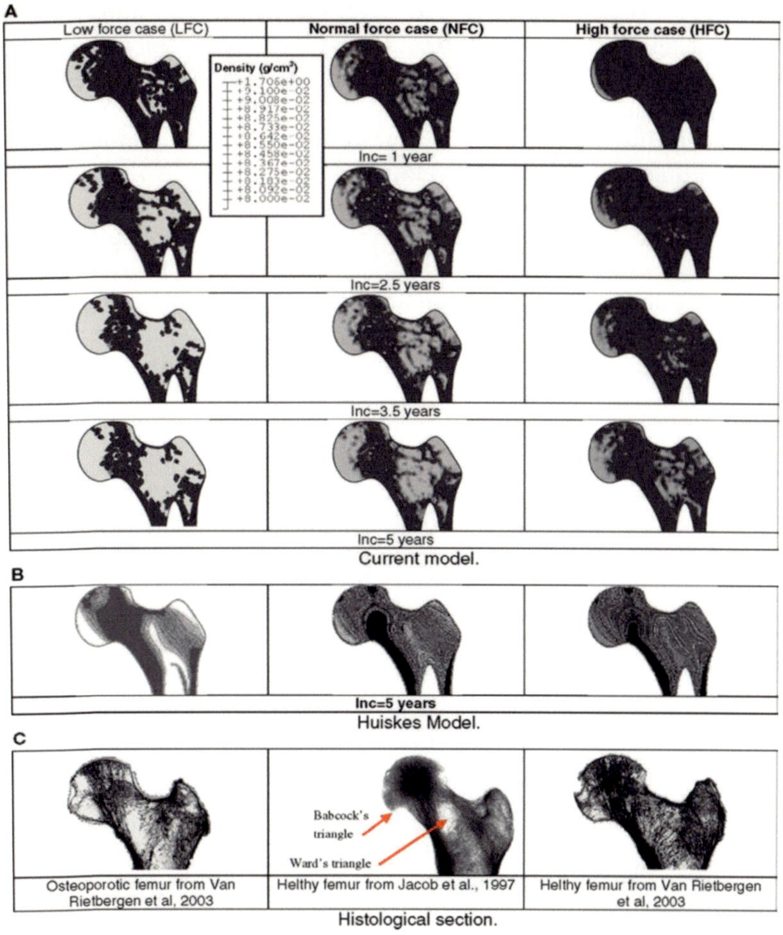

Figure 13.
Sequences of predicted density distributions (gray level) for three different remodeling load levels [18].

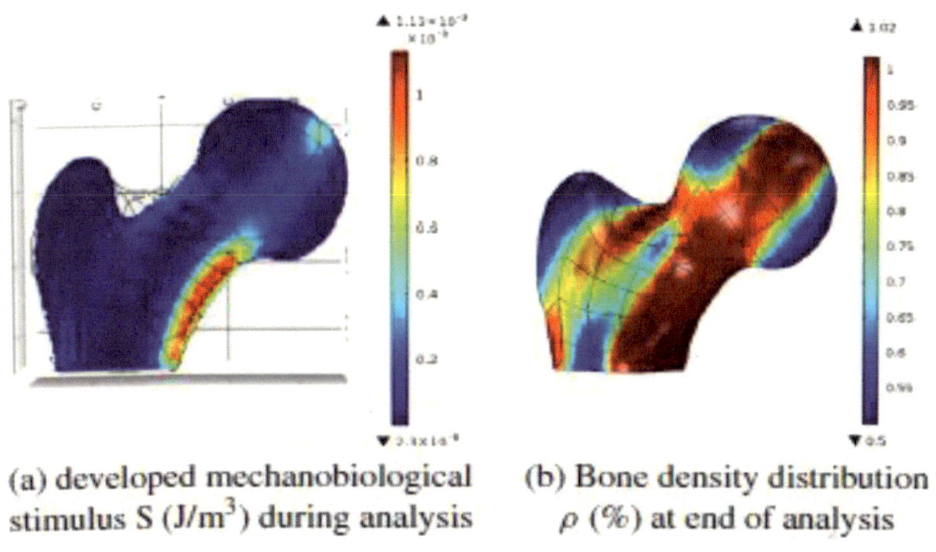

Figure 14.
Macroscopic evolution from applied external mechanical boundary conditions [19].

function of local mechanobiology (**Figure 14**). The hypotheses and the approaches used are well mastered to discover and understand the mechanical-biological phenomena, as well as a clear vision for different life periods of biological changes and their use for industrial applications.

Comparable studies, taking into account local mechanics to biology, have been developed by Ruimermann [20] to develop specific techniques of bone remodeling of patients for 3D micro-architectures but no study has shown a real link with medical applications. Real. The model of this study will allow coupling between these different scales to be able to obtain a macroscopic mechanobiological model predictive of bone changes as a function of local biological constituents.

Figure 15 shows a complementary analysis, which was carried out based on different boundary conditions. Through a triangular compressive load applied to

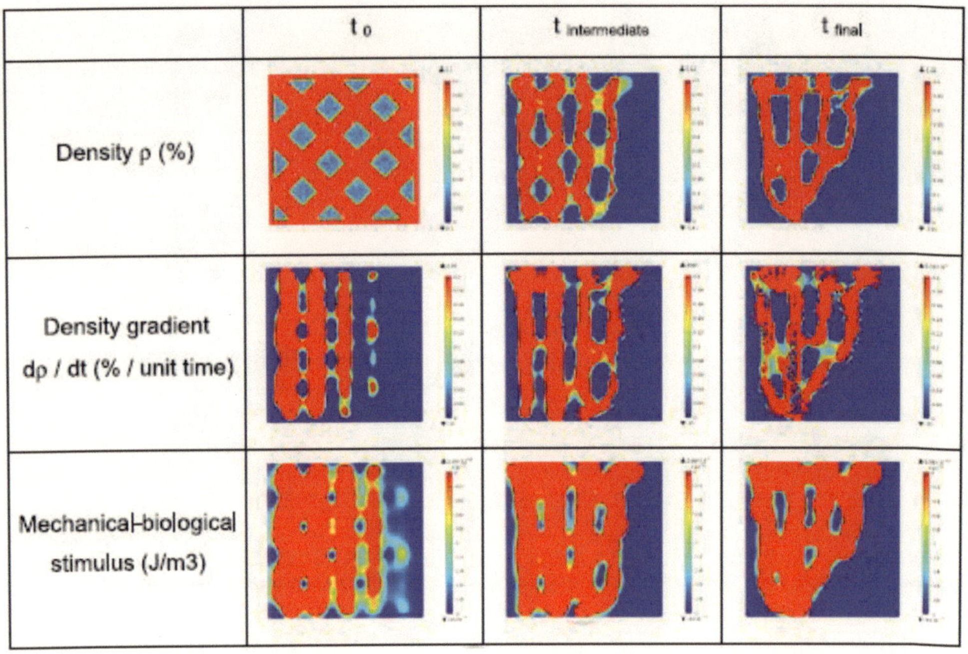

Figure 15.
Mesoscopic (trabecular size) evolution for the triangular load condition [20]. (a) Trabecular bone density obtained with current 3D model and cell activation. (b) Schematic of trabecular bone density obtained froma 2D phenomenological model with same loading conditions from Weinans [21].

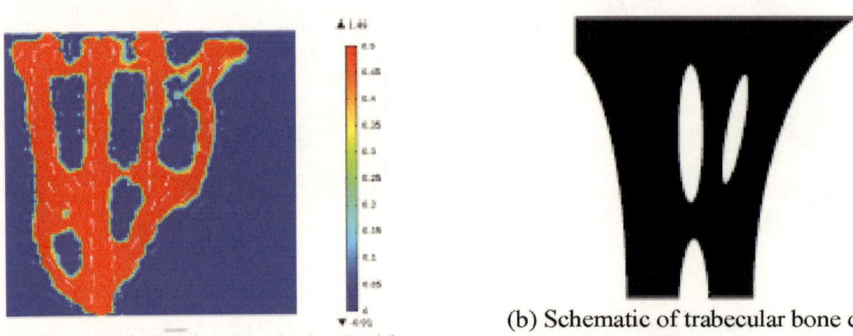

(a) Trabecular bone density obtained with current 3D model and cell activation

(b) Schematic of trabecular bone density obtained froma 2D phenomenological model with same loading conditions from Weinans [21]

Figure 16.
Comparison of bone density distribution between current mechanobiological model and phenomenological model after applying triangular compressive mechanical load.

the entire basic bone microstructure. As a result, the trabeculae are mostly directed along the main load directions with an increasingly smaller size and less intense loads. The localization of cell activation is linked to the calculated mechanobiological stimulus and its quantification is done in the same way.

The results obtained are compared with data extracted from a phenomenological model developed in the literature [21]. Here, comparable results are observed at the level of bone density distribution (**Figure 16**). As a result, the model developed has a good estimate of biological activations and a consistency more adaptable to the patient. The microstructural properties of the bone obtained is strongly related to mechanical and quantifiable biological parameters. Mechanical stability is obtained by provocation and localization of biological cells, and can be physically close to real cases.

7. Conclusion

In this study, three 3D FE model for each nano-scopic struc- ture of bone ultrastructure (MCM, MCF and MCFR) were proposed. Different numerical simulations were performed to identify the apparent behavior for each structure (global homogenized) and to identify the corresponding apparent mechanical properties. The proposed 3D geometric models were used to perform para- metric studies to see the influence of geometrical and mechanical properties of the elementary constituents (HA crystals, TC molecules and cross-links) on the equivalent properties. In a second step, a multiscale approach using neural networks was developed. This approach uses the results of the finite element analysis for the training phase. It allows us to generalize the results obtained by finite element and do the transition between the different scale levels. The results were compared and vali- dated by other studies from the literature and a good agreement was observed. This hybrid multiscale approach allows deter- mining quickly (a few seconds) the mechanical equivalent properties as a function of the entered parameters. Here the method was only used to determine the elastic properties but can be approved to identify mechanical equivalent properties related to fracture behavior.

Otherwise, the proposed bone remodeling model can be enriched by the integration of transduction processes in addition to cellular activities and the explicit integration of the effects of RANKL/RANK/OPG regulation. It would also be useful to study the behavior of the bone remodeling model on heterogeneous 2D and 3D femurs. The scenarios (age, sex, physical activities, etc.) illustrated in this study are not exhaustive and others (medication, calcium content, etc.) can be incorporated.

Nomenclature

MCMs	the mineralized collagen microfibrils
MCFs	the mineralized collagen fibrils
MCFRs	the mineralized collagen fibers

Author details

Brahim Tlili[1]*, H. Guizani[1], K. Aouadi[2] and M. Nasser[1]

1 Laboratory of Applied Mechanics and Engineering (LR-MAI): National School of Engineers of Tunis, University of Tunis El Manar, Tunisia

2 Applied Mechanics and Systems Research Laboratory, Tunisia Polytechnic School, University of Carthage, Tunisia

*Address all correspondence to: tlilii_brahim@yahoo.fr

References

[1] TOPPETS V, PASTORET V, De BEHRV, ANTOINE N, DESSY C, Morphologie GABRIELA. croissance et remaniement du tissu osseux. Ann. Méd. Vét. 2004;**148**:1-13

[2] WOLFF J.L. The law of bone remodeling (traducted by Marquet P., Furlong R.) Springer, Berlin; 1986.

[3] FROST H.M. Skeletal structural adaptations to mechanical usage: 2. Redefining Wolff's law: the remodeling problem. Anat. Rec. 1990; 226: 414-22.

[4] E. Hamed, E. Novitskaya, J. Li, P.-Y. Chen, I. Jasiuk, J. McKittrick. Elastic moduli of untreated, demineralized and deproteinized cortical bone: Validation of a theoretical model of bone as an interpenetrating composite material. Acta Biomaterialia 8 (2012) 1080-1092.

[5] COURET I. Biologie du remodelage osseux. Médécine Nucléaire - Imagérie Fonctionnelle et Métabolique. vol. 28-n° 2, 2004.

[6] A. Madeo, D. George and Y. Rémond, Second gradient models for some effects of micro-structure on reconstructed bone remodeling, Computer Methods in Biomechanics and Biomedical Engineering 16 (2013), S260–S261. doi:10.1080/ 10255842.2013.815856.

[7] Y. Lu and T. Lekszycki, A novel coupled system of non-local integro-differential equations modelling Young's modulus evolution, nutrients' supply and consumption during bone fracture healing, Zeitschrift fur Angewandte Mathematik und Physik 67 (2016), 111. doi: 10.1007/s00033-016-0708-1

[8] D. George, C. Spingarn, A. Madeo and Y. Rémond, in: Effects of Mechanical Loading Conditions on 3D Bone Reconstruction: A Theoretical Numerical Study for Application to Maxillo-Facial Surgery, 9th European Solid Mechanics Conference, Madrid, Spain, 2015.

[9] Dessouter, J. Le remodelage osseux normal et pathologique. Revue francophone des laboratoires. 2012. vol. 2012, no 446, p. 33-42.

[10] Servier TechBlog. L'os un tissu vivant - Le remodelage osseux : du normal au pathologique. [Vidéo en ligne]. 2013. Cité le 12 nov. 2017.

[11] Charbonnier, B. Développement de procédés de mise en forme et de caractérisation pour l'élaboration de biocéramiques en apatites phosphocalciques carbonatées. [Thèse de doctorat]. Lyon. France. ED SIS Saint-Étienne. 2016.

[12] A. Barkaoui, R. Hambli, Nanomechanical properties of mineralised collagen microfibrils based on finite elements method: biomechanical role of cross-links, Comput. Methods Biomech. Biomed. Engin. 17-14 (2014) 1590-1601.

[13] F. Yuan, S.R. Stock, D.R. Haeffner, J.D. Almer, D.C. Dunand, L. Catherine Brinson, A new model to simulate the elastic properties of mineralized collagen fibril, Biomech. Model. Mechanobiol. 10 (2011) 147-160.

[14] M. Nierenberger, G. Fargier, S. Ahzi and Y. Rémond, Evolution of the three-dimensional collagen structure in vascular walls during deformation: An in situ mechanical testing under multiphoton microscopy observation, Biomechanics and modeling in mechanobiology 14 (2015), 693-702. doi:10.1007/s10237-014-0630-4.

[15] Jason Coquim, Joseph Clemenzi, Mohsen Salahi. Biomechanical Analysis Using FEA and Experiments of Metal Plate and Bone Strut Repair of a Femur Midshaft Segmental Defect. BioMed

Research International, Volume 2018, 11 pages.

[16] T. Lekszycki, Modeling of bone adaptation based on an optimal response hypothesis, Meccanica 37 (2002), 343-354. doi:10.1023/A:1020831519496.

[17] M. Nierenberger, Y. Rémond and S. Ahzi, A new multiscale model for the mechanical behavior of vein walls, Journal of the mechanical behavior of biomedical materials 23 (2013), 32-43. doi:10.1016/j.jmbbm.2013.04.001.

[18] S. Jaramillo-Isaza, P.E. Mazeran, K. El-Kirat and M.C. Ho Ba Tho, Effects of bone density in the time-dependent mechanical properties of human cortical bone by nanoindentation, Computer Methods in Biomechanics and Biomedical Engineering 17 (2014), 34-35. doi:10.1080/10255842.2014.931090.

[19] George, Daniel et al. 'Examples of Multiscale and Multiphysics Numerical Modeling of Biological Tissues'. Bio-Medical Materials and Engineering 28 (2017) S15-S27 S15. DOI 10.3233/BME-171621.

[20] R. Ruimerman, P. Hilbers, B. van Rietbergen and R. Huiskes, A theoretical framework for strain-related trabecular bone maintenance and adaptation, Journal of Biomechanics 38 (2005), 931-941. doi:10.1016/j.jbiomech.2004.03.037.

[21] H. Weinans, R. Huiskes and H.J. Grootenboer, The behavior of adaptative bone remodeling simulation models, Journal of Biomechanics 25 (1992), 1425-1441. doi:10.1016/0021-9290 (92) 90056 -7.

Chapter 2

Mechanobiological Behavior of a Pathological Bone

Imane Ait Oumghar, Abdelwahed Barkaoui and Patrick Chabrand

Abstract

Bone density and bone microarchitecture are two principle parameters needed for the evaluation of mechanical bone performance and consequently the detection of bone diseases. The mechanobiological behavior of the skeletal tissue has been described through several mathematical models. Generally, these models fingerboard different length scale processes, such as the mechanical, the biological, and the chemical ones. By means of the mechanical stimulus and the biological factors involved in tissue regeneration, bone cells' behavior and bone volume changes are determined. The emergence of bone diseases leads to disrupt the bone remodeling process and thus, induces bone mechanical properties' alteration. In the present chapter, an overview of bone diseases and their relationship with bone density alteration will be presented. Besides, several studies treating bone diseases' effect on bone remodeling will be discussed. Finally, the mechanobiological models proposed to treat bone healing and drugs' effect on bone, are going to be reviewed. For this sake, the chapter is subdivided into three main sequences: (i) Bone remodeling, (ii) Bone deterioration causes, (iii) Mathematical models of a pathological bone, and (iv) Mechanobiological models treating bone healing and drugs effect.

Keywords: mechanobiological modeling, bone remodeling, mathematical models, bone diseases, bone healing, drugs

1. Introduction

An adult body skeleton is renewed once each 10 years as a median frequency. The renewing is the result of a biological process, persisting in the human body, known as bone remodeling. This biological phenomenon has been defined, for the first time, as a dynamic process [1]. It permits to maintain the mechanical bone strength by preserving the most important minerals' homeostasis. It consists of a spatial and temporal coupling of two main phases: (i) old bone resorption and (ii) new bone formation. This process is controlled by a variety of signaling mechanisms that orchestrate bone cells functioning. These cells are: (i) osteoblasts, (ii) osteoclasts, and (iii) osteocytes. Osteoblasts are mononucleated cells that derive from mesenchymal stem cells (MSCs), which originate in the bone marrow. These lasts are responsible of bone formation. Then, osteoclasts are multinucleated cells that derive from hematopoietic stem cells, which are notably produced in the bone marrow. These lasts are the only cells able to degrade bone [2, 3]. Eventually, osteocytes are the cells type that represent the highest amount of bone cells in the body (90–95%) [4]. They are the result of the last differentiation of the osteogenic lineage and have a mechanosensing feature that allow them to feel the mechanical loading applied on the bone matrix and release various signaling factors that triggers the other bone cells to start their activity. During bone remodeling process, these cells are interacting with each other and various biochemical and mechanical factors are orchestrating their functioning [5]. Bone diseases emerge when the normal process of bone remodeling is interrupted. This result is generally occurring when the balance of the biochemical factors controlling the process is lost. Indeed, there are many types of bone diseases. Yet, some of them are more common than the others. The most prevalent types of bone problems are osteoporosis, Paget's disease of bone, and cancer-associated bone loss. Three cancer types are affecting a large slice of society and induce bone degradation and fracturs: Multiple myeloma, Breast cancer, and Prostate cancer. Several studies have been interested in analyzing these bone diseases' effect and also drugs' effect on bone remodeling process [5–8] to predict the bone behavior after getting affected by the disease and determine to which extent a treatment's type or specific dose are reducing the effect of the disease. In the present chapter we are going to provide a description of bone remodeling and some diseases feature, then to present the different mechanobiological models dealing with bone diseases and drugs' effect on bone remodeling. The chapter is subdivided into three main sequences: (ii) Bone deterioration causes, (ii) Mathematical models of a pathological bone, and (iii) Mechanobiological models treating bone healing and drugs effect.

2. Bone remodeling

2.1 Generalities

The cell activity leading to bone renewing has been identified by Frost [9] as a bone multicellular unit (BMU). A mature BMU contains a group of osteoclast and osteoblast cells, in addition to blood supply associated with the connective tissue. Knowing that the lifespan of a BMU is higher than the cells one, new osteoclasts and osteoblasts have to continually adhere to the BMU space in order to maintain its operation [10]. The bone multicellular units are presented in our skeletal under the form of discrete foci that could take different shapes, such as the unidirectional, the branched, and the clustered forms [11]. These foci move forward in all bone compartment to assure the renewing of concerned places with a longitudinal advance rate of 25 μm/day [12].

In order to characterize and discover precisely the movement of bone cells during the remodeling process, researchers have identified four phases of this biological phenomenon. First, the activation phase where osteoblasts are excited to release resorbing cytokines, after receiving the biological signal transmitted by osteocytes. Osteocytes are a bone cells that are embedded in the bone matrix and have the ability to sense the mechanical force applied upon the bone. Resorbing cytokines are responsible of the osteoclasts' recruitment. The involvement of these cells engenders the start of resorption phase. During this remodeling step, active osteoclasts erode the damaged bone matrix by means of ions, acid, and enzymes [13, 14]. Thereafter, macrophages appear into the gap created and clean the surface from the remaining bone debris. This step is called the reversal phase and it is essential to prepare a clean surface for matrix formation. In order to fill in the bone lacunae, active osteoblasts migrate into the concerned surface and produce the osteoid, which gets gradually mineralized [15]. The final result of bone remodeling is, thus, a new, healthy, and stronger bone matrix.

2.2 Bone cells regulation

As shown above, osteoblast, osteoclast, and osteocytes are predominantly controlling the bone turnover. Thus, it is essential to understand the different steps of these cells differentiation and how biological factors are regulating their activity.

2.2.1 Regulation of osteoblasts

Osteoblasts are mononucleated cells that derive from mesenchymal stem cells (MSCs), which originate in the bone marrow. Those cells are multipotent stromal cells that have the ability to differentiate into a multitude of different cells thanks to their gene expression program. Among these cells, we can find osteoblasts, fibroblasts, adipocytes, and chondrocytes [16, 17]. The first step of osteoblastogenesis is regulated by Wingless-int (Wnt), specifically the Wnt10b protein coding gene. In [18], the authors proved that Wnt plays a key role in the stimulation of MSCs differentiation into osteo/chondro progenitors and the inhibition of preadipocyte commitment. Several other biological factors are involved in MSC differentiation into active osteoblast. Among which we can cite Runt-related transcriptor factor (Runx2), Osterix (Osc), Alkaline Phosphatase (ALP), type 1 parathyroid receptor (PTH1R), Osteopontin, and sialoprotein 2 (BSP II) (**Figure 1**). The process is described in details in [19].

Based on these information, we can deduct that osteoblastogenesis is a couple of complex biological interactions involving various factors where a simple alteration could destroy the whole system. For instance, Runx2, plays an important role in skeletal development. However, high amount of this transcription factor could inhibit the osteoblast maturation process and lead consequently to osteopenia disease [20]. Concurrently, other factors such as bone morphogenetic proteins (BMPs), transforming growth factor beta (TGFβ), parathyroid hormone (PTH), and fibroblast growth factor (FGF) have been judged as critical regulator factors of Runx2 [21]. Aside from Runx2, Wnt/β-catenin and BMPs have also a huge impact on bone formation and precisely on osteoblastogenesis regulation [22–24].

2.2.2 Regulation of osteoclasts

Osteoclasts are the only cells able to degrade the bone [2, 3]. They derive from hematopoietic stem cells, which are produced in the bone marrow. By dint of the macrophage colony stimulating factor (M-CSF), these stem cells are differentiated into macrophages and osteoclast progenitors. M-CSF is known as one of the main stimulator factors of osteoclastogenesis as it stimulates preosteoclasts proliferation and their expression of receptor activator of NFkB (RANK), that represents a key

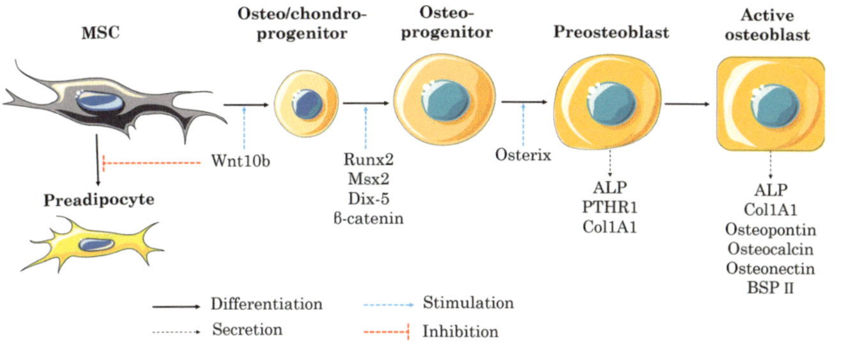

Figure 1.
Schematic representation of oteoblastogenesis process.

factor in osteoclasts maturation. Indeed, additionally to its principal function of bone synthesize, osteoblasts have been reported to regulate osteoclastogenesis through its secretion of the M-CSF and the receptor activator of NFkB Ligand (RANKL). According to the literature, RANKL is also secreted by osteocytes [25]. This ligand expression is stimulated by various types of hormones and factors such as PTH, prostaglandin E2 (PGE2) and 1.25-dihydroxyvitamin D3 (1.25$(OH)_2D_3$). Indeed, RANKL's interaction with its receptor RANK is mandatory for osteoclasts' differentiation, maturation and activation as it induces the recruitment of many hormones inside the preosteoclasts. RANK/RANKL binding simulates the recruitment of the tumor necrosis factor receptor associated factor 6 (TRAF6), which triggers a succession of interactions leading to osteoclastogenesis transcription. During osteoclastogenesis the osteoclast progenitors get differentiated into preosteoclasts. Then as a result of preosteoclasts fusion, mature multinucleated osteoclasts are created, where the nuclei's number can variate between four to twenty nuclei [26].

2.2.3 Regulation of osteocytes

Osteocytes represent the highest amount of bone cells in the body (90–95%) [4]. They are the result of the last differentiation of the osteogenic lineage. Indeed, during bone gap filling, some osteoblasts get trapped into the osteoid and differentiate into osteocytes [27]. Some authors have distinguished between several stages of osteocytogenesis. Based on [28], it has been mentioned that the transition from osteoblasts into osteocytes is governed by seven stages: (i) osteoblast, (iii) osteoblastic osteocyte (Type 1 preosteocyte), (vi) osteoid osteocyte (Type 2 preosteocyte), (v) Type 3 preosteocyte, (vi) young osteocyte, and (vii) old osteocyte. Throughout the transition, a multitude of actions took place. Actually, during all these differential stages, the cell undergoes many morphological changes to become a cell with dendritic extensions [29, 30]. In contrary to MSC to osteoblast transition, the signaling mechanisms during the process governing osteoblast to osteocyte transition is poorly understood. However, some authors have recently found some regulating factors impacting the process such as PTH and insulin-like growth factor type 1 (IGF-1) as, according to [31], they enhance osteoblast-osteocyte differentiation. The osteocytes surround the blood vessels in a cylindrical way and are organized in parallel to the bone surface. They are interconnected between each other by means of their dendritic extensions that occupy tiny canals called canaliculi. These canaliculi permit the transduction of biochemical signals to other osteocytes and bone cells located in the surface [32, 33]. Thanks to their characteristics, osteocytes are the best known for their ability to sense the mechanical loadings and transmit the information to the other bone cells in such a way the bone remodeling process can start.

2.3 Bone remodeling cycle

Bone remodeling process (**Figure 2**) as mentioned before is a succession of events governed by many biochemical factors. In this section, the most important interactions, actions and reactions are described in summary to show the bone cells dynamics and their effect on the bone mass changes.

2.3.1 Activation

1. Mechanical loading applied on the skeletal

2. Osteocytes are excited

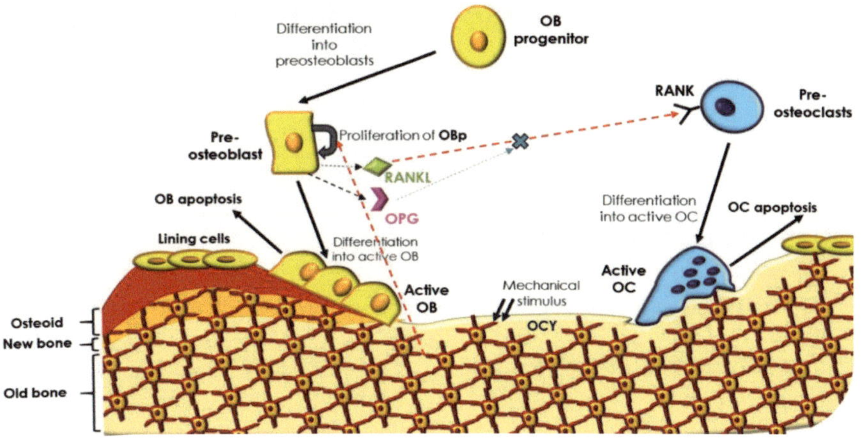

Figure 2.
Schematic representation of bone cells main biochemical interactions during bone remodeling process.

3. Osteocytes release biochemical factors stimulating osteoblasts and osteoclasts (e.g. nitric oxide (NO), sclerostin (SCLR), M-CSF and RANKL) promoting osteoblast proliferation and osteoclasts differentiation.

4. MSCs release biochemical factor stimulating osteoclastogenesis (e.g. M-CSF and RANKL)

2.3.2 Formation

1. Differentiation, proliferation, and activity of osteoclasts. The osteoclastogenesis is mediated by RANK-RANKL binding.

2. Active osteoclasts secrete hydrogen ions and acid phosphatases

3. Mineral phase of the bone matrix is dissolved

4. Active osteoclasts secrete enzymes

5. Organic phase of the bone is resorbed, and embedded biochemical factors are released (e.g. TGFβ and BMP)

6. Osteoblastogenesis is stimulated and osteoprotegerin (OPG) amount increases inducing RANKL decrease

7. Osteoclasts undergo apoptosis

2.3.3 Reversal

1. Macrophages clean the bone lacunae from bone matrix debris

2. Active osteoblasts adhere to bone lacunae

2.3.4 Formation

1. Active osteoblasts synthetize the collagen to produce the osteoid that gets gradually mineralized.

2. At the end osteoblasts differentiate into osteocyte, lining cells or undergo apoptosis

2.3.5 Termination

1. Signals exciting bone cells decreases in the area

2. BMU recruitment gets smaller

Any interruption of the biological pathways, during remodeling process, can lead to enormous consequences on the bone cells functioning, which in its turn leads to very dangerous diseases.

2.4 Bone mechanobiology

The mechanobiology particularity of bone tissue is the base source of its renewing ability and its capacity to be adapted to external charges. Based on many experimentations, researchers have found noticeable changes in bone mass, while variating the external applied charges on the skeleton [34–39]. Thanks to the bone microarchitecture and its tissue composition, the mechanical loads are transmitted at the cells' level as a combination of fluid shear stress and extracellular strain matrix [40]. Then, thanks to the osteocytes' mechanosensing mechanisms like ion channels, integrins, gap junction, and actin cytoskeleton, these cells become able to release biochemical components (e.g. proteins and cytokines) that regulates osteoblasts and osteoclasts' activity (e.g. increasing their proliferation/differentiation and inhibiting their apoptosis). For the sake of illustration, we mention the most known biochemical factors involved: PGE2 [41], NO [42], and SCLR [43]. In addition to osteocytes, osteoblasts have also been classified as a mechanosensory cell as their respond to the mechanical signal mediated by the fluid flow by upregulating the cyclooxygenase-2 (Cox-2) and c-fos and producing intracellular calcium (Ca^{2+}).

3. Bone deterioration causes

3.1 Normal bone diseases

3.1.1 Osteoporosis

Osteoporotic bone is a fragile bone characterized by a low mass (**Figure 3**) and deteriorated microstructure. These features are making this bone highly susceptible to fractures. Osteoporosis is a biochemical problem resulted from both osteoblast and osteoclast behaviors' dysregulation that leads to excessive bone resorption. It affects a large slice of the world's population, especially women, and it causes physical debilitation and frequent fracture incidence in patients. Osteoporotic fractures are generally occurring in the spine, hips, femur, and forearm; and they can be detected in case of a drop in the bone mineral density (BMD) value in the fractured area [44]. Based on the disease type, scientists have subdivided osteoporosis into two categories: (i) the primary osteoporosis, which is related to age and hormonal dysregulation, or unknown causes. This latter case is called idiopathic primary osteoporosis [45]. Then, (ii) the secondary osteoporosis, which is related to other diseases appearance (e.g. cancer, hematologic, and gastrointestinal diseases), or to some treatments use (e.g. Cancer chemotherapeutic drugs, glucocorticoids, and anticonvulsants [45]).

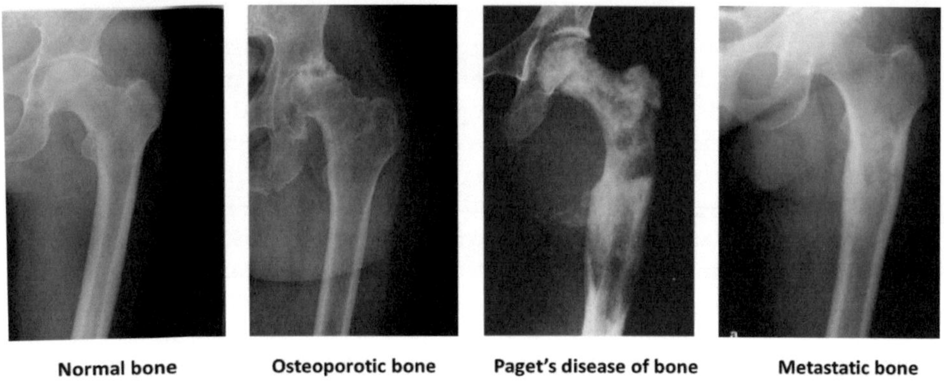

Figure 3.
Difference between normal proximal femur and femur affected by osteoporosis, Paget's disease, and cancer, based on medical images.

3.1.2 *Paget's disease of bone*

Paget's disease of bone is a chronic bone disease, that affect either a single or multiples parts of the skeletal. The concerned areas are characterized by increased bone resorption accompanied with increased but disorganized bone formation [46] (**Figure 3**). These problems in the bone remodeling process causes deformed and weak bones. Generally, this disease affect men and the elderly more than women and young people [47]. The real etiology of this disease is still unknown, however, 40% of patient affected by Paget's disease have been detected to have a family history of SQSTM1 gene mutation with a protein regulating osteoclasts called p62 [48]. Advanced Paget's disease of bone could cause several complication to the patient, among which, bone pain, bone fractures, and hypercalcemia [49].

3.1.3 *Osteogenesis imperfecta*

Also known as brittle bone disease, osteogenesis imperfecta is a group of rare bone diseases characterized by heterogeneous disturbance of the cognitive tissue. All these diseases are associated with bone mass diminution, increased bone fragility, bone disfigurement, and bone formation insufficiency [50]. Osteogenesis imperfecta etiology-associated differ from a disease to another as it depends mainly on the onsets and intensity of each one. Genetic, phenotypic and functional classification have been adopted to find out the new causative mutation of osteogenesis imperfecta onset [51]. The most commonly known osteogenesis imperfecta diseases are: (i) X-linked hyposphantaemia (XLH), which is characterized by a mutation of phosphate regulating endopeptidase (PHEX) leading to dysregulate 1,25 OH vitamin D levels; (ii) Hypoparathyroidism, which is characterized by PTH deficit that regulate calcium homeostasis; (iii) Hypophosphatasia, which results from mutation of a responsible gene of encoding ALP called ALPL. The dysregulation of the enzyme disrupts its function to prompt adequate mineralization at an appropriate time in bone tissue; and (vi) Osteopetrosis caused by gene mutation code for RANK and RANKL, leading to an impairment of osteoclasts and thus increased bone mass with a deterioration of bone quality resulting in atraumatic fractures.

3.2 Metastatic bone diseases

Bone degradation is related to several different factors among which, cancer is the most discussed issue. Regardless of the cancer type, cancer patients have a higher risk of bone loss than the rest of the population [52]. In fact, bone microenvironment enables tumor cells to home, proliferate, and colonize [5]. Thus, generally, cancer cells migrate form their inherent location to bone microenvironment, were osteoblasts and osteoclasts secrete important biochemical factors for their survival [53]. Each cancer type secretes special biochemical factors affecting bone environment and stimulating their growth. The spread of tumor causes the so-called bone metastasis disease either if it is a solid tumor (e.g. prostate cancer, breast cancer) or a liquid tumor (e.g. multiple myeloma). Bone metastasis incidence is mostly occurring in multiple myeloma patients (95–70%), breast cancer patients (75–65%), and prostate cancer patients (75–65%) [54].

3.2.1 Multiple myeloma

Multiple myeloma is a blood cancer disease characterized by an abnormal growth of B-lymphocytes, while differentiating into plasma cells. This cancer is characterized by renal impairment (creatinine >2 mg/dL), hypercalcemia (calcium >11 mg/dL) anemia (hemoglobin <10 mg/dL), the infiltration of clonal plasma, and end organ damage such as lytic lesions in the bone [55, 56]. As mentioned before, this disease is tightly related to bone degradation. Located in the bone marrow, multiple myeloma cells are able to interact with bone remodeling cells by means of adhesion molecules to proliferate and survive [57]. Indeed, multiple myeloma adhesion incite osteoblastic cells to release interleukin- 6 (IL-6), which has an essential role in tumor growth and survival [5, 58]. Studies found that multiple myeloma growth affect both bone formation and bone resorption. On one hand, they stimulate the differentiation and activity of osteoclasts by secreting RANKL, the interleukins IL-1, IL-3, IL-6, and the parathyroid hormone-related protein (PTHrP) that in turn stimulate RANKL expression by osteoblasts. Additionally, they express syndecan-1, which is a type 1 transmembrane proteoglycan, that binds OPG [59]. This multiple effects on RANK/RANKL/OPG pathway enhances osteoclastogenesis and consequently bone resorption. On the other hand, multiple myeloma cells inhibit the osteoblastogenesis by expressing some biochemical factors such like Wnt and dickkopf-related protein 1 (DKK-1) [60].

3.2.2 Breast cancer

Breast cancer is a common disease among postmenopausal women. It is characterized by an abnormal growth of breast epithelial cells. Multiple factors are related to this disease incidence including age, as advancing age increases the risk of getting breast cancer, gender, as women are the most concerned, personal or family history of breast cancer, and exogenous hormone use, as some treatments increasing sex hormones notably estrogen and progesterone [61]. Brest cancer develops because of DNA damage that could be the result of sex hormones exposure [62]. Epithelial tumor cells tend as well as the other cancer types, to migrate into the bone microenvironment and interact with bone cells. Actually, breast cancer tumor cells stimulate RANKL expression and inhibit the OPG one by expressing a multitude of biochemical factors, among which we note the interukins IL-1, IL-6, IL-8, IL-11, M-CSF, BMP, DKK-1, PGE2, PTHrP [63]. As a consequence, tumor prevalence in the bone area induces bone loss.

3.2.3 Prostate cancer

Prostate cancer is a common disease among elderly men, which usually leads to death as it is the case in the USA [64]. It is characterized by an abnormal growth of the prostate basal and luminal epithelial cells [65]. The real etiology of prostate cancer is still unknown, however, there is some factors related to its incidence. For instance, age, as advancing age increases the risk of getting prostate cancer, family history of prostate cancer, and using dietary supplement rich of vitamin E [66]. Similarly to multiple myeloma and breast cancer, prostate tumor cells also adhere to bone microenvironment and interact with bone cells. It has been reported that prostate tumor cells secrete PTHrP, Wnt and DKK-1 that regulates osteoblast and osteoclast behavior once settled in the bone [67, 68]. Thereafter, when prostate cancer cells adapt to the new environment, they start secreting the prostate- specific antigen (PSA), that inhibit PTHrP. The high amount of Wnt stimulate osteoblasts differentiation, and thus RANKL amount increase. When RANKL increases, bone resorptions is enhanced as result, and the biochemical factors incorporated in the old bone are released stimulating tumor cells proliferation [7].

4. Mathematical models of a pathological bone

Several studies have been interested in bone diseases' effect on bone remodeling process [5]. A large number of the mathematical models, developed in this regard have been concentrated on the biological aspect related to bone remodeling, so that they can provide a better understanding of the disease biological effect on the process.

4.1 Normal bone diseases

Osteoporosis, as it is the most widespread bone disease and the most known bone problem, it has captured the attention of many authors, especially those developing bone remodeling mathematical models. Through their mathematical models, the authors try to schematize as best as possible the osteoporosis disease in such a way the results could fit the experimental data.

In their study [69], Lemaire and co-authors have investigated the effect of osteoporosis on the normal biochemical interactions during remodeling process. They opted for the implementation of three osteoporosis causes: (i) estrogen deficiency, (ii) vitamin D hormone calcitriol ($1.25(OH)_2D_3$) deficiency, and (iii) glucocorticoid excess. These osteoporosis' causes have been implemented by changing some parameters' value in the principal bone remodeling mathematical model. According to authors, estrogen deficiency could be represented by decreasing OPG's production rate parameter until osteoclast to osteoblast concentration ratio reaches 5 in the steady state. Then, concerning vitamin D deficiency, it could be represented by increasing the PTH production rate, while glucocorticoid excess could be schematized by decreasing osteoblast progenitors' differentiation rate. The choices made by the authors are inspired from the literature: (i) authors have choose to decrease PTH production, as originally estrogen expression is stimulating OPG production [70], (ii) PTH effect on bone cells changes with vitamin D3 deficiency, thus PTH production rate alteration has been based on experimental observations [71], and (iii) Glucocorticoid induces a decrease in the core binding factor A1 (Cbfa) that is important for osteoblast differentiation, thus, the rate of preosteoblast differentiation has been reduced to mimic the glucocorticoid excess effect osteoblastogenesis [72].

Targeting the same objective, Pivonka et al. [73] have studied the RANK-RANKL-OPG signaling pathway to model osteoporosis disease in postmenopausal women. In their research study, the catabolic bone disease has been represented firstly by decreasing the OPG production value, then by testing a combination of changed parameter related to the components RANK-RANKL-OPG. The combination used in the model is based on [74]'s work, where RANK responsiveness and RANKL production are up-regulated, while OPG production is down-regulated. These changes enhanced osteoclasts' response comparably to the osteoblasts' one. However, the intensity of bone resorption resulted is different from changing one parameter to three parameters. Indeed, it has been observed that a change in one single parameter leads to less sever bone resorption. Overall, the obtained numerical results were qualitatively consistent with the experimental observation related to RANK/RANKL/OPG system changes in the case of postmenopausal osteoporosis (PMO) bone disorder.

Apart from osteoporosis, Paget's disease has also interested some researchers, but another time the model developed considering this bone problem have only treated the biological side of the remodeling process. The work of Komarova et al. [75] have illustrated the bone cells dynamics in the presence of Paget's disease. To proceed, authors have altered the parameters representing the normalized activity of resorption and formation parameters in addition to the autocrine parameters. Their model has demonstrated more sensitivity to changes made on the autocrine parameters' values. These changes lead to increase bone resorption succeeded by increased bone formation and represented nearly the same effect of Paget's disease of bone. Nevertheless, the real biological process or the particular effects inducing this type of bone diseases have not been deemed.

4.2 Metastatic bone diseases

Being one of bone metastasis causes, cancer seems to be an important subject to treat for the clinical interest. As shown before, different types of cancer are causing bone loss, that could be sometimes escorted by bone formation. These bone changes are due to the cancer cells growing inside the bone, that represents a rich area assuring their expansion.

The paper of [76] have treated the problem of cancer's effect on bone health independently of the cancer type. Based on a mathematical model composed of differential equations, authors have calculated bone cells number's variation, which depend either from a normal biological process or a disrupted process controlled by tumor cells growth. According to the tumor growth, the type of bone disorder (i.e. osteolysis or osteosclerosis) is deducted. Therefore, the types of biochemical released factors controlling the process are identified (i.e. TGFβ and PTHrP for osteolysis case/TGFβ and IGF for osteosclerosis case).

In more detailed studies, authors have opted for specific cancer's type effect on the remodeling process. For instance, a mathematical model have been described by Farhat et al. [7] to quantifying bone remodeling changes within the existence of prostate tumor cells in the bone microenvironment. Based on a large literature study, the authors managed to detect the main biological factor controlling the interactions between bone cells and the tumor's one. In summary, authors have made the following assumptions:

- Uncommitted osteoblast differentiation into preosteoblasts is governed by either TGFβ and Wnt.

- Preosteoblasts' differentiation is controlled not only by TGFβ, but also by the Wnt. Wnt is playing an activator role in the process, while TGFβ is inhibiting the differentiation.

- Active osteoclasts apoptosis is variating from a given base rate, then, it follows TGFβ's concentration as it performs as a stimulator factor of active osteoclasts' death.

- Bone formation is controlled by calcium concentration, which plays a stimulating function, rather than being only relied to active osteoblast concentration.

Through this article, prostate cancer growth's impact on the bone remodeling process has been properly established as each influencing factor has been simply explained. According to the results, prostate cancer cells existence induces an increase of RANKL-OPG ratio and bone production. Besides, they found that there are two osteogenic states over the course of disease.

Multiple myeloma's influence on bone remodeling has captured more attention than the other cancers. The research article [6] has provided a model schematizing multiple myeloma cells' growth impact on bone cells dynamics. The model has not clearly shown the biochemical effect of these malignant cells on the normal process. Although, it has shown their effect on the autocrine and paracrine parameters described previously in [75]. Authors have suggested a tumor density differential equation to schematize the metastasis evolution, and they have implemented it mathematically into the paracrine and autocrine variables to disrupt the normal oscillation of bone cells during remodeling cycles. This study findings have completely represented multiple myeloma effect on bone mass evolution. However, the biological interaction occurring between tumor cells and bone cells have not been explicitly shown. Thus, the effect of biochemical factors is not clearly presented.

One year later, a study considered precisely the main biological interactions occurring during a remodeling process affected by multiple myeloma's actions. In the model suggested by Wang et al. [77], multiple myeloma cells behavior have been modeled by differential equations, which permit to calculate the concentration of the principal biochemical factors affecting the bone cells. These factors are the interleukin 6 IL-6, which is secreted by uncommitted osteoblasts promoting multiple myeloma tumor cells' proliferation, and the very-late antigen 4 (VLA-4), which mediate Multiple myeloma-Bone marrow-derived mesenchymal stem cells adhesion and promote IL-6 expression. This antigen effect appears after VLA-4 binding vascular cell adhesion molecule 1 (VCAM-1) expressed by the uncommitted osteoblasts. A further investigation of the problem has been done by [78], where, additionally to the previous biochemical factors incorporated in the model of [77], they have added the effect of small leucine-rich proteoglycan (SLRPs). This regulator is secreted by active osteoblasts. Its main function, in the case on multiple myeloma tumor cells existence, is to inhibit their proliferation. Through this work, the biochemical mechanism controlling the bone remodeling is clearly described and properly established by means of the proposed system of differential equations.

5. Mechanobiological mathematical models of a pathological bone

In contrary to strictly biological mathematical models, bone diseases have been also incorporated into mechanobiological mathematical models, where the mechanical aspect is taken into consideration. Nevertheless, very few bone diseases have been discussed through these models. In this chapter, we are going to present the mechanobiological models treating osteoporosis problem. All the presented models are based on biological bone remodeling models that represent bone cell population through differential Equations [79]. These equations permit to determine bone cells' concentration variation over time. The behavior of these cells is controlled by the most influencing biochemical factors that exist in bone area within remodeling process.

In the work [80], authors were interested in explaining the experimentally changes of bone mass in postmenopausal women suffering from osteoporosis, without neglecting the mechanical influence on the process. Indeed, bone cells concentration variation over time has been controlled by biochemical factors and also by the mechanical strains in the extravascular cortical bone matrix. An activation function $\Pi^{mech}_{act,OBa}$ (Eq. (1)), representing strains in the extravascular area, was used to promote preosteoblast proliferation and RANKL production. The mechanical stimulus represented by strain energy density (SED) has a minimum and maximum values that correspond respectively to the threshold SED values $\Psi_{bm,min}$ and $\Psi_{bm,max}$. Indeed, according to the literature, RANKL/OPG ratio is affected by hydraulic pressure at the microscopic level [81]. Therefore, RANKL production function has been formulated as a function of the SED sensed at the bone matrix's level. On the other hand, the effect of postmenopausal osteoporosis has been implemented by considering the effect of mechanical feedback on the progress of PMO. First, authors have fixed a production rate of PTH that reflect the PMO and then they variated the maximum proliferation rate of preosteoblasts depending on the mechanical stimulus' level. Based on this, various PMO-scenarios have been established by changing the value of the strength of anabolic strength parameter . This parameter represents the slope of the activation function. Hence, it determines the degree of which the SED should be increased to reach the maximum value of the activation function that allows a maximum proliferation rate to the preostoblasts.

$$\Pi^{mech}_{act,OBa} = \begin{cases} 1/2 & \Psi_{bm} < \Psi_{bm,min} \\ 1/2\left(1+\lambda\left(\dfrac{\Psi_{bm}}{\Psi_{bm,min}}-1\right)\right) & \Psi_{bm,min} < \Psi_{bm} < \Psi_{bm,max} \\ 1 & \Psi_{bm,max} \le \Psi_{bm} \end{cases} \quad (1)$$

Based on the results, bone porosity, calculated based on the bone remodeling mathematical model, was able to show the severity of PMO evolution over time. According to the authors, the negligence of the mechanical feedback in the presence of PMO disease, lead to unbounded bone resorption, which doesn't reflect the reality. Thus, every study dealing with biological aspects of bone remodeling should take into consideration the mechanical aspect as well. With the same perspective, Pivonka et al. [82], have addressed the geometrical feedback effect upon bone volume evolution throughout the remodeling process and its capacity of accelerating osteoporotic porosity evolution. In this study, the osteoporosis origin has not been mentioned. Yet, its effect has been incorporated by increasing the PTH concentration by applying a continuous PTH administration rate of 500 pM/day, as previously done in [69], which induces an increase of RANKL/OPG's ratio and perturbs consequently its homeostatic steady-state.

Several other studies have been interested in osteoporosis effect on bone remodeling. For instance, [83, 84] are studies where the mechanobiological model developed by [80] has been modified to include PMO disease effect on bone remodeling process. RANKL production P_{RANKl} has been modified by adding the RANKL produced because of the PMO P^{PMO}_{RANKL} (Eq. (2)). This term leads to increase RANKL concentration and enhance preosteoclasts differentiation. The excess of RANKL production is defined by (Eq. (3)), where $P^{PMO,ini}_{RANKL}$ is PMO-initiating excess production rate of RANKL and φ^{RANKL}_{PMO} is reduced factor of $P^{PMO,ini}_{RANKL}$ which is formulated as presented in (Eq. (4)). In (Eq. (4)), ξ represents the characteristic time of the RANKL production decrease, t_{PMO}^{RANKL} determine the shape of Lorentz-type function (Eq. (4)), and $t_{PMO,ini}$ the time corresponding to PMO onset.

$$P_{RANKl} = P_{RANKL}^{mech} + P_{RANKL}^{PMO} \tag{2}$$

$$P_{RANKL}^{PMO} = P_{RANKL}^{PMO,ini}\varphi_{PMO}^{RANKL} \tag{3}$$

$$\varphi_{PMO}^{RANKL} = \frac{\xi^2}{\xi^2 + \left(\frac{t - t_{PMO,ini}}{t_{PMO}^{RANKL}}\right)2} \tag{4}$$

Furthermore, PMO effect has been mediated by decreasing the anabolic strength parameter, as previously done in [80].

Recently, PMO problem has been further investigated in the mechanobiological model described in [85]. PMO effect has been incorporated while taking into consideration the mechanical loading applied on the bone. Indeed, the model mechanical aspect has been similar to the previous discussed work of [80] and PMO effect was incorporated in a similar way to the work [86], where authors have imposed an increase in RANKL concentration by including a dosage term that increases RANKL production. This term is derived from experimental data of ovariectomized rats.

6. Mechanobiological models treating bone healing and drugs effect

Mechanobiological mathematical models of bone remodeling are not only used to present diseases and mechanical effects on the process. Actually, the main target of all researchers, by developing these models, is to provide ideas and therapeutic solutions that could be applied in the real life after a clinical validation. Hence, in this section, some models considering bone healing and the effect of some bone diseases' treatments are discussed.

A mathematical model integrating the biological and mechanical aspects to describe the process of osteointegration has been described in [87]. The osteointegration is the direct structural and functional connection between a living bone and an artificial implant surface [88]. Knowing that many factors are involved into healing the interface between the non-biological material and bone, a mechanobiological modeling of the concerned surface is mandatory. In this study, authors have subdivided the bone healing process into four stages: (i) Blood clotting, (ii) Cell migration, (iii) Granulation tissue, and finally (iv) bone formation. The formulated mathematical model, describing the process, took into consideration all the stages of bone-implant healing. Yet, in this chapter, we have only shed the light on bone formation phase. Researchers have suggested a differential equation to schematize the osteogenesis stage, that depends on ontogenetic cells' migration and the osteogenic chemical variables. These two component values have been calculated based on previous equations describing the former phases. Concerning the mechanical stimulus, it has been presented through a displacement matrix.

In another study, authors have developed a mathematical bone remodeling model gathering the biological factors and the mechanical stimuli's effect on bone cells dynamics [89]. This research has been devoted to assess the bone mechanobiological response and the cellular activity variation over time depending on specific types of physical activities. Based on the previous works [88, 89], the bone cells concentrations have been calculated. The mechanical stimuli have been added to promote the proliferation of the preosteoblast and to regulate RANKL production. As well as the majority of studies [80, 90, 91], the SED has been used to schematize the biomechanical stimuli's influence on cellular dynamics. The SED is calculated based on the stress and deformation tensors. In this study, these tensors were decomposed into deviatoric and hydrostatic parts, in order to get both hydrostatic and deviatoric SED quantities. Considering three stimuli in different remodeling periods, researchers have performed their finite element isotropic models. Seeking to know the formation performance, cortical and trabecular bone densities in the diaphysis and epiphysis regions of a proximal femur have been investigated. The comparison between the three mechanical stimuli (SED, deviatoric SED, and hydrostatic SED) revealed that: the formation of cortical and trabecular bone is higher for hydrostatic SED, followed by deviatoric SED, and finally by the whole SED stimuli. It has been remarked that the thickness of cortical bone was more significant applying Hydrostatic SED compared with the other stimulus type, while the trabecular density was higher under deviatoric SED stimulus. This study investigated then many mechanical stimuli and their particularity and effect on the development of bone density in many regions. Thus, it gave some insight about bone remodeling especially bone formation phase, which is also a primordial phase in bone healing process.

Concerning, the investigation of drugs dose effect on bone remodeling, the traditional mathematical models were not widely used in the literature. Instead, researchers opted for pharmacokinetic pharmacodynamic (PK/PD) models, which permit to predict the behavior of the treatment in different compartment of the body before reaching the blood. The results are then coupled with a traditional bone remodeling mathematical model. Various studies have been done in this respect, but which mostly treat the same type of drugs used for bone reparation such as denosumab. Studding denosumab effect on bone remodeling, this treatment has been generally included by modifying the function dedicated to calculate RANKL concentration in such a way the RANKL-binding denosumab is taken into consideration [82, 92]. In the work of [83], the mechanobiological feedback function has been incorporated to regulate preosteoclasts proliferation as previously done in [80] and the denosumab effect has been added by adjusting RANKL concentration. Other studies have been interested in PTH drug's effect, which is usually used for postmenopausal women. In the work of [86] for example, authors have created an equation representing PTH amount in the blood depending on the serum concentration injected. Based on the outcomes, they formulated another function that will control preosteoblast proliferation, lining cells differentiation, and active osteoclast apoptosis. Another recent study [85] has been based on [86], have investigated the same thing, which is PTH effect on bone density. This time, authors have included PTH into their bone remodeling mathematical model by modifying active osteoblasts apoptosis rate multiplying the normal parameter value by the function representing PTH drug concentration. In contrary to the work of [86], this model considered the mechanical feedback triggering preosteoblast proliferation. The term representing this mechanical feedback is the same used in [80].

7. Conclusion

To maintain the multiple functions of a skeletal, this last should be regularly renewed in such a way the old bone tissue is substituted with a new one. Applying cyclic mechanical loading on the bone helps to trigger the bone remodeling. Thus, people doing physical activities generally have stronger bones. On the other hand, the occurrence of some diseases because of age, hormonal deficiency or bad dietary habits leads to bone deterioration. The present chapter shed the light on the most popular bone diseases and the different mechanobiological bone remodeling that investigate the evolution of these diseases and some drugs effect on the evolution of bone mass over time. Based on the forgoing reviewed articles, some conclusions could be extracted:

- Further studies should be elaborated to treat additional bone diseases effect on bone, especially the prostate and breast cancer.
- Further studies should be elaborated to treat several drugs effect on bone repairing such as bisphosphonates and estrogen drugs.
- The mechanical aspect is extremely important while investigating the bone remodeling process as bone is always in touch with the external environment and the loading effects are not negligible.

Acknowledgements

This work was supported by the Partenariat Hubert Curien FrancoMoroccan TOUBKAL (PHC Toubkal) N° TBK/20/102 - CAMPUS N°43681QG.

Conflict of interest

The authors declare no conflict of interest.

Author details

Imane Ait Oumghar[1,2]*, Abdelwahed Barkaoui[2] and Patrick Chabrand[1]

1 Aix Marseille Univ, CNRS, ISM Inst Mouvement Sci, Marseille, France

2 Laboratoire des Energies Renouvelables et Matériaux Avancés (LERMA), Université Internationale de Rabat, Rabat-Sala El Jadida, Morocco

*Address all correspondence to: imane.aitoumghar@uir.ac.ma

References

[1] L. C. Johnson, “Morphologic analysis in pathology: the kinetics of disease and general biology of bone,” Bone Biodyn., pp. 543–654, 1964.

[2] T. Ono and T. Nakashima, “Recent advances in osteoclast biology,” Histochemistry and Cell Biology. pp. 325–341, 2018, doi: 10.1007/s00418-018-1636-2.

[3] I. Nakamura, N. Takahashi, E. Jimi, N. Udagawa, and T. Suda, “Regulation of osteoclast function,” Modern Rheumatology. pp. 869–879, 2012, doi: 10.1007/s10165-011-0530-8.

[4] C. V. B. de Gusmão and W. D. Belangero, “HOW DO BONE CELLS SENSE MECHANICAL LOADING?,” Rev. Bras. Ortop. (English Ed., pp. 299–305., 2009, doi: 10.1016/s2255-4971(15) 30157-9.

[5] I. Ait Oumghar, A. Barkaoui, and P. Chabrand, “Toward a Mathematical Modeling of Diseases’ Impact on Bone Remodeling: Technical Review,” Frontiers in Bioengineering and Biotechnology. p. 1236, 2020, doi: 10.3389/fbioe.2020.584198.

[6] B. P. Ayati, C. M. Edwards, G. F. Webb, and J. P. Wikswo, “A mathematical model of bone remodeling dynamics for normal bone cell populations and myeloma bone disease,” Biol. Direct, pp. 1–17, 2010, doi: 10.1186/1745-6150-5-28.

[7] A. Farhat, D. Jiang, D. Cui, E. T. Keller, and T. L. Jackson, “An integrative model of prostate cancer interaction with the bone microenvironment,” Math. Biosci., vol. 294, pp. 1–14, 2017, doi: 10.1016/j.mbs.2017.09.005.

[8] R. Hambli, M. H. Boughattas, J. L. Daniel, and A. Kourta, “Prediction of denosumab effects on bone remodeling: A combined pharmacokinetics and finite element modeling,” J. Mech. Behav. Biomed. Mater., pp. 492–504, 2016, doi: 10.1016/j.jmbbm.2016.03.010.

[9] H. M. Frost, “Tetracycline-based histological analysis of bone remodeling,” Calcif. Tissue Res., vol. 3, pp. 211–237, 1969, doi: 10.1007/bf02058664.

[10] S. C. Manolagas, “Birth and death of bone cells: Basic regulatory mechanisms and implications for the pathogenesis and treatment of osteoporosis,” Endocrine Reviews. pp. 115–137, 2000, doi: 10.1210/er.21.2.115.

[11] D. M. L. Cooper, C. D. L. Thomas, J. G. Clement, and B. Hallgrímsson, “Three-dimensional microcomputed tomography imaging of basic multicellular unit-related resorption spaces in human cortical bone,” Anat. Rec. - Part A Discov. Mol. Cell. Evol. Biol., vol. 288, no. 7, pp. 806–816, 2006, doi: 10.1002/ar.a.20344.

[12] Z. F. G. Jaworski, “Haversian systems and haversian bone,” Bone Metab. Miner., vol. 4, pp. 21–45, 1992.

[13] H. K. Väänänen, H. Zhao, M. Mulari, and J. M. Halleen, “The cell biology of osteoclast function,” Journal of Cell Science. pp. 377–381, 2000.

[14] K. Väänänen, “Mechanism of osteoclast mediated bone resorption - Rationale for the design of new therapeutics,” Advanced Drug Delivery Reviews. pp. 959–971, 2005, doi: 10.1016/j.addr.2004.12.018.

[15] D. J. Hadjidakis and I. I. Androulakis, “Bone remodeling,” Ann. N. Y. Acad. Sci., vol. 1092, no. October 2018, pp. 385–396, 2006, doi: 10.1196/annals.1365.035.

[16] A. E. Grigoriadis, J. N. M. Heersche, and J. E. Aubin, "Differentiation of muscle, fat, cartilage, and bone from progenitor cells present in a bone-derived clonal cell population: Effect of dexamethasone," J. Cell Biol., vol. 106, pp. 2139–2151, 1988, doi: 10.1083/jcb.106.6.2139.

[17] A. Yamaguchi and A. J. Kahn, "Clonal osteogenic cell lines express myogenic and adipocytic developmental potential," Calcif. Tissue Int., vol. 49, pp. 221–225, 1991, doi: 10.1007/BF02556122.

[18] C. N. Bennett et al., "Regulation of osteoblastogenesis and bone mass by Wnt10b," Proc. Natl. Acad. Sci. U. S. A., pp. 3324–3329, 2005, doi: 10.1073/pnas.0408742102.

[19] N. Rucci, "Molecular biology of bone remodelling," Clin. Cases Miner. Bone Metab., vol. 5, no. 1, pp. 49–56, 2008.

[20] W. Liu et al., "Overexpression of Cbfa1 in osteoblasts inhibits osteoblast maturation and causes osteopenia with multiple fractures," J. Cell Biol., pp. 157–166, 2001, doi: 10.1083/jcb.200105052.

[21] H. Kaneki et al., "Tumor necrosis factor promotes Runx2 degradation through up-regulation of Smurf1 and Smurf2 in osteoblasts," J. Biol. Chem., pp. 4326–4333, 2006, doi: 10.1074/jbc.M509430200.

[22] G. Rawadi and S. Roman-Roman, "Wnt signalling pathway: A new target for the treatment of osteoporosis," Expert Opinion on Therapeutic Targets. pp. 1063–1077, 2005, doi: 10.1517/14728222.9.5.1063.

[23] J. J. Westendorf, R. A. Kahler, and T. M. Schroeder, "Wnt signaling in osteoblasts and bone diseases," Gene. pp. 19–39, 2004, doi: 10.1016/j.gene.2004.06.044.

[24] D. M. Kingsley et al., "The mouse short ear skeletal morphogenesis locus is associated with defects in a bone morphogenetic member of the TGFβ superfamily," Cell, vol. 71, pp. 399–410, 1992, doi: 10.1016/0092-8674(92)90510-J.

[25] B. F. Boyce and L. Xing, "Biology of RANK, RANKL, and osteoprotegerin," Arthritis Research and Therapy. pp. 1–7, 2007, doi: 10.1186/ar2165.

[26] N. Udagawa et al., "Origin of osteoclasts: Mature monocytes and macrophages are capable of differentiating into osteoclasts under a suitable microenvironment prepared by bone marrow-derived stromal cells," Proc. Natl. Acad. Sci. U. S. A., vol. 87, pp. 7260–7264, 1990, doi: 10.1073/pnas.87.18.7260.

[27] H. M. FROST, "In vivo osteocyte death.," J. Bone Joint Surg. Am., pp. 138–143., 1960, doi: 10.2106/00004623-196042010-00011.

[28] T. A. Franz-Odendaal, B. K. Hall, and P. E. Witten, "Buried alive: How osteoblasts become osteocytes," Developmental Dynamics. pp. 176–190, 2006, doi: 10.1002/dvdy.20603.

[29] S. L. Dallas and L. F. Bonewald, "Dynamics of the transition from osteoblast to osteocyte," in Annals of the New York Academy of Sciences, 2010, p. 437, doi: 10.1111/j.1749-6632.2009.05246.x.

[30] S. L. Dallas, M. Prideaux, and L. F. Bonewald, "The osteocyte: An endocrine cell . . . and more," Endocrine Reviews. pp. 658–690, 2013, doi: 10.1210/er.2012-1026.

[31] T. Qiu, J. L. Crane, L. Xie, L. Xian, H. Xie, and X. Cao, "IGF-I induced phosphorylation of PTH receptor enhances osteoblast to osteocyte transition," Bone Res., vol. 6, pp. 1–12, 2018, doi: 10.1038/s41413-017-0002-7.

[32] L. E. Lanyon, "Amplification of the Osteogenic Stimulus of Load-Bearing as a Logical Therapy for the Treatment and Prevention of Osteoporosis," in Novel Approaches to Treatment of Osteoporosis, 1998, pp. 199–209.

[33] C. H. Turner, R. L. Duncan, and F. M. Pavalko, "Mechanotransduction: An Inevitable Process for Skeletal Maintenance," in Novel Approaches to Treatment of Osteoporosis, 1998, pp. 157–177.

[34] D. R. Carter, "Mechanical loading histories and cortical bone remodeling," Calcif. Tissue Int., vol. 36, pp. S19–S24, 1984, doi: 10.1007/BF02406129.

[35] M. R. Forwood and C. H. Turner, "Skeletal adaptations to mechanical usage: results from tibial loading studies in rats," Bone, vol. 17, pp. S197–S205, 1995, doi: 10.1016/8756-3282(95)00292-L.

[36] W. S. S. Jee, X. J. Li, and M. B. Schaffler, "Adaptation of diaphyseal structure with aging and increased mechanical usage in the adult rat: A histomorphometrical and biomechanical study," Anat. Rec., vol. 230, pp. 332–338, 1991, doi: 10.1002/ar.1092300306.

[37] J. R. Mosley and L. E. Lanyon, "Strain rate as a controlling influence on adaptive modeling in response to dynamic loading of the ulna in growing male rats," Bone, vol. 23, pp. 313–318, 1998, doi: 10.1016/S8756-3282(98)00113-6.

[38] J. A. O'Connor, L. E. Lanyon, and H. MacFie, "The influence of strain rate on adaptive bone remodelling," J. Biomech., vol. 15, pp. 767–781, 1982, doi: 10.1016/0021-9290(82)90092-6.

[39] S. L. Y. Woo et al., "The effect of prolonged physical training on the properties of long bone: A study of Wolff's law," J. Bone Jt. Surg. - Ser. A, vol. 63, pp. 780–787, 1981, doi: 10.2106/00004623-198163050-00013.

[40] S. W. Verbruggen and L. M. McNamara, "Bone mechanobiology in health and disease," in Mechanobiology in Health and Disease, 2018, pp. 157–214.

[41] J. Klein-Nulend et al., "Sensitivity of osteocytes to biomechanical stress in vitro," FASEB J., vol. 9, pp. 441–445, 1995, doi: 10.1096/fasebj.9.5.7896017.

[42] A. Liedert, D. Kaspar, P. Augat, A. Ignatius, and L. Claes, Mechanobiology of Bone Tissue and Bone Cells. 2005.

[43] G. L. Galea, L. E. Lanyon, and J. S. Price, "Sclerostin's role in bone's adaptive response to mechanical loading," Bone, vol. 96, pp. 38–44, 2017, doi: 10.1016/j.bone.2016.10.008.

[44] National Institute for Health and Care Excellence (Great Britain), "Clinical audit tool. Osteoporosis: assessing the risk of fragility fracture," 2012.

[45] Rockville, Bone health and osteoporosis: a report of the Surgeon General. 2004.

[46] J. L. Shaker, "Paget's disease of bone: A review of epidemiology, pathophysiology and management," Therapeutic Advances in Musculoskeletal Disease. pp. 107–125, 2009, doi: 10.1177/1759720X09351779.

[47] J. F. Charles, E. S. Siris, and G. D. Roodman, "Paget disease of bone," in Primer on the Metabolic Bone Diseases and Disorders of Mineral Metabolism, 2018, pp. 657–668.

[48] S. H. Ralston and R. Layfield, "Pathogenesis of paget disease of bone," Calcified Tissue International. pp. 97–113, 2012, doi: 10.1007/s00223-012-9599-0.

[49] S. H. Ralston, "Paget's disease of bone," N. Engl. J. Med., vol. 368, pp.

644–650, 2013, doi: 10.1056/NEJMcp 1204713.

[50] A. Forlino and J. C. Marini, "Osteogenesis imperfecta," The Lancet. pp. 1657–1671, 2016, doi: 10.1016/ S0140-6736(15)00728-X.

[51] S. Bacon and R. Crowley, "Developments in rare bone diseases and mineral disorders," Therapeutic Advances in Chronic Disease. pp. 51–60, 2018, doi: 10.1177/2040622317739538.

[52] M. Reuss-Borst, U. Hartmann, C. Scheede, and J. Weiß, "Prevalence of osteoporosis among cancer patients in Germany Prospective data from an oncological rehabilitation clinic," Osteoporos. Int., vol. 23, pp. 1437–1444, 2012, doi: 10.1007/s00198-011-1724-9.

[53] G. D. Roodman, "Mechanisms of Bone Metastasis," New England Journal of Medicine. pp. 1655–1664, 2004, doi: 10.1056/NEJMra030831.

[54] R. Rizzoli et al., "Cancer-associated bone disease," Osteoporos. Int., vol. 24, pp. 2929–2953., 2013, doi: 10.1007/ s00198-013-2530-3.

[55] S. V. Rajkumar and S. Kumar, "Multiple Myeloma: Diagnosis and Treatment," Mayo Clinic Proceedings. pp. 1371–1382, 2016, doi: 10.1016/j. mayocp.2015.11.007.

[56] R. A. Kyle and S. V. Rajkumar, "Criteria for diagnosis, staging, risk stratification and response assessment of multiple myeloma," Leukemia. pp. 3–9, 2009, doi: 10.1038/leu.2008.291.

[57] R. E. Walker, M. A. Lawson, C. H. Buckle, J. A. Snowden, and A. D. Chantry, "Myeloma bone disease: Pathogenesis, current treatments and future targets," Br. Med. Bull., vol. 111, no. 1, pp. 117–138, 2014, doi: 10.1093/ bmb/ldu016.

[58] K. Gadó, G. Domján, H. Hegyesi, and A. Falus, "Role of interleukin-6 in the pathogenesis of multiple myeloma," Cell Biol. Int., vol. 24, pp. 195–209, 2000, doi: 10.1006/cbir.2000.0497.

[59] E. Terpos, I. Ntanasis-Stathopoulos, M. Gavriatopoulou, and M. A. Dimopoulos, "Pathogenesis of bone disease in multiple myeloma: From bench to bedside," Blood Cancer Journal. pp. 1–12, 2018, doi: 10.1038/ s41408-017-0037-4.

[60] Y. Tanaka et al., "Myeloma cell-osteoclast interaction enhances angiogenesis together with bone resorption: A role for vascular endothelial cell growth factor and osteopontin," Clin. Cancer Res., vol. 13, pp. 816–823, 2007, doi: 10.1158/1078-0432.CCR-06-2258.

[61] Fadi M. Alkabban; Troy Ferguson, "Cancer, Breast," in StatPearls, StatPearls Publishing, 2020.

[62] A. Muhammad, M. Ibrahim, O. Erukainure, I. Malami, H. Sani, and H. Mohammed, "Metabolism and Toxicological Implications of Commonly Used Chemopreventive Drugs Against Breast Cancer/ Carcinogenesis," Curr. Drug Metab., vol. 17, pp. 930–936, 2017, doi: 10.2174/ 1389200218666161116121225.

[63] P. Clézardin, "Therapeutic targets for bone metastases in breast cancer," Breast Cancer Res., vol. 13, no. 2, pp. 1–9, 2011, doi: 10.1186/bcr2835.

[64] G. Galletti, L. Portella, S. T. Tagawa, B. J. Kirby, P. Giannakakou, and D. M. Nanus, "Circulating tumor cells in prostate cancer diagnosis and monitoring: An appraisal of clinical potential," Mol. Diagnosis Ther., vol. 18, pp. 389–402, 2014, doi: 10.1007/s40291-014-0101-8.

[65] J. W. Park et al., "Prostate epithelial cell of origin determines cancer differentiation state in an organoid transformation assay," Proc. Natl. Acad.

Sci. U. S. A., vol. 113, pp. 4482–4487, 2016, doi: 10.1073/pnas.1603645113.

[66] E. A. Klein et al., "Vitamin E and the risk of prostate cancer: The selenium and vitamin E cancer prevention trial (SELECT)," JAMA - J. Am. Med. Assoc., vol. 306, pp. 1549–1556, 2011, doi: 10.1001/jama.2011.1437.

[67] C. L. Hall, S. D. Daignault, R. B. Shah, K. J. Pienta, and E. T. Keller, "Dickkopf-1 expression increases early in prostate cancer development and decreases during progression from primary tumor to metastasis," Prostate, vol. 68, pp. 1396–1404, 2008, doi: 10.1002/pros.20805.

[68] F. Asadi, M. Farraj, R. Sharifi, S. Malakouti, S. Antar, and S. Kukreja, "Enhanced expression of parathyroid hormone-related protein in prostate cancer as compared with benign prostatic hyperplasia," Hum. Pathol., vol. 27, pp. 1319–1323, 1996, doi: 10.1016/S0046-8177(96)90344-5.

[69] V. Lemaire, F. L. Tobin, L. D. Greller, C. R. Cho, and L. J. Suva, "Modeling the interactions between osteoblast and osteoclast activities in bone remodeling," J. Theor. Biol., vol. 229, no. 3, pp. 293–309, 2004, doi: 10.1016/j.jtbi.2004.03.023.

[70] L. C. Hofbauer, S. Khosla, C. R. Dunstan, D. L. Lacey, T. C. Spelsberg, and B. L. Riggs, "Estrogen stimulates gene expression and protein production of osteoprotegerin in human osteoblastic cells," Endocrinology, vol. 140, pp. 4367–4370, 1999, doi: 10.1210/endo.140.9.7131.

[71] E. Slatopolsky, A. Dusso, and A. Brown, "New analogs of vitamin D3," Kidney Int. Suppl., vol. 56, pp. S46–S51, 1999, doi: 10.1046/j.1523-1755.1999.07305.x.

[72] T. Komori et al., "Targeted disruption of Cbfa1 results in a complete lack of bone formation owing to maturational arrest of osteoblasts," Cell, vol. 89, pp. 755–764, 1997, doi: 10.1016/S0092-8674(00)80258-5.

[73] P. Pivonka et al., "Theoretical investigation of the role of the RANK-RANKL-OPG system in bone remodeling," J. Theor. Biol., vol. 262, pp. 306–316, 2010, doi: 10.1016/j.jtbi.2009.09.021.

[74] L. C. Hofbauer, C. A. Kühne, and V. Viereck, "The OPG/RANKL/RANK system in metabolic bone diseases," J. Musculoskelet. Neuronal Interact., vol. 4, p. 268, 2004.

[75] S. V. Komarova, R. J. Smith, S. J. Dixon, S. M. Sims, and L. M. Wahl, "Mathematical model predicts a critical role for osteoclast autocrine regulation in the control of bone remodeling," Bone, vol. 33, no. 2, pp. 206–215, 2003, doi: 10.1016/S8756-3282(03)00157-1.

[76] D. A. Garzón-Alvarado, "A mathematical model for describing the metastasis of cancer in bone tissue," Comput. Methods Biomech. Biomed. Engin., vol. 15, pp. 333–346, 2012, doi: 10.1080/10255842.2010.535522.

[77] Y. Wang, P. Pivonka, P. R. Buenzli, D. W. Smith, and C. R. Dunstan, "Computational modeling of interactions between multiple myeloma and the bone microenvironment," PLoS One, vol. 6, p. e27494, 2011, doi: 10.1371/journal.pone.0027494.

[78] B. Ji, P. G. Genever, R. J. Patton, and M. J. Fagan, "Mathematical modelling of the pathogenesis of multiple myeloma-induced bone disease," Int. j. numer. method. biomed. eng., vol. 30, pp. 1085–1102, 2014, doi: 10.1002/cnm.2645.

[79] P. Pivonka et al., "Model structure and control of bone remodeling: A theoretical study," Bone, vol. 43, no. 2, pp. 249–263, 2008, doi: 10.1016/j.bone.2008.03.025.

[80] S. Scheiner, P. Pivonka, and C. Hellmich, "Coupling systems biology with multiscale mechanics, for computer simulations of bone remodeling," Comput. Methods Appl. Mech. Eng., vol. 254, pp. 181–196, 2013, doi: 10.1016/j.cma.2012.10.015.

[81] C. Liu, Y. Zhao, W. Y. Cheung, R. Gandhi, L. Wang, and L. You, "Effects of cyclic hydraulic pressure on osteocytes," Bone, vol. 46, pp. 1449–1456, 2010, doi: 10.1016/j.bone.2010.02.006.

[82] P. Pivonka, P. R. Buenzli, S. Scheiner, C. Hellmich, and C. R. Dunstan, "The influence of bone surface availability in bone remodelling-A mathematical model including coupled geometrical and biomechanical regulations of bone cells," Eng. Struct., vol. 47, pp. 134–147, 2013, doi: 10.1016/j.engstruct.2012.09.006.

[83] J. Martínez-Reina and P. Pivonka, "Effects of long-term treatment of denosumab on bone mineral density: insights from an in-silico model of bone mineralization," Bone, vol. 125, pp. 87–95, 2019, doi: 10.1016/j.bone.2019.04.022.

[84] S. Scheiner, P. Pivonka, D. W. Smith, C. R. Dunstan, and C. Hellmich, "Mathematical modeling of postmenopausal osteoporosis and its treatment by the anti-catabolic drug denosumab," Int. j. numer. method. biomed. eng., vol. 30, pp. 1–27, 2014, doi: 10.1002/cnm.2584.

[85] M. Lavaill, S. Trichilo, S. Scheiner, M. R. Forwood, D. M. L. Cooper, and P. Pivonka, "Study of the combined effects of PTH treatment and mechanical loading in postmenopausal osteoporosis using a new mechanistic PK-PD model," Biomech. Model. Mechanobiol., vol. 19, pp. 1765–1780, 2020, doi: 10.1007/s10237-020-01307-6.

[86] S. Trichilo, S. Scheiner, M. Forwood, D. M. L. Cooper, and P. Pivonka, "Computational model of the dual action of PTH — Application to a rat model of osteoporosis," J. Theor. Biol., vol. 473, pp. 67–79, 2019, doi: 10.1016/j.jtbi.2019.04.020.

[87] J. C. Vanegas-Acosta, N. S. Landinez P., D. A. Garzón-Alvarado, and M. C. Casale R., "A finite element method approach for the mechanobiological modeling of the osseointegration of a dental implant," Comput. Methods Programs Biomed., vol. 101, pp. 297–314, 2011, doi: 10.1016/j.cmpb.2010.11.007.

[88] R. K. Schenk and D. Buser, "Osseointegration: A reality," Periodontol. 2000, vol. 17, pp. 22–35, 1998, doi: 10.1111/j.1600-0757.1998.tb00120.x.

[89] E. G. F. Mercuri, A. L. Daniel, M. B. Hecke, and L. Carvalho, "Influence of different mechanical stimuli in a multi-scale mechanobiological isotropic model for bone remodelling," Med. Eng. Phys., vol. 38, pp. 904–910, 2016, doi: 10.1016/j.medengphy.2016.04.018.

[90] M. I. Pastrama, S. Scheiner, P. Pivonka, and C. Hellmich, "A mathematical multiscale model of bone remodeling, accounting for pore space-specific mechanosensation," Bone, vol. 107, no. May 2018, pp. 208–221, 2018, doi: 10.1016/j.bone.2017.11.009.

[91] M. Ashrafi, J. E. Gubaua, J. T. Pereira, F. Gahlichi, and M. Doblaré, "A mechano-chemo-biological model for bone remodeling with a new mechano-chemo-transduction approach," Biomech. Model. Mechanobiol., vol. 19, pp. 2499–2523, 2020, doi: 10.1007/s10237-020-01353-0.

[92] A. Marathe, M. C. Peterson, and D. E. Mager, "Integrated cellular bone homeostasis model for denosumab pharmacodynamics in multiple myeloma patients," J. Pharmacol. Exp. Ther., vol. 326, pp. 555–562, 2008, doi: 10.1124/jpet.108.137703.

Chapter 3

Cell Interaction and Mechanobiological Modeling of Bone Remodeling Process

Rabeb Ben Kahla, Abdelwahed Barkaoui, Fatma Zohra Ben Salah and Moez Chafra

Abstract

According to the structural and metabolic demands of the body, proportionate and accurate bone quantities are resorbed and formed, establishing what is known as bone remodeling process. This physiological process requires a highly coordinated regulation through a complex interconnected network involving several cells from diverse origins, in addition to various hormones, cytokines, growth factors and signaling pathways. One of the main factors initiating the remodeling process is the mechanotransduction mechanism, through which osteocytes translate the mechanical stimuli subjected to the bone into biochemical signals, generating thereby the activation of osteoclasts and osteoblasts that govern bone resorption and formation. This mechanically-induced behavior of bone tissue has been the target of computational modeling and numerical simulations, to address biomechanical questions and provide information that is not amenable to direct measurements. In this context, the current chapter aims to review the coupling and mechanotransduction mechanisms spearheading the remodeling process, in addition to the main mathematical models developed over recent years and their use in bone numerical simulations based on the finite element method.

Keywords: bone remodeling, mechanical stimulus, cell interaction, mechanotransduction, finite element method

1. Introduction

Bone is a living composite material, providing various mechanical and homeostatic functions and characterized by a constant adaptation of its structure according to the metabolic and physical demands of the body. This self-adaptation property is governed by the complementary activities of resorption and formation, establishing what is known as bone remodeling process. This process requires a highly coordinated regulation over time and space to consistently maintain the proper quality and quantity of bone forming the skeleton. This coordination mainly incorporates two types of cells: bone-resorbing osteoclasts and bone-forming osteoblasts, representing the two major players of the remodeling event and providing a delicate balance between the removed bone amount and the subsequent deposited amount, which is carried out by generating the appropriate number of osteoblasts, a phenomenon known as the coupling mechanism. The coordination between osteoblast and osteoclast activities also involves other cells of various origins, in addition to several hormones, cytokines and growth factors that tightly connect the osteoblast- and osteoclast-lineages through a complex communication network during the remodeling cycle.

The remodeling process maintains the calcium homeostasis and provides a crucial mechanism for old bone removal, as well as for damage repair and adaptation to physical stress, which helps preserving the mechanical integrity of the skeleton. The remodeling process takes place at an anatomically distinct sites called bone mass units (BMUs), with each BMU operating asynchronously and independently of other BMUs throughout the skeleton. Notably, BMUs in the cortical bone greatly differ from those in the trabecular bone, in terms of structure, but also of the resorption and formation activities. Bone remodeling is initiated in a canopy, defining what is called the bone remodeling compartment (BRC), where intercellular communication occurs among the component bone cells, from vascular and endothelial cells and probably from immune cells reaching the remodeling sites through the blood supply. To better understand bone behavior and biomechanics, several research have been conducted using clinical investigations, as well as numerical modeling.

Computational modeling and numerical simulation of represent an interesting tool to address biomechanical questions, particularly those targeting the biomechanical behavior of bone, allowing to provide information that is not amenable to direct measurements, such as bone strength and joint load. This kind of information is required for several clinical applications, including fracture prevention, implant design, and pathology analysis. In recent years, partition of unity methods, explicitly using finite element (FE) mesh, has become popular due to its easy applicability. The FE method is one of the most widely used numerical analysis techniques based on FE mesh. It provides approximate solutions to a wide range of engineering problems. Recently, the FE method has experienced a phenomenal expansion in the field of bone biomedical engineering, owing to its flexibility and diversity as an analysis tool, but also because it easily manages complex and evolving cellular domains, and can be generalized to multidimensions with little complication. Particularly, the FE method has been widely used to analyze and predict the mechanical behavior of bones, under physiologic and pathologic conditions, based on mathematical models that describe the cellular mechanisms governing the remodeling process. These mathematical models are including more and more factors and actors, to attempt affording a more realistic description of bone cell interactions.

In this context, the current paper provides a review of the processes of bone remodeling and cell interactions, as well as the recent findings about the mechanotransduction mechanisms, in addition to the mechanobiological models targeting bone dynamics and the main generated FE results in recent years.

2. Bone cells and coupling mechanisms

Osteoblasts are cuboidal cells located on the newly synthesized bone interface and have two types of functions: a bone building function, through which they produce matrix proteins, and endocrine functions, through which they release a wide range of regulatory factors that influence energy metabolism, male fertility and cognition [1, 2]. Osteoblasts originate from mesenchymal stromal cells (MSCs) according to two distinct embryonic populations: the first one is when osteoblast-lineage cells derive from the neural ectoderm, the mesenchymal progenitors directly differentiate into preosteoblasts and the subsequent mature osteoblasts form the calvarian bones and clavicles through intramembranous ossification, whereas the second one is when the MSCs differentiate into perichondral cells and chondrocytes, a subsequent chondrocyte hypertrophy drives the perichondral cell differentiation into preosteoblasts, and mature osteoblasts form bone in the extremities and in the axial skeleton through endochondral ossification [3–5].

Osteoclasts are giant multinucleated cells that hydrolyze and solubilize both of the inorganic and organic components of bone, owing to their polarized secretion of acid and proteolytic enzymes. Thus, osteoclasts provide bone with a unique characteristic of being the only tissue in the body able to undergo a self-destruction, fulfilling thereby a crucial physiologic process for bone homeostasis [6]. Osteoclasts originate from the fusion of monocyte–macrophage [7] precursors that derive from hematopoietic stem cells (HSCs) in the marrow [8]. The hematopoietic precursors required for osteoclast formation are provided through the capillary blood supply closely associated with and penetrating the BRC [9], as well as from nearby marrow precursors [10]. Interestingly, the programming of osteoclast formation involve the actions of osteoblast-lineage cells, endothelial cells, and BRC microenvironment [9].

Osteocytes are the most abundant and the dominant mechanosensory cells of bone and are easily identified in a bone section, owing to the matrix in which they are completely embedded during skeletal maturation of previous remodeling cycles [1, 11]. These long-living cells are characterized by a stellar/spider shape, due to which they form and extensive interconnected network of long branched cellular processes within a fluid-filled canalicular system [12]. These processes contact each other, and probably other cell populations through gap junctions, providing thereby a cell–cell interaction by an intercellular exchange of small signaling molecules. This network plays a crucial role in regulating bone material turnover, by coordinating bone response to mechanical signals, as well as to endocrine and paracrine biological signals [13, 14]. Osteocytes have both local and systemic effects through responding to the strains generated by mechanical stimuli and translating the load into biochemical signals via a mechanotransduction mechanism [11, 15], which is one of the main factors initiating the remodeling process. Osteocytes emerge from the differentiation of a subset of osteoblasts that are trapped in the newly synthetized osteoid matrix before its mineralization [16], by undergoing a four-stage differentiation process to become mature osteocytes: (i) type I preosteocytes, named osteoblastic osteocytes, (ii) type II preosteocytes, named osteoid-osteocytes, (iii) type III preosteocytes, named young osteocytes, and (iv) old osteocytes [17].

Reversal cells were found to belong to osteoblast-lineage cells that seem to particularly be preosteoblasts [18] that progressively mature into bone-forming osteoblasts and play a crucial role in the resorption-to-formation coupling mechanism [19, 20]. The intermediate position of the reversal cells between osteoblasts and osteoclasts suggests their obvious contribution to the osteoblast–osteoclast interplay [21]. Interestingly, the early reversal cells located proximal to osteoclasts are less mature than the late ones located proximal to osteoblasts [18] and appear to be morphologically, ultrastructurally and immunohistochemically quite different from the late ones located next to osteoid surfaces. These differences reflect their diverse cellular interactions, varied functions, and distinct differentiation states [18–20].

Bone lining cells are an osteoblast subpopulation and their interaction with osteoclasts attached to bone, due to close contact, is tightly associated with the initiation of osteoclastogenesis [22, 23]. Besides, the lining cells establish physical homotypic connections with osteocytes through gap functions, which suggests that these lining cells form a functional membrane separating bone from interstitial fluids [24]. Particularly during the remodeling cycle, bone lining cells persist over the remodeling sites to isolate osteoblasts and osteoclasts from the bone marrow [25].

Indeed, at the very beginning of a remodeling cycle, the lining cells separate and raise from the underlying bone surface, forming a canopy above the site to be resorbed. This initiating phenomenon might result from osteocyte signaling to surface cells through their canaliculae when they recognize the need for replacing a specific bone area [26]. Subsequent signals could come from osteocyte apoptosis or from the lining cells themselves, generating the release of paracrine factors and chemokines, which attract the precursors of both osteoblasts and osteoclasts, as well as other required vascular elements [27].

3. Coupling mechanism

The spatial and temporal arrangement of bone cells within the BMU is crucial to the remodeling process, ensuring its distinct and sequential phase coordination, under the control of several hormones, cytokines, and growth factors. The communication between bone cells is led through at least three modes: (i) a communication through a direct cell–cell contact, (ii) a communication through gap junction formation, and (iii) a communication through diffusible paracrine factors.

Indeed, osteoblasts regulate osteoclast formation, differentiation, and maturation. In turn, osteoclasts exert positive and negative regulatory effects on osteoblast activity. Moreover, osteocytes, reversal cells, lining cells and bone matrix are all actors in the osteoblast–osteoclast crosstalk, among others. The interplay between osteoblasts and osteoclasts is also mediated by bidirectional signaling pathways, including Eph/ephrin pathways, Semaphorins/Plexins pathways, as well as RANKL/W9/RANK pathway. **Figure 1** summarizes the communication network between bone cells.

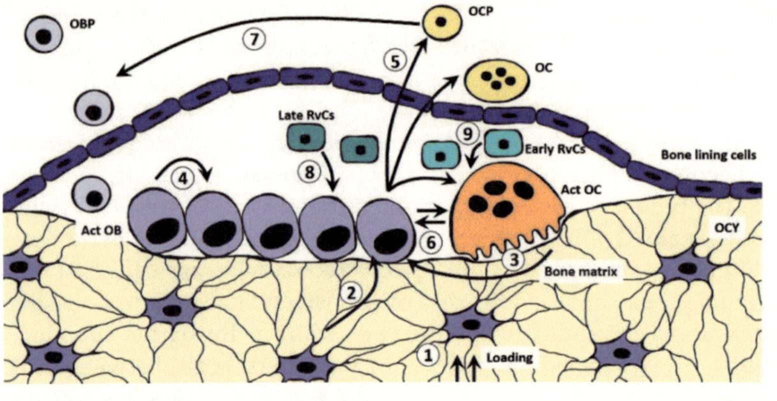

Figure 1.
Intercellular communication pathways within the BMU whereby the remodeling process takes place. (1) mechanical stimulus affecting OCY (osteocytes). (2) stimulatory effects from OCY to act OB (active osteoblasts). (3) bone matrix signals to act OB. (4) signaling within osteoblast-lineage cells. (5) Stimulatory and inhibitory signaling from act OB to OCP (osteoclast precursors), OC (osteoclasts), and act OC (activated osteoclasts). (6) bidirectional signaling between act OB and act OC. (7) Stimulatory and inhibitory signals from OCP to OBP (osteoblast precursors). (8) stimulatory signals from late RvCs (reversal cells) to act OB. (9) Stimulatory signals from early RvCs to act OC.

4. Mechanotransduction mechanisms

As mentioned above, osteocytes are the dominant mechanosensory cells in bone, owing to their location in the matrix and their complex dendritic network. However, the lining cells were also suggested to be important mechanosensory cells in the adult skeleton, which thereby needs more investigation to clarify their exact role in bone biology. Unlike in vivo loading, where the ideal intensity, frequency, and timing to increase bone mass [28–30] are well characterized, in vitro experiments to identify these parameters and replicate in vivo results remain a major challenge. The fact that in vivo osteocyte gene expression changes under mechanical loading and unloading shows that the load affects osteocyte function [31–34].

Early in vitro experiments were based on hydrostatic pressure and substrate stretching, whereas current ones are based on fluid flow shear stress (FFSS), owing to the higher sensitivity of primary osteocytes to shear stress than to substrate stretching [35, 36].

Mechanosensation ability allows osteocytes to orchestrate osteoblast activation and osteoclast partial suppression under increased loading, and osteoblast partial suppression and osteoclast activation under reduced loading [37]. However, the way external forces are transmitted at the cellular and molecular levels is still unclear. Mechanical stressors include hydrostatic pressure, FFSS, and direct cellular deformation [38]. These mechanical stresses are driven by microstrain of bone matrix generated by loading and gravitational forces. Cell responses are also influenced by the specific components of these stressors, such as amplitude, frequency and rate.

Although the calcified bone matrix is a mechanically rigid material, mechanical loading induces poro-elastic interactions and microstrains of the matrix, of up to 0.2% [39, 40]. These microstrains drive the interstitial fluid flow (IFF) within the lacunocanalicular spaces [41, 42]. Indeed, real-time measurement of load-induced solute transport has been demonstrated, which suggested a peak shear stress of 5 Pa on osteocyte processes [43]. Loading of long bones also increases the pressure at the intramedullary cavity and induces IFF at the endosteal surface, as well as within the lacunocanalicular network [41]. Moreover, intramedullary pressurization-derived IFF can induce fluid shear stress-related responses not only in osteocytes but also in osteoblasts and osteoclasts on the endosteal surface, which suggests that osteoblast and osteoclasts are also mechanosensitive [44, 45]. Several research works have shown that osteocytes are connected to the canalicular wall through transverse tethering elements and transmembrane molecules that provide physical connections between the extracellular matrix, the intracellular protein complexes and cytoskeletal structures [46–49].

Several mechanosensors have been identified in bone, including cilia, integrins, calcium channels and G-protein coupled receptors (GPCRs). Integrins, among which $\alpha v\beta 3$ is highly expressed in osteocytes, are composed of an α and β dimer and FFSS generates conformational changes in the β-subunit and the cascade signaling activation [46, 47]. The primary cilium is a non-motile structure needed for both mechano- and chemosensation, and represents another cellular moiety required to perceive FFSS. According to physical laws, FFSS occurs around the cell processes and not on the cell body where the primary cilium is located. The latter was proposed to perceive hydrostatic pressure applied on the cell body and not FFSS [50]. TAZ/YAP was also found to be an important signaling pathway for mechanosensation. Furthermore, glycocalyces on the dendritic process surfaces, but not on the cell body, were found to play a crucial role in mechanotransduction, whereas a different mechanosensing mechanism is active on the cell body [51]. Moreover, osteocytes sense load through cilia, which are single flagellar-like structures found on every cell [52, 53] and have specific functions. Particularly, cilia in bone cells induce the PGE2 release [53]. It was also reported that polycystin 1 (PC-1) in osteocytes is important for the anabolic response of bone to load [54]. Indeed, applying 2000 microstrain to bone sample at the macroscopic scale induced over 30,000 microstrain surrounding the osteocyte lacunae [55]. Besides, osteocyte processes are extremely responsive to mechanical loadings of piconewton-level, which is not the case for their cell body and processes with no local attachments [56].

In osteocytes, among other cells, biophysical stressors are transmitted to the cells by coupling the extracellular matrix to the actin cytoskeleton through focal adhesions. The actin cytoskeleton transmits mechanical forces from a focal adhesion site to a mechanosensing site within the cell and to the neighboring ones. Focal adhesion kinases (FAK) are major components of focal adhesions and are required for the mechanotransduction mechanism by osteocytes. Besides, a structural cytoskeletal protein named spectrin is required for osteoblast-to-osteocyte differentiation and was recently identified as a mechanosensitive element within the osteocyte [11, 57]. Other potential mechanosensors are ephrins, Connexin 43 (Cx43) hemichannels and ion channels, as well as gap junctions. A response of bone to mechanical loading and unloading also requires the action of an intact axis of parathyroid hormone (PTH)-related peptide (PTHrP) and its receptor (PTHR), or PTH-PTHrP-PTHR axis [58].

Mechanotransduction is the mechanism of transducing the mechanical signal sensed by osteocytes via the mechanosensation mechanism into biological cues. Ca++, ATP, NO, PGE2 and Wnts are the best described mechanically-induced pathways. Deleting one of these molecules inhibits the anabolic response of bone to mechanical stimulation.

Ca++ is an exclusively intracellular signal and the opening of stretch-activated calcium channel (TRPV6) results in a quick increase in intracellular Ca++, subsequently followed by cellular response to mechanical cues. Ca++ is also required for ATP response and ATP concentration rapidly increases upon mechanical forces. However, the exact mechanism by which Ca++ regulates ATP release is still not completely elucidated [49]. ATP can be released from osteocytes in response to whether mechanical stimulation or extracellular calcium [59, 60]. An ATP-gated ion channel, known as P2X7 nucleotide receptor, is expressed in many cell types and significantly influences the mechanosensation mechanisms, and P2X7 receptor is suggested to be essential for PGE2 release in response to mechanical strain [11].

In turn, NO and PGE2 are also expressed in and affect osteoblasts and osteoclasts. In bone, NO suppresses bone resorption and promotes its formation. Indeed, both osteoblasts and osteocytes release NO in response to mechanical strain or FFSS [61], but osteoblasts are less sensitive to FFSS than osteocytes [35, 36]. Under mechanical forces, osteocytes synthetize and release PGE2, which has been known to be one of the earliest responses to loading [62–65]. FFSS promotes gap junction-mediated intercellular communication and stimulates Cx43 expression, which in turn forms hemichannels, allowing thereby to release PGE2 [62]. The latter acts in an autocrine fashion and activates EP2-EP4 receptors expressed on osteocytes, while acting in a paracrine fashion to modulate osteoblast and osteoclast activities. The activation of EP2-EP4 is associated with increased intracellular cAMP and activated protein kinase A (PKA), which regulates the expression of many downstream effectors, including RANKL, Dmp1, and Sost. In vivo, new bone formation is induced by PGE2 and anabolic loading effects are blocked by indomethacin [66]. PGE2 seem to be released in response to shear stress through hemichannels unopposed halves of gap-junction channels [62]. These hemichannels in osteocytes exert multiple functions, including the protection of cell viability and the release of signaling factors [67, 68].

The canonical Wnt-signaling plays a significant role in bone homeostasis and mainly targets osteocytes among bone cells. Wnt activity increases under mechanical loading and decreases during unloading. Most of these effects are, indeed, mediated by sclerostin [49]. Mechanical transduction is also associated with sex hormones that are estrogens and androgens, and a close relationship has been determined between them and skeletal mechanobiology [69–71]. Insulin-like growth factor 1 (IGF-1) was also found to form another signaling pathway required for proper mechanotransduction [72].

5. Mathematical models

5.1 Main biological approaches of bone cell dynamics

Komarova et al. [73] developed a first mathematical model for the interaction between osteoblasts and osteoclasts, where the temporal osteoblast and osteoclast population dynamics and the associated changes in bone mass at a single BMU, were constructed. The originality of this work was the incorporation of autocrine and paracrine interactions among osteoblasts and osteoclasts, allowing to investigate the cooperative roles of both of these regulation mechanisms in bone remodeling control. The cell population dynamics were described using the following system of differential equations:

$$\frac{dx_1}{dt} = \alpha_1 x_1^{g_{11}} x_2^{g_{21}} - \beta_1 x_1 \tag{1}$$

$$\frac{dx_2}{dt} = \alpha_2 x_1^{g_{12}} x_2^{g_{22}} - \beta_2 x_2 \tag{2}$$

where 1 and 2 denote the osteoclasts and osteoblasts, respectively, x_i the cell number, α_i the cell production activity, β_i the cell removal activity, and g_{ij} the net effectiveness of osteoclast- or osteoblast-derived autocrine or paracrine factors.

The changes in bone mass was determined using the following equation:

$$\frac{dz}{dt} = -k_1 y_1 + k_2 y_2 \tag{3}$$

where z denotes the total bone mass, k_i the normalized resorption and formation activities, and y_i the active cell numbers, which is calculated according to the following conditions, with $\overline{x}_i$ being the cell number at steady state.

The findings revealed that the remodeling dynamic behavior mode mainly depends on osteoclast autocrine regulation parameter and the model suggests that preosteoblast availability may be a limiting factor in bone formation under certain conditions. This study revealed that modeling the simultaneous processes of osteoblast and osteoclast regulations and interactions, even in a simplistic form, results in a highly complex nonlinear behavior, and that the intrinsic properties of the osteoblast–osteoclast system can generate complex remodeling modes observed in vivo. However, only two cell types were taken into account, local autocrine and paracrine factors were supposed to only regulate osteoblast and osteoclast formation, and the parameters describing the autocrine and paracrine regulation effectiveness included actions of several factors.

Then, Lemaire et al. [74] developed a theoretical framework able to explain the experimental observations of bone biology. In their paper, a mathematical model of bone remodeling cellular control was proposed to particularly examine the biochemical control network failures leading to bone diseases, such as osteoporosis. The model consists of a synthetic system including the cellular and biomechanical feedback mechanisms that spearhead bone turnover regulation, taking into account the PTH action in the remodeling process. The originality of this model was the incorporation of the RANK-RANKL-OPG pathway, representing an essential regulation mechanism of osteoclast formation.

The reaction scheme of PTH binding with its receptor was formulated as follows, without taking osteoblastic interactions into account:

$$\begin{array}{l} p_P \\ \downarrow \\ P \; + P_r \underset{k_6}{\overset{k_5}{\rightleftharpoons}} P_r \diamond P \\ \downarrow \\ d_P \end{array} \tag{4}$$

where P denotes PTH, P_r the PTH receptor, p_P and d_P are the PTH production and dissociation fluxes, respectively, and $P_r \diamond P$ is the complex formed by PTH and its receptor.

The reaction schemes of the bindings of RANKL with RANK and of OPG with RANKL were giving by (Eq. 9) and (Eq. 10), respectively:

$$\begin{array}{l} p_L \\ \downarrow \\ L \; + K \underset{k_4}{\overset{k_3}{\rightleftharpoons}} K \diamond L \\ \downarrow \\ d_L \end{array} \tag{5}$$

$$\begin{array}{ccccc} p_O & & p_L & & \\ \downarrow & & \downarrow & k_1 & \\ O & + & L & \rightleftharpoons & O \diamond L \\ \downarrow & & \downarrow & k_2 & \\ d_O & & d_L & & \end{array} \tag{6}$$

where K denotes the RANK receptor, L, the RANKL cytokine, O the OPG protein, $K \diamond L$ the RANK-RANKL complex, and $O \diamond L$ the OPG-RANKL complex.

The model was able to simulate the coupling mechanism between osteoblasts and osteoclasts, the catabolic effect related to PTH continuous administration, the RANKL catabolic action and the OPG anti-catabolic action, in addition to metabolic bone diseases, such as glucocorticoid excess, senescence, vitamin D deficiency, and estrogen deficiency. The model also confirmed that bone formation therapies yielded better results that anti-resorptive therapies in restoring bone loss, and that combining anabolic and anti-resorptive therapies may provide better benefits than monotherapy.

Later, Pivonka et al. [75] developed a model to investigate and incorporate an optimal model structure for RANKL and OPG expression on osteoblast lineage at different maturation stages. Afterwards, the investigation dealt with optimal changes in differentiation rates able to provide effective functional control within an active BMU. The cell population model proposed in this study was mainly based on that of Lemaire et al. [74], but incorporating a rate equation describing changes in bone volume, a rate equation describing TGF-β concentration in terms of the resorbed bone volume, RANKL and OPG expressions on osteoblast-lineage cells at different maturation stages, as well as activator/repressor functions based on enzyme kinetics. The model does not refer to a single BMU. It includes spatial averages of cell numbers over a finite bone volume that contains many BMUs. But, it may be contrasted in the case of studying a single BMU, since temporal and spatial sequences define the type of the present bone cells.

The cell population dynamics were described by the following cell balance equations:

$$\frac{dOB_p}{dt} = D_{OB_u} \cdot \pi_{act,OB_u}^{TGF-\beta} - D_{OB_p} \cdot OB_p \cdot \pi_{act,OB_p}^{TGF-\beta} \tag{7}$$

$$\frac{dOB_a}{dt} = D_{OB_p} \cdot OB_p \cdot \pi_{rep,OB_p}^{TGF-\beta} - A_{OB_a} \cdot OB_a \tag{8}$$

$$\frac{dOC_a}{dt} = D_{OC_p} \cdot OC_p \cdot \pi_{act,OC_p}^{RANKL} - A_{OC_a} \cdot OC_a \cdot \pi_{act,OC_p}^{TGF-\beta} \tag{9}$$

where OB_u denotes the uncommitted osteoblast progenitors, OB_p the preosteoblast cells, OC_p the preosteoclast cells, OB_a, the active osteoblasts, OC_a the active osteoblasts, D_i the cell differentiation rate, A_i the cell apoptosis rate, $\pi_{act,OB_u}^{TGF-\beta}$, $\pi_{rep,OB_p}^{TGF-\beta}$, and $\pi_{act,OC_p}^{TGF-\beta}$ the activator/repressor functions related to the binding of TGF-β to its receptors on osteoblasts and osteoclasts, and π_{act,OC_p}^{RANKL} the activator function related to the binding of RANKL to its RANK on preosteoclasts. The above cell balance equations represent the changes in each cell population owing to the addition and removal of the respective cell lineage. Several activator and repressor function regulate the differentiation and apoptosis rates. For instance, the binding of TGF-β on its receptors expressed on uncommitted osteoblast progenitors promotes their differentiation, whereas its binding on its receptors expressed on preosteoblasts inhibits their differentiation.

The evolution, over time, of bone volume, BV was later formulated as follows, assuming that bone resorption and formation rates are proportional to the active cell numbers:

$$\frac{dBV}{dt} = -k_{res}\tilde{OC}_a + k_{form}\tilde{OB}_a \tag{10}$$

where BV here denotes the percentage of normalized bone volume, k_{res} the relative bone resorption rate, and k_{form} the relative bone formation rate, with $\tilde{OC}_a = OC_a(t) - OC_a(t_0)$ and $\tilde{OB}_a = OB_a(t) - OB_a(t_0)$, where $OC_a(t_0)$ and $OC_a(t_0)$ denote the numbers of active osteoclasts and osteoblasts at the initial state, t_0. This formulation allows to link the evolution of cell numbers to the changes in bone volume.

The outcomes of this study suggested that RANKL expression profile provides BMUs with a best functional responsiveness, and that TGF-β is included in the up-regulation of osteoblast progenitor differentiation rate, in the down-regulation of preosteoblast differentiation rate, and in the up-regulation of active osteoclast apoptosis rate, which partially explains the particular suitability of TGF-β physiological actions in bone.

5.2 Main mechanical models of bone remodeling

Miller et al. [76] used an orthotropic material model to provide a 2D representation of the effective properties of the trabecular bone, with the aim of explaining its structure in the proximal femur. The proposed model explained the directionality of the trabecular bone and provided a quite well prediction of the directional material properties, which supported the consideration of anisotropy in adaptation algorithms. However, the study was based on a 2D plane stress assumption, which cannot reflect the 3D reality, the investigated problem was simplified, and the number of elastic constants per element was reduced.

Bonfoh et al. [77] proposed a bone remodeling model based on an external mechanical stimulus and tested its predictions for simple loading scenarios. Their approach allowed to describe osteoblast and osteoclast interactions when bone is subjected to external loading. The latter was expressed in terms of strain energy density ω detected by an osteocyte i at its location $\vec{x}^{(i)}$:

$$\omega\left(\vec{x}^{(i)}\right) = \frac{1}{2}\underline{\underline{\sigma}}\left(\vec{x}^{(i)}\right) : \underline{\underline{\varepsilon}}\left(\vec{x}^{(i)}\right) \tag{11}$$

where $\underline{\underline{\sigma}}$ and $\underline{\underline{\varepsilon}}$ are the tensors of stress and strain, respectively.

The model predictions provided a coherent remodeling description. Applied to the dental implant osseointegration simulation, the model forecasted plausible results. However, the comparison of the obtained results with previous ones from literature showed significant differences regarding the remodeling area and the stress/strain fields.

Geraldes et al. [78] proposed an orthotropic strain-driven adaptation algorithm to assess the distribution of the volumetric material properties at the femur and the directionality of its internal structures within a continuum. The proposed algorithm included multiple load cases (**Figure 2**) and the maximum strain components across all frames from the daily physical activities were selected to generate a strain field

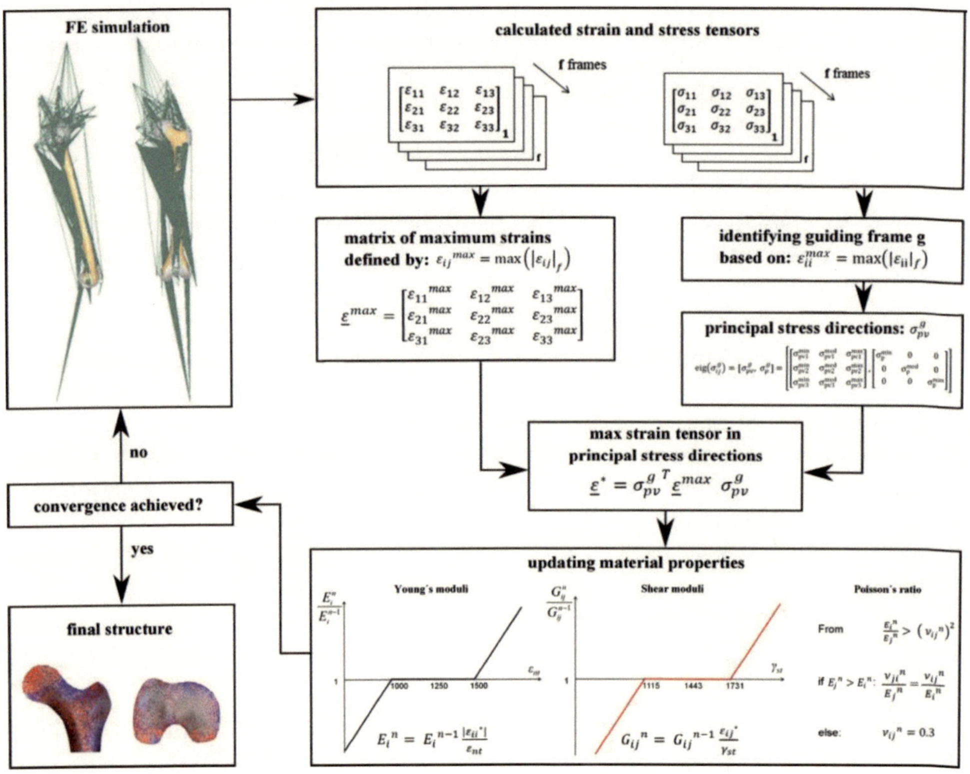

Figure 2.
Key steps in updating the orthotropic material properties and directionality for the multiple load case adaptation process [78].

envelope involving the maximum driving stimuli for the material properties and orientations.

The study particularly highlighted the importance of stair climbing in the evolution of the properties of the fracture-prone femoral neck region, with implications for prevention strategies of non-pharmacological fracture based on exercise. However, the model was based on geometrical definition of certain muscles through straight lines, which may result in non-physiological lines of action and moment arms. Besides, the used femur geometry is not personalized for the studied case, but extracted from the muscle standardized femur, which may contribute to overassessment of the hip contact forces. The proposed multiple loading scenario did not take into account any impact activity and the performed analysis did not consider time- or frequency-dependent adaptation.

6. Finite element simulations

The primary results (**Figure 3**) of the study of Miller et al. [76] are the two local Young's moduli E_1 and E_2, as well as the predicted density distribution. The model converged after 25 iterations. The results show the predicted properties of the trabecular elements, with the cortical shell shown as an outline.

The results generated by the model of Bonfoh et al. [77] showed that the magnitude of the signal received by pre-osteoblasts and pre-osteoclasts depends on the load intensity the osteocyte concentration that varies according to the age, sex, type of the considered bone, etc. Bone density is also related to the type of the considered bone and mainly to its initial apparent density. For the considered load case, the tops of the threads of the simulated implant are the most loaded areas where the stimulus is sufficient to lead the cell activity into an opposition. However, the strain energy density for the other zones remains deficient. Therefore, the concerned areas are in resorption or in a steady state.

Among the obtained results of Geraldes et al. [78], **Figure 4** shows the predicted density (right) and dominant material orientations (middle) for coronal section of the proximal femur, compared to μCT slices of the same regions (left).

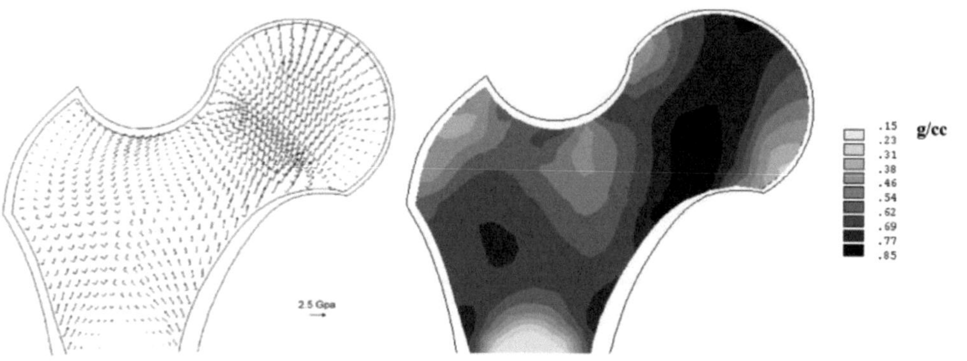

Figure 3.
(Top) Predicted material properties after model converged. The arrow directions show the material axes of each element, which are the predicted trabecular directions. The lengths of the arrows represent the effective elastic moduli E1 and E2 of each element. The legend arrow represents a Young's modulus of 2.5 GPa. (Bottom) Predicted density distribution. Density was estimated from the average elastic modulus of each element. All recognized major features of the proximal femur are visible. Maximal density is 0.88 g/cm3, which corresponds to a volume fraction of approximately 48%. The division of the model into constant cortical elements and variable trabecular elements prevents unrealistic densities in regions that are close to the cortices. [76].

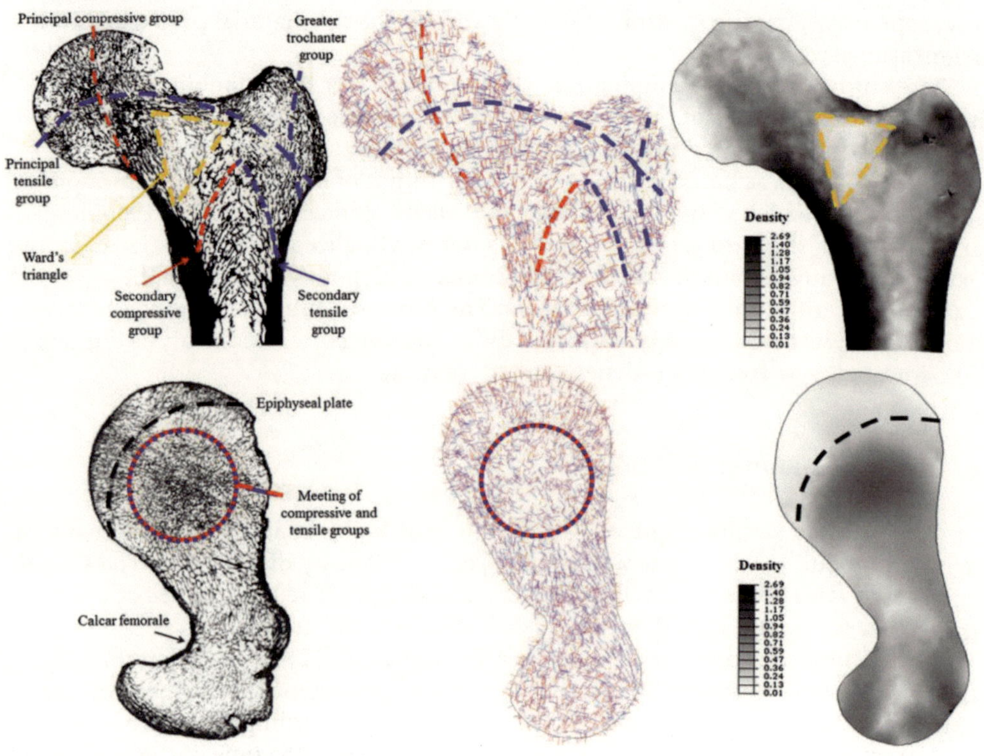

Figure 4.
Predicted density (right, in g/cm³) and dominant material orientations (middle) for a coronal (top) and transverse (bottom) section of the converged proximal femur undergoing multiple load cases. Legends highlighting the most interesting features identified by Singh et al. [79] (top, left) and Tobin [80] (bottom, left) were superimposed onto a μCT slice of the same region. The material orientations associated with E_1 *are shown in red and* E_3 *in blue [78].*

7. Conclusion

The BMU, previously seen as a changing structure where homogenous cell populations enter, act, and leave, is now revealed to be a tiny microenvironment where heterogeneous cell types mingle and interact with each other to provide a delicate preservation of bone quality and quantity, with highly coordinated activities between the different actors through a complex communication network. Besides, the integrity of bone homeostasis is significantly based on a proper detection and transduction of the mechanical stimulus to biochemical signals. This is mainly performed by osteocytes that were found to be the major mechanosensory and most abundant cells in an adult skeleton. However, the precise mechanisms by which osteocytes perceive and transduce mechanical forces are still unclear. What have emerged is the complexity and multiplicity of the signaling systems activated by subjecting bone to mechanical strains. Owing to the unique in vivo environment of an osteocyte, it is difficult to establish in vitro models that faithfully replicate the required processes. Still, recent technological advances have demonstrated an impressive progress in understanding osteocyte biology and functions, and further elucidation on the mechanobiological mechanisms of osteocytes holds promises of biological and medical implications.

Mathematical models have recently been widely largely used in biomechanical engineering to better understand bone dynamics and mechanical behavior, and to prevent thereby bone pathologies and fractures. Mathematically describing bone cellular and biomechanical behavior is not an easy task to perform, since bone is a living heterogeneous composite material and attempting to model it strongly depends on numerous mechanical and biochemical factors. It should be noted that accurate predictions are tightly linked to realistic characterization of the material behavior. Many of these models are currently combined with FE method to numerically investigate specific scenarios. Although the FE method presents several limitations, the accuracy of numerical results may be improved due to emerging advancing techniques and FE analysis still provides an important tool for assessing bone properties and understanding its behavior. It also offers a personalized analysis of bone stiffness based on specific measurements. The development of the FE method could successfully prevent and treat age- and disease-related bone fractures. The accurate assessment of bone structure and mechanical properties, with a more realistic prediction of applied stresses, should significantly improve the outcome of FE modeling and make this method effective in treating patients and developing new implant designs.

Author details

Rabeb Ben Kahla[1], Abdelwahed Barkaoui[2,3]*, Fatma Zohra Ben Salah[4] and Moez Chafra[1]

1 Laboratoire de Systèmes et de Mécanique Appliquée (LASMAP), Ecole Polytechnique de Tunis Université De Carthage, 2078, La Marsa, Tunisie

2 Laboratoire des Energies Renouvelables et Matériaux Avancés (LERMA), Université Internationale de Rabat, Rocade Rabat Salé 11100, Rabat-Sala El Jadida, Morocco

3 Laboratoire de Mécanique Appliquée etIngénierie (LR-MAI), Ecole Nationale d'Ingénieurs de Tunis Université Tunis El Manar, BP 37,1002, Tunis, Tunisie

4 Faculté de médecine de Tunis, Université de Tunis El Manar, Tunis, Tunisie

*Address all correspondence to: abdelwahed.barkaoui@uir.ac.ma

References

[1] M. Capulli, R. Paone, and N. Rucci, "Osteoblast and osteocyte: games without frontiers," *Arch. Biochem. Biophys.*, vol. 561, pp. 3–12 , 2014.

[2] A. Rutkovskiy, K.-O. Stensløkken, and I. J. Vaage, "Osteoblast differentiation at a glance," *Med. Sci. Monit. Basic Res.*, vol. 22, p. 95, 2016.

[3] R. Nishimura, K. Hata, T. Matsubara, M. Wakabayashi, and T. Yoneda, "Regulation of bone and cartilage development by network between BMP signalling and transcription factors," *J. Biochem.*, vol. 151, no. 3, pp. 247–254, 2012.

[4] L. Yang, K. Y. Tsang, H. C. Tang, D. Chan, and K. S. E. Cheah, "Hypertrophic chondrocytes can become osteoblasts and osteocytes in endochondral bone formation," *Proc. Natl. Acad. Sci.*, vol. 111, no. 33, pp. 12097–12102, 2014.

[5] N. S. Fedarko, "Osteoblast/osteoclast development and function in osteogenesis imperfecta," in *Osteogenesis Imperfecta*, Elsevier, 2014, pp. 45–56.

[6] J. F. Charles and A. O. Aliprantis, "Osteoclasts: more than 'bone eaters,'" *Trends Mol. Med.*, vol. 20, no. 8, pp. 449–459, 2014.

[7] C. Heinemann, S. Heinemann, H. Worch, and T. Hanke, "Development of an osteoblast/osteoclast co-culture derived by human bone marrow stromal cells and human monocytes for biomaterials testing," *Eur Cell Mater*, vol. 21, pp. 80–93, 2011.

[8] L. Wang *et al.*, "Osteoblast-induced osteoclast apoptosis by fas ligand/FAS pathway is required for maintenance of bone mass," *Cell Death Differ.*, vol. 22, no. 10, pp. 1654–1664, 2015.

[9] H. B. Kristensen, T. L. Andersen, N. Marcussen, L. Rolighed, and J. Delaisse, "Increased presence of capillaries next to remodeling sites in adult human cancellous bone," *J. Bone Miner. Res.*, vol. 28, no. 3, pp. 574–585, 2013.

[10] N. A. Sims and T. J. Martin, "Coupling the activities of bone formation and resorption: a multitude of signals within the basic multicellular unit," *Bonekey Rep.*, vol. 3, 2014.

[11] L. F. Bonewald, "The amazing osteocyte," *J. bone Miner. Res.*, vol. 26, no. 2, pp. 229–238, 2011.

[12] P. R. Buenzli and N. A. Sims, "Quantifying the osteocyte network in the human skeleton," *Bone*, vol. 75, pp. 144–150, 2015.

[13] R. Civitelli, "Cell–cell communication in the osteoblast/ osteocyte lineage," *Arch. Biochem. Biophys.*, vol. 473, no. 2, pp. 188–192, 2008.

[14] M. B. Schaffler, W.-Y. Cheung, R. Majeska, and O. Kennedy, "Osteocytes: master orchestrators of bone," *Calcif. Tissue Int.*, vol. 94, no. 1, pp. 5–24, 2014.

[15] B. S. Noble, "The osteocyte lineage," *Arch. Biochem. Biophys.*, vol. 473, no. 2, pp. 106–111, 2008.

[16] M. L. K. Tate, J. R. Adamson, A. E. Tami, and T. W. Bauer, "The osteocyte," *Int. J. Biochem. Cell Biol.*, vol. 36, no. 1, pp. 1–8, 2004.

[17] T. A. Franz-Odendaal, B. K. Hall, and P. E. Witten, "Buried alive: how osteoblasts become osteocytes," *Dev. Dyn. an Off. Publ. Am. Assoc. Anat.*, vol. 235, no. 1, pp. 176–190, 2006.

[18] M. E. Abdelgawad *et al.*, "Early reversal cells in adult human bone remodeling: osteoblastic nature, catabolic functions and interactions

with osteoclasts," *Histochem. Cell Biol.*, vol. 145, no. 6, pp. 603–615, 2016.

[19] H. B. Kristensen, T. L. Andersen, N. Marcussen, L. Rolighed, and J.-M. Delaisse, "Osteoblast recruitment routes in human cancellous bone remodeling," *Am. J. Pathol.*, vol. 184, no. 3, pp. 778–789, 2014.

[20] T. L. Andersen *et al.*, "Understanding coupling between bone resorption and formation: are reversal cells the missing link?," *Am. J. Pathol.*, vol. 183, no. 1, pp. 235–246, 2013.

[21] J.-M. Delaisse, "The reversal phase of the bone-remodeling cycle: cellular prerequisites for coupling resorption and formation," *Bonekey Rep.*, vol. 3, 2014.

[22] K. Matsuo and N. Irie, "Osteoclast–osteoblast communication," *Arch. Biochem. Biophys.*, vol. 473, no. 2, pp. 201–209, 2008.

[23] V. Everts *et al.*, "The bone lining cell: its role in cleaning Howship's lacunae and initiating bone formation," *J. Bone Miner. Res.*, vol. 17, no. 1, pp. 77–90, 2002.

[24] M. N. Wein, "Bone Lining Cells: Normal Physiology and Role in Response to Anabolic Osteoporosis Treatments," *Curr. Mol. Biol. Reports*, vol. 3, no. 2, pp. 79–84, 2017.

[25] A. M. Parfitt, "The bone remodeling compartment: a circulatory function for bone lining cells," *J. Bone Miner. Res.*, vol. 16, no. 9, pp. 1583–1585, 2001.

[26] O. Verborgt, G. J. Gibson, and M. B. Schaffler, "Loss of osteocyte integrity in association with microdamage and bone remodeling after fatigue in vivo," *J. bone Miner. Res.*, vol. 15, no. 1, pp. 60–67, 2000.

[27] N. A. Sims and K. W. Ng, "Implications of osteoblast-osteoclast interactions in the management of osteoporosis by antiresorptive agents denosumab and odanacatib," *Curr. Osteoporos. Rep.*, vol. 12, no. 1, pp. 98–106, 2014.

[28] C. T. Rubin, "Skeletal strain and the functional significance of bone architecture," *Calcif. Tissue Int.*, vol. 36, no. 1, pp. S11–S18, 1984.

[29] C. H. Turner, M. R. Forwood, and M. W. Otter, "Mechanotransduction in bone: do bone cells act as sensors of fluid flow?," *FASEB J.*, vol. 8, no. 11, pp. 875–878, 1994.

[30] A. G. Robling, F. M. Hinant, D. B. Burr, and C. H. Turner, "Shorter, more frequent mechanical loading sessions enhance bone mass.," *Med. Sci. Sports Exerc.*, vol. 34, no. 2, pp. 196–202, 2002.

[31] A. G. Robling *et al.*, "Mechanical stimulation of bone in vivo reduces osteocyte expression of Sost/sclerostin," *J. Biol. Chem.*, vol. 283, no. 9, pp. 5866–5875, 2008.

[32] T. M. Skerry, L. E. Lanyon, L. Bitensky, and J. Chayen, "Early strain-related changes in enzyme activity in osteocytes following bone loading in vivo," *J. Bone Miner. Res.*, vol. 4, no. 5, pp. 783–788, 1989.

[33] J. Gluhak-Heinrich, D. Pavlin, W. Yang, M. MacDougall, and S. E. Harris, "MEPE expression in osteocytes during orthodontic tooth movement," *Arch. Oral Biol.*, vol. 52, no. 7, pp. 684–690, 2007.

[34] J. Gluhak-Heinrich *et al.*, "Mechanical loading stimulates dentin matrix protein 1 (DMP1) expression in osteocytes in vivo," *J. Bone Miner. Res.*, vol. 18, no. 5, pp. 807–817, 2003.

[35] J. Klein-Nulend *et al.*, "Sensitivity of osteocytes to biomechanical stress in vitro," *FASEB J.*, 1995.

[36] J. Kleinnulend, C. M. Semeins, N. E. Ajubi, P. J. Nijweide, and E. H. Burger, "Pulsating fluid flow increases nitric oxide (NO) synthesis by osteocytes but not periosteal fibroblasts-correlation with prostaglandin upregulation," *Biochem. Biophys. Res. Commun.*, vol. 217, no. 2, pp. 640–648, 1995.

[37] S. Tatsumi *et al.*, "Targeted ablation of osteocytes induces osteoporosis with defective mechanotransduction," *Cell Metab.*, vol. 5, no. 6, pp. 464–475, 2007.

[38] T. Takano-Yamamoto, "Osteocyte function under compressive mechanical force," *Jpn. Dent. Sci. Rev.*, vol. 50, no. 2, pp. 29–39, 2014.

[39] S. C. Cowin, L. Moss-Salentijn, and M. L. Moss, "Candidates for the mechanosensory system in bone," 1991.

[40] S. Weinbaum, S. C. Cowin, and Y. Zeng, "A model for the excitation of osteocytes by mechanical loading-induced bone fluid shear stresses," *J. Biomech.*, vol. 27, no. 3, pp. 339–360, 1994.

[41] R. Y. Kwon *et al.*, "Skeletal adaptation to intramedullary pressure-induced interstitial fluid flow is enhanced in mice subjected to targeted osteocyte ablation," *PLoS One*, vol. 7, no. 3, p. e33336, 2012.

[42] E. H. Burger and J. Klein-Nulend, "Mechanotransduction in bone—role of the lacunocanalicular network," *FASEB J.*, vol. 13, no. 9001, pp. S101–S112, 1999.

[43] C. Price, X. Zhou, W. Li, and L. Wang, "Real-time measurement of solute transport within the lacunar-canalicular system of mechanically loaded bone: direct evidence for load-induced fluid flow," *J. Bone Miner. Res.*, vol. 26, no. 2, pp. 277–285, 2011.

[44] B. D. Riehl, J. S. Lee, L. Ha, I. K. Kwon, and J. Y. Lim, "Flowtaxis of osteoblast migration under fluid shear and the effect of RhoA kinase silencing," *PLoS One*, vol. 12, no. 2, p. e0171857, 2017.

[45] C. Liu, S. Li, B. Ji, and B. Huo, "Flow-induced migration of osteoclasts and regulations of calcium signaling pathways," *Cell. Mol. Bioeng.*, vol. 8, no. 1, pp. 213–223, 2015.

[46] F. A. A. Weyts, Y. Li, J. van Leeuwen, H. Weinans, and S. Chien, "ERK activation and αvβ3 integrin signaling through Shc recruitment in response to mechanical stimulation in human osteoblasts," *J. Cell. Biochem.*, vol. 87, no. 1, pp. 85–92, 2002.

[47] M. P. Yavropoulou and J. G. Yovos, "The molecular basis of bone mechanotransduction," *J. Musculoskelet. Neuronal Interact.*, vol. 16, no. 3, p. 221, 2016.

[48] S. Weinbaum, Y. Duan, M. M. Thi, and L. You, "An integrative review of mechanotransduction in endothelial, epithelial (renal) and dendritic cells (osteocytes)," *Cell. Mol. Bioeng.*, vol. 4, no. 4, pp. 510–537, 2011.

[49] Y. Uda, E. Azab, N. Sun, C. Shi, and P. D. Pajevic, "Osteocyte mechanobiology," *Curr. Osteoporos. Rep.*, vol. 15, no. 4, pp. 318–325, 2017.

[50] A. Bell, "The pipe and the pinwheel: is pressure an effective stimulus for the 9+ 0 primary cilium?," *Cell Biol. Int.*, vol. 32, no. 4, pp. 462–468, 2008.

[51] S. Burra *et al.*, "Dendritic processes of osteocytes are mechanotransducers that induce the opening of hemichannels," *Proc. Natl. Acad. Sci.*, vol. 107, no. 31, pp. 13648–13653, 2010.

[52] Z. Xiao *et al.*, "Cilia-like structures and polycystin-1 in osteoblasts/ osteocytes and associated abnormalities in skeletogenesis and Runx2

expression," *J. Biol. Chem.*, vol. 281, no. 41, pp. 30884–30895, 2006.

[53] A. M. D. Malone *et al.*, "Primary cilia mediate mechanosensing in bone cells by a calcium-independent mechanism," *Proc. Natl. Acad. Sci.*, vol. 104, no. 33, pp. 13325–13330, 2007.

[54] Z. Xiao *et al.*, "Conditional deletion and/or disruption of Pkd1 in osteocytes results in a significant reduction in anabolic response to mechanical loading," *J Bone Min. Res*, vol. 24, 2009.

[55] C. R. Jacobs, S. Temiyasathit, and A. B. Castillo, "Osteocyte mechanobiology and pericellular mechanics," *Annu. Rev. Biomed. Eng.*, vol. 12, pp. 369–400, 2010.

[56] M. M. Thi, S. O. Suadicani, M. B. Schaffler, S. Weinbaum, and D. C. Spray, "Mechanosensory responses of osteocytes to physiological forces occur along processes and not cell body and require αVβ3 integrin," *Proc. Natl. Acad. Sci.*, vol. 110, no. 52, pp. 21012–21017, 2013.

[57] X.-T. Wu, L.-W. Sun, X. Yang, D. Ding, D. Han, and Y.-B. Fan, "The potential role of spectrin network in the mechanotransduction of MLO-Y4 osteocytes," *Sci. Rep.*, vol. 7, no. 1, pp. 1–12, 2017.

[58] J. Delgado-Calle *et al.*, "Control of bone anabolism in response to mechanical loading and PTH by distinct mechanisms downstream of the PTH receptor," *J. Bone Miner. Res.*, vol. 32, no. 3, pp. 522–535, 2017.

[59] H. Kamioka *et al.*, "Extracellular calcium causes the release of calcium from intracellular stores in chick osteocytes," *Biochem. Biophys. Res. Commun.*, vol. 212, no. 2, pp. 692–696, 1995.

[60] D. C. Genetos, D. J. Geist, D. Liu, H. J. Donahue, and R. L. Duncan, "Fluid shear-induced ATP secretion mediates prostaglandin release in MC3T3-E1 osteoblasts," *J. Bone Miner. Res.*, vol. 20, no. 1, pp. 41–49, 2005.

[61] A. D. Bakker, K. Soejima, J. Klein-Nulend, and E. H. Burger, "' 'The Production of Nitric Oxide and Prostaglandin E 2 by Primary Bone Cells is Shear Stress Dependent"by Bakker et al.," *J. Biomech.*, vol. 3, no. 35, p. 389, 2002.

[62] P. P. Cherian *et al.*, "Mechanical strain opens connexin 43 hemichannels in osteocytes: a novel mechanism for the release of prostaglandin," *Mol. Biol. Cell*, vol. 16, no. 7, pp. 3100–3106, 2005.

[63] L. Bonewald, "Osteocytes as multifunctional cells," *J. Musculoskelet. Neuronal Interact.*, vol. 6, no. 4, p. 331, 2006.

[64] B. Cheng *et al.*, "PGE2 is essential for gap junction-mediated intercellular communication between osteocyte-like MLO-Y4 cells in response to mechanical strain," *Endocrinology*, vol. 142, no. 8, pp. 3464–3473, 2001.

[65] B. Cheng, S. Zhao, J. Luo, E. Sprague, L. F. Bonewald, and J. X. Jiang, "Expression of functional gap junctions and regulation by fluid flow in osteocyte-like MLO-Y4 cells," *J. Bone Miner. Res.*, vol. 16, no. 2, pp. 249–259, 2001.

[66] M. R. Forwood, "Inducible cyclo-oxygenase (COX-2) mediates the induction of bone formation by mechanical loading in vivo," *J. Bone Miner. Res.*, vol. 11, no. 11, pp. 1688–1693, 1996.

[67] J. X. Jiang, A. J. Siller-Jackson, and S. Burra, "Roles of gap junctions and hemichannels in bone cell functions and in signal transmission of mechanical stress," *Front. Biosci. a J. virtual Libr.*, vol. 12, p. 1450, 2007.

[68] L. F. Bonewald, “Osteocytes,” *Prim. Metab. bone Dis. Disord. Miner. Metab.*, vol. 7, pp. 32–38, 2008.

[69] K. Lee, H. Jessop, R. Suswillo, G. Zaman, and L. Lanyon, “Bone adaptation requires oestrogen receptor-α,” *Nature*, vol. 424, no. 6947, p. 389, 2003.

[70] C. Ciani, D. Sharma, S. B. Doty, and S. P. Fritton, “Ovariectomy enhances mechanical load-induced solute transport around osteocytes in rat cancellous bone,” *Bone*, vol. 59, pp. 229–234, 2014.

[71] M. Sinnesael *et al.*, “Androgens inhibit the osteogenic response to mechanical loading in adult male mice,” *Endocrinology*, vol. 156, no. 4, pp. 1343–1353, 2015.

[72] K.-H. William Lau *et al.*, “Osteocyte-derived insulin-like growth factor I is essential for determining bone mechanosensitivity,” *Am. J. Physiol. Metab.*, vol. 305, no. 2, pp. E271–E281, 2013.

[73] S. V. Komarova, R. J. Smith, S. J. Dixon, S. M. Sims, and L. M. Wahl, “Mathematical model predicts a critical role for osteoclast autocrine regulation in the control of bone remodeling,” *Bone*, vol. 33, no. 2, pp. 206–215, 2003.

[74] V. Lemaire, F. L. Tobin, L. D. Greller, C. R. Cho, and L. J. Suva, “Modeling the interactions between osteoblast and osteoclast activities in bone remodeling,” *J. Theor. Biol.*, vol. 229, no. 3, pp. 293–309, 2004.

[75] P. Pivonka *et al.*, “Model structure and control of bone remodeling: A theoretical study,” *Bone*, 2008.

[76] Z. Miller, M. B. Fuchs, and M. Arcan, “Trabecular bone adaptation with an orthotropic material model,” *J. Biomech.*, vol. 35, no. 2, pp. 247–256, 2002.

[77] N. Bonfoh, E. Novinyo, and P. Lipinski, “Modeling of bone adaptative behavior based on cells activities,” *Biomech. Model. Mechanobiol.*, vol. 10, no. 5, pp. 789–798, 2011.

[78] D. M. Geraldes, L. Modenese, and A. T. M. Phillips, “Consideration of multiple load cases is critical in modelling orthotropic bone adaptation in the femur,” *Biomech. Model. Mechanobiol.*, vol. 15, no. 5, pp. 1029–1042, 2016.

[79] M. Singh, A. Nagrath, and P. S. Maini, “Changes in trabecular pattern of the upper end of the femur as an index of osteoporosis,” *JBJS*, vol. 52, no. 3, pp. 457–467, 1970.

[80] W. J. Tobin, “The internal architecture of the femur and its clinical significance: the upper end,” *JBJS*, vol. 37, no. 2, p. 434, 1955.

Section 2

Stem Cells and Functional Tissue Engineering

Chapter 4

Prologue: Oro-Dental-Derived Stromal Cells for Cranio-Maxillo-Facial Tissue Engineering - *Past, Present and Future*

Sebastián E. Pérez and Ziyad S. Haidar

1. Introduction

Stomal/Stem Cells (SCs) can be classified as either embryonic (ESCs) or adult stem cells (ASCs), depending on origin. Embryonic stem cells (ESCs) can be derived from the inner cell mass of blastocyst stage embryos [1–4] after fertilization. ESCs are potent and have un-limited self-renewal capacity, and can differentiate into cells of all three germinal layers of the organism; mesoderm, endoderm and ectoderm [2, 3]. While their characteristics are extraordinary and attractive for further investigation, the use of human ESCs is limited by an ethical controversy. Hence, ASCs have emerged, with no ethical debate (s) orbiting their study. ASCs can be harvested from many bodily tissues, and do fulfill all the criteria necessary to be considered as SCs, since they are long-lived, have a significant self-renewal capacity, can differentiate toward a set of various cellular types (such as chondrocytes, adipocytes, osteoblasts, among others) and have potential need/use in regenerative and reparative medicine [5, 6].

Mesenchymal Stem Cells (MSCs) are one of the most controversial groups, not because ethical concerns regarding their harvesting, but for the proper utilization of the term. MSCs were first described by Arnold Caplan in 1991, taking their name from the Greek terms "meso" (middle) and "enchyme" (infusion, related to cellular tissue) making a relation with the embryonic mesoderm layer, establishing their capacity to differentiate toward skeletal tissues (cartilage, bone, marrow stroma, connective tissue, etc) as one of their principal characteristics [7]. Despite the amount of evidence of their existence, characteristics and functionality, there is controversy around them with respect to the nuances of the term MSCs, and what specific characteristics do all MSCs share.

To solve this situation, the International Society for Cellular Therapy (ISCT) stated minimum criterions to classify a potential lineage as MSCs. The first criterion is to display plastic-adherence capacity. Second, they must express certain biomarkers, such as the surface membrane protein Thy-1, usually denominated CD90 (Cluster of Differentiation 90), or the membrane gluco-protein Endoglin (also called CD105). Besides from the presence of the already mentioned CD90 and CD105, MSCs must be at least CD73+, CD14-, CD34-, CD44- and HLA-DR-. Finally, should be capable to differentiate to chondrocytes, adipocytes and osteoblasts, to be classified as MSCs [8, 9].

Since the year 2000, several MSC types have been identified and isolated from oral tissues, including the teeth, dental pulp, gingival, periodontal and supporting structures (**Figure 1**) [10–12]. This has provoked cellular biologists and dentists to bridge and strengthen their relation, communication and collaboration even more,

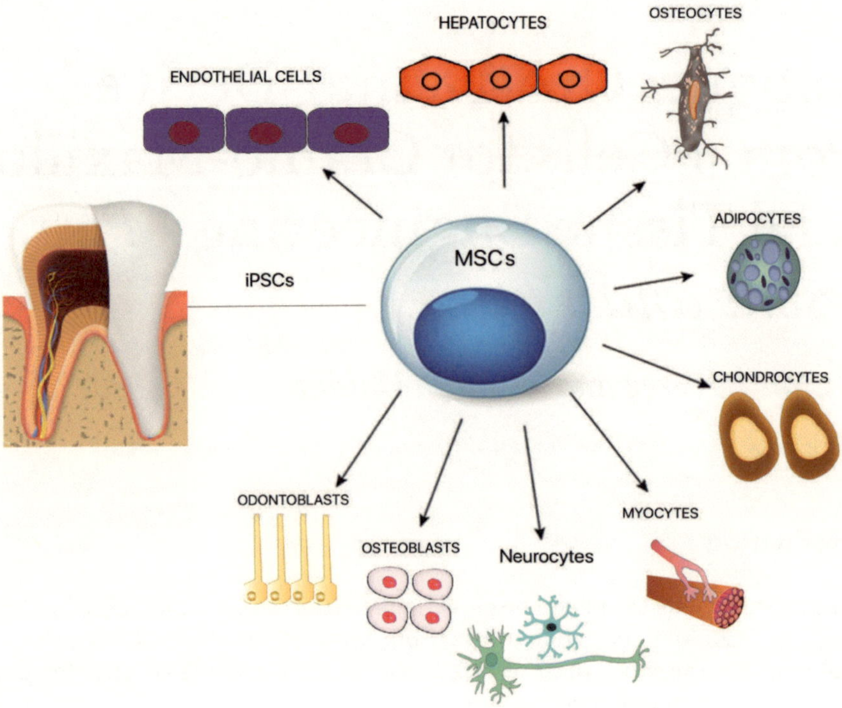

Figure 1.
Dental stem cells and their multi-lineage differentiation capability. Abbreviations; iPSCs: Induced pluripotent stem cells; MSCs: Mesenchymal stem cells.

as a thorough understanding of the cellular mechanisms underlying these oro-dental MSCs must come along or go in parallel with the expected development of their use in different and wide range of therapies and/or therapeutic strategies.

The aim of this introductory chapter is to provide a practically-comprehensive, systematic and updated SC overview (PRISMA flow-chart for the conducted literature e-search is illustrated in **Figure 2**) directed to general dentists, oral and maxillofacial surgeons and head and neck health students and professionals interested in oral cavity-derived MSCs, their reported characteristics and the possible uses/applications in oro-dental tissue engineering, regeneration and repair, and beyond.

1.1 Dental pulp stem cells

Dental Pulp Stem Cells (DPSCs) are one of the most attractive oro-dental derived stem cells, as they are highly clonogenic and rapidly proliferative, exhibit self-renewal, multiple differentiation capabilities, and have the potential for being used on tissue regeneration and immunotherapy [13]. DPSCs can differentiate into osteoblasts, chondrocytes, myocytes, cardiomyocytes, active neurons, Schwann's cells, melanocytes, and hepatocyte-like cells (**Table 1**) [12, 14].

Several studies have shown that DPSCs have immuno-modulatory capabilities, which include T cell-proliferation suppression [15], inhibition of the proliferation of peripheral blood mononuclear cells [16] and induction of T cell apoptosis *in vitro*, ameliorating inflammation-related tissue injuries in mice with colitis [17]. Regarding *in vivo* studies, there has been extensive research using DPSCs to promote tissue regeneration in animal models. A systematic review, (that focused in the use of DPSCs and SHED to repair non-dental tissues) concluded that the use of both of these MSCs on bone tissue repair/regeneration seems to be effective.

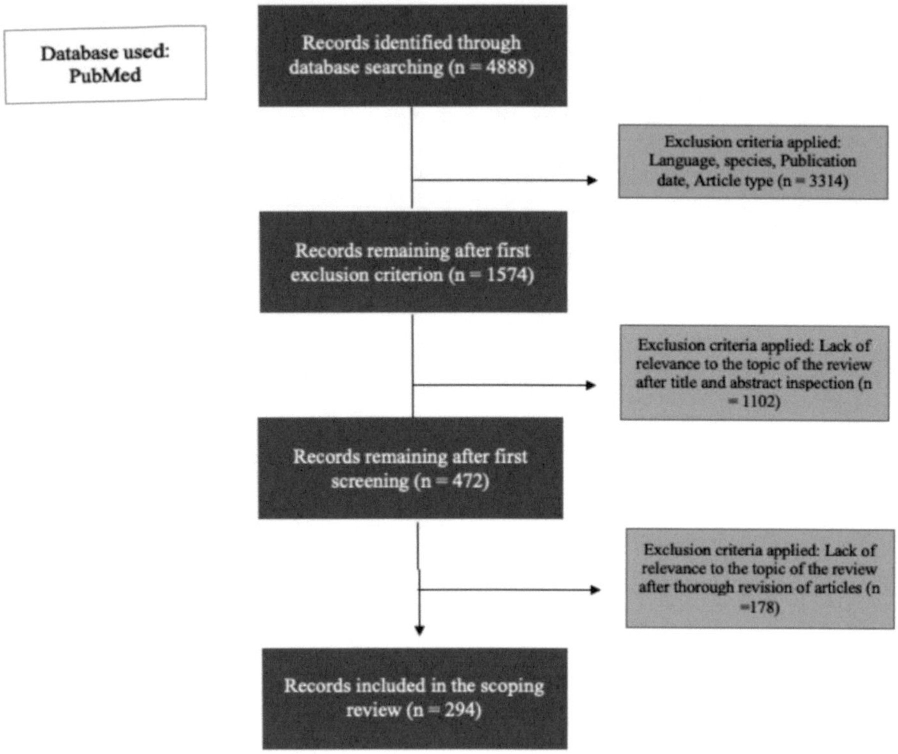

Figure 2.
PRISMA flow diagram for the bibliographic electronic search conducted on PubMed central.

Nevertheless, much more tests are needed to assess whether this effectivity/efficiency extends to the promotion of functional recovery of other types of tissue(s), such as: neuronal tissue, blood vessels, muscle or cartilage [18].

DPSCs have been used in regenerative therapies in clinical trials. Nakashima *et al.* [18] disclosed an experiment performed on five patients, diagnosed with irreversible pulpitis, and no periapical radiolucency in the X-ray analysis. These pulps were isolated and then a fraction of them were separated through the addition of granulocyte colony-stimulating factor (G-CSF). This fraction called mobilized dental pulp stem cells (MDPSCs). These MDPSCs were transplanted with G-CSF in an atelocollagen scaffold into devitalized teeth. Patients were followed up at 1, 2, 4, 12 and 24/28/32 weeks after MDPSCs transplantation. No adverse events or toxicity were detected after clinical and laboratory evaluations. The electric pulp test (EPT) after 4 weeks demonstrated a positive response. The signal intensity of magnetic resonance imaging (MRI) of the regenerated tissue after 24 weeks was similar to those in control group. Finally, cone beam computed tomography demonstrated functional dentin formation in three of the five patients [19]. In another study, DPSCs were isolated from inflammatory dental pulp tissue (thus renaming them as DPSCs-IPs), loaded with a β-tricalcium phosphate scaffold, and engrafted into the periodontal intrabone defect area in the root furcation of two patients, with combined periodontal–endodontic lesions with pocket depth from 5 to 6 mm. Nine months after the surgical procedure, DPSCs-IPs engraftment and regenerative effect was detected on both patients [20]. In a different study, 17 systemically healthy patients (7 assisted to the 1-year follow-up) were subjected to extraction of their third molars for isolation of DPSCs. After this the cells were seeded onto a collagen sponge scaffold, which was then used to fill the injury site left by the

Name	Niche	Biomarkers expressed	Biomarkers not expressed	Differentiation *in vitro*	Tissue Formation *in vivo*	Clinical Trials *human*
DPSCs	Dental pulp, can be harvested from wisdom teeth or other teeth removed from orthodontic reason	CD13, CD29, CD44, CD70, CD73, CD90, CD105, CD146 and CD166	CD14, CD31, CD34, CD35, CD45, CD117, CD133, CD144, CD271 and HLA-DR	Osteoblasts, chondrocytes, myocytes, cardiomyocytes, active neurons, melanocytes, and hepatocyte-like cells.	Transplantation of DPSCs seeded to fibroin scaffolds along with human amniotic fluid stem cells into rats to promote regeneration of critical-size calvarial defects showed bone-regeneration and higher expression of dental markers DPSCs cultured onto human treated dentin and transplanted into the dorsum of mice showed generation of dentin-like tissue and expression of dentin markers DSPP and BMP-1 Dentin/pulp-like structures are generated after transplantation of CD146-positive, CD146-negative and unsorted DPSCs into immunocompromised rats, with a higher degree of generation displayed by the first group.	Dentin formation after transplantation with an atelocollagen matrix and a G-CSF supplementation into a pulpectomized teeth.
						Engraftment and regenerative effect after transplantation of DPSCs isolated from inflammatory dental tissue mixed with a β-tricalcium phosphate matrix.
						Alveolar bone and periodontal tissue reparation after transplantation of autologous DPSCs into the injury site left by the extraction of mandibular third molars.
DFSCs	Dental follicle, ecto-mesenchymal tissue that surrounds the developing tooth germ prior to eruption	CD29, CD44, CD73, CD90, CD105, CD146, HLA-1, NOTCH-1, STRO-1 and Nestin	CD14, CD25, CD28, CD34, and CD45	Osteoblasts, chondrocytes, adipocytes, fibroblasts, cementoblasts and hepatocyte-like cells.	New bone formation when transplanted to a surgically-created cranial bone defect on immunosuppressed rats.	N/A
					Dentin-pulp like tissue and cementum-periodontal ligament complex formed after transplantation of DFSCs co-cultured with treated dental matrix.	
					New bone formation when a DFSCs – Demineralized bone matrix scaffold biocomplex was transplanted into mandibular defects of miniature pigs and subcutaneous tissue of mice.	

Name	Niche	Biomarkers expressed	Biomarkers not expressed	Differentiation *in vitro*	Tissue Formation *in vivo*	Clinical Trials *human*
SHED	Living pulp obtained from the remaining crown of exfoliated deciduous teeth	CD29, CD44, CD73, CD90, CD105, CD146, STRO-1 and Nestin	CD34 and CD271	Osteoblasts, adipocytes, chondroblasts, angiogenic endothelial cells, hepatocyte-like cells and neuron-like cells.	Substantial bone formation after transplantation of SHED-HA/TCP biocomplex in critical-size calvarial defects in mice.	An interventional clinical trial using scaffold-free SHED-derived pellets for the revitalization of young immature permanent teeth with necrotic pulps is yet to be published.
					Transplantation of SHED seeded in tooth slice/scaffolds differentiated into functional odontoblasts that generated tubular dentin.	

Abbreviations: ***DPSCs:*** *Dental Pulp Stem Cells;* ***DFSCs:*** *Dental Follicle Stem Cells;* ***SHED:*** *Stem Cells from Human Exfoliated Deciduous Teeth;* ***N/A:*** *not applicable or determined.*

Table 1.
Principal characteristics of Oro-dental-derived MSCs: DPSCs, DFSCs and SHED.

extraction of the mandibular third molars. The progression of the treatment was evaluated after three months, with a vertical alveolar bone repair and a complete reparation of the periodontal tissue. Furthermore, after histological analysis it was clear that complete regeneration of bone occurred at the injury site, and optimal bone regeneration was evident one year after the grafting [21]. Beyond the evident supporting the use of DPSCs on dental regeneration applications, it has been described that DPSCs could aid in the regeneration of tissues non-related with oro-dental structures, such as corneal epithelium, central nervous system tissues, craniofacial bone, among other examples [22–25].

1.2 Dental follicle stem cells

The dental follicle, has been identified as a source of stem cells and lineage-committed progenitor cells for cementoblasts, odontoblasts and periodontal ligament cells [12]. During cementogenesis, the inner and outer enamel epithelia fuse to form the bi-layered Hertwig's epithelial root sheath (HERS), which induces the differentiation of the dental follicle stem cells (DFSCs) into cementoblasts and odontoblasts [26]. DFSCs are thought to be the origin of the periodontum, (including cementum, periodontal ligament and alveolar bone) (**Table 1**). DFSCs are plastic adherent cells that are positive for the MSCs biomarkers CD29, CD44, CD73, CD90, CD105, CD146, HLA-1, NOTCH-1, STRO-1 and Nestin, while being negative for the hematopoietic markers CD14, CD25, CD28, CD34, and CD45 [27–29]. Yildrim *et al.* [26] proved the capacity of DFSCs to differentiate *in vitro* into osteoblasts, chondrocytes, adipocytes, and other cell types too, such as fibroblasts, cementoblasts and hepatocyte-like cells [27, 30, 31]. Regarding to *in vivo* experimentation, DFSCs have been reported to support new bone formation after the transplantation to a surgically cranial bone defect on immunosuppressed rats [26]. In another study, a treated-dentin matrix (TDM) was obtained from extracted premolars, and used as a scaffold for isolated and cultured DFSCs, from extracted wisdom teeth in humans. An *in vitro* experiment, showed an increase of the expression of DMP-1 and BSP the co-culture with TDM liquid extract in comparison with DFSCs co-cultured groups with HA/TCP liquid extract and DFSCs without co-culture, reflecting an up-regulation of formation and mineralization of dentin. Results have also been seen on a *in vivo* experiment, that showed the implantation of the TDM-DFSCs biocomplex resulted in the formation of dentin-pulp like tissue and cementum-periodontal ligament complex, with the expression of tooth root-related antibodies on the regenerated tissues.

The presence of human mitochondria in a model mouse indicates that the presence of TDM-DFSCs biocomplex could participate in tooth regeneration [32]. Kang *et al.*, [32] transplanted a biocomplex of a demineralized bone matrix scaffold and human DFSCs, both isolated from fresh dental follicle and cryopreserved, into mandibular defects of miniature pigs and subcutaneous tissues of mice. Eight weeks after, the transplanted DFSCs generate bones when it was compared to the original size of the mandibular defects, with a high expression of osteocalcin and VEGF (Vascular endothelial growth factor). Furthermore, a decrease of CD4 expression was measured on the DFSCs-transplanted tissues compared to the control model, this could demonstrate the existence of an immunomodulatory capability [33].

1.3 Stem cells from human exfoliated deciduous teeth

In 2003, a team formed by Dr. Miura's, demonstrate the presence of stem cells population on an isolated deciduous tooth. These stem cells were named stem cells from human exfoliated deciduous teeth (SHED) [34].

As long as it exists the deciduous teeth, as biologically discarded tissues, their collection and isolation are far from ethical concerns around the scientific community. Miura *et al.* [33] discovered that SHED showed a significantly proliferation and number of populations compared to bone marrow mesenchymal stem cells (BMMSCs) and DPSCs.

SHED express biomarkers such as CD29, CD31, CD44, CD73, CD90, CD105, CD146, STRO-1 and Nestin [34–37]. A complete proteomic landscaping was conducted on these oro-dental derived stem cells, with the identification of 2032 proteins, with 1516 of them expressed also on periodontal ligament stem cells (PDLSCs). Furthermore, a more in-depth analysis of the proteomic profile on SHED, showed that they predominantly expressed molecules that are involved in organizing the cytoskeletal network, cellular migration and adhesion. This corresponds with more results presented on the same research, where SHED proved to have a strong migration capacity during wound-healing assays [38].

SHED can differentiate *in vitro* into osteoblasts, adipocytes, chondroblasts, angiogenic endothelial cells, hepatocyte-like cells and neuron-like cells [35, 36], and it has been proven that they can differentiate *in vivo* into adipogenic, chondrogenic and odontogenic lineages in mice models (**Table 1**) [39–41]. A large quantity of research has been conducted about the capacity displayed by SHED to aid on regenerative therapy. Seo *et al.* [41] performed an experiment to elucidate if SHED-mediated bone reparation could be used for therapeutic purposes, generating critical-size calvarial defects in immune-compromised mice and later transplanting a SHED-HA/TCP biocomplex into the defect areas. The defects were repaired after the treatment with bone formation [42]. This kind of research has been conducted in swine deciduous teeth, with similar results, after 6 months of the surgical procedure [43]. In another research, SHED was seeded on tooth slice/scaffolds and implanted into immunodeficient mice subcutaneously. The results showed the capacity of SHED to differentiate into functional odontoblasts, while *in vitro* tests studies, demonstrate, that they can organized into capillary-like sprouts and expressed endothelial markers such as CD31, vascular endothelial cadherin (VE-cadherin) and vascular endothelial growth factor receptor – 2 (VEGFR-2, when are inducted vascular endothelial growth factor (VEGF) [35]. Despite the lack of clinical trials; a recent study showed that the preparation of a biocomplex comprising SHED and a Polyhydroxybutyrate (PHB)/ Chitosan /Nano-bioglass (nBG) scaffold fabricated through electrospinning allowed SHED to differentiate into odontoblast-like cells after the induction with Bone Morphogenetic Protein – 2 (BMP-2), with a 6-fold increase in the expression of DSPP genes and collagen type-1 and a 2-fold expression of alkaline phosphatase (ALP) compared to the control [44]. This type of investigation shows promising results for the use of SHED in oral regenerative therapies, however, more studies are needed in this field [45].

1.4 Periodontal ligament stem cells

The periodontal ligament (PDL), a specialized connective tissue, is developed from dental follicle tissue during tooth formation and is the responsible for the regeneration of the adjacent periodontal structures. Although this regeneration process involves and depends of the recruitment of stem cells that differentiate into fibroblasts, cementoblasts or osteoblasts [46, 47]. Periodontal ligament stem cells (PDLSCs) were first isolated from third molars and since then, they have shown to be able to differentiate into periodontal cells, cementoblasts, adipocytes, collagen-producing cells and retinal ganglion-like cells [48–50]. PDLSCs express biomarkers such as CD13, CD29, CD44, CD73, CD90, CD105, CD166 and Nestin (**Table 2**). The expression of the MSCs biomarker CD146 is disputed, as some sources detected

Name	Niche	Biomarkers expressed	Biomarkers not expressed	Differentiation *in vitro*	Tissue Formation *in vivo*	Clinical Trials *human*
PDLSCs	Periodontal ligament, soft connective tissue between the cementum and the inner wall of the alveolar bone socket	CD13, CD29, CD44, CD73, CD90, CD105, CD166 and Nestin. CD46 expression is disputed	CD14, CD19, CD34, CD45, CD117, CD133, CD144, CD271, STRO-1 and HLA-DR	Periodontal cells, cementoblasts, adipocytes, collagen-producing cells, retinal ganglion-like cells, cells of neurogenic, cardiomyogenic, chondrogenic and osteogenic lineages.	A cementum/PDL-like complex was generated after subcutaneous transplantation into the dorsal surface of mice. PDL-like tissue with PDLSCs closely associated to alveolar bone was observed 8 weeks after transplantation of a PDLSCs-HA/TCP biocomplex into two periodontal defects surgically created in the buccal cortex of rat's mandibular molar. Osteogenic repair of calvarial defects on rats was detected after implantation of a collagen membrane with PDLSCs and conditioned medium.	The transplantation of a biocomplex comprising PDLSCs and the bone grafting material CALCITITE 4060–2 into deep intrabony defects generated through the removal of inflammatory periodontal tissues resulted in periodontal tissue regain, along with decrease in probing depth, increase in gingival recession and attachment gain.
SCAP	Root apical papilla tissue on the exterior of the root foramen area	CD13, CD44, CD73, CD90, CD105, CD146, DSPP, Osteocalcin, Nestin, Neurofilament M, FGFR-1 and TGF-β-RI. STRO-1 expression is disputed	CD34, CD45 and HLA-DR	Odontoblast, adipocytes and hepatocyte-like cells.	A 3-D nerve-like tissue with axon and myelin structures can be obtained culturing SCAP using an integrated bioprocess composed of polyethylene glycol microwell-mediated cell spheroid formation and subsequent dynamic culture in a high aspect ratio vessel bioreactor. Hard tissue of uncertain characteristics is formed after transplantation of a SCAP/HA biocomplex into immuno-compromised mice. A pulp-like tissue with well-established vascularity and a continuous layer of dentin-like tissue were induced after insertion of SCAP in tooth fragments and subsequent transplantation into immuno-deficient mice.	N/A

Name	Niche	Biomarkers expressed	Biomarkers not expressed	Differentiation *in vitro*	Tissue Formation *in vivo*	Clinical Trials *human*
TGPCs	Tooth germ of third molars	CD29, CD31, CD73, CD90, CD105, CD166, VEGFR2, VE-Cadherin, vWF, Cytokeratin-17, Cytokeratin-19 and STRO-1	CD14, CD34, CD45, CD133 and CD144	Osteoblasts, neural cells, adipocytes, chondrocytes and hepatocytes.	New bone matrix formation was observed, along with osteocytes and an active osteoblast lining in on the matrix surface, after transplantation of a TGPCs/HA biocomplex into immunocompromised mice	N/A

Abbreviations: TGPCs: *Tooth-Germ Progenitor Cells;* ***SCAP:*** *Stem Cells from the Apical Papilla;* ***PDLSCs:*** *Periodontal Ligament Stem Cells;* ***N/A:*** *not applicable or determined.*

Table 2.
Principal characteristics of Oro-dental-derived MSCs: PDLSCs, SCAP and TGPCs.

it, while other sources did not [46, 47]. In the previously mentioned proteomic landscape performed by Taraslia *et al.*, [37] 3235 proteins were identified on PDLSCs, where 1721 were found only in PDLSCs and 1516 were shared with SHED. It is interesting that researchers who performed this proteomic profile found that the recorded proteins found on PDLSCs, are tightly involved in cellular growth, proliferation and in the replication, recombination and repair of the DNA [38]. To explore the regenerative potential of these stem cells, PDLSCs were mixed with HA/TCP ceramic particles, and transplanted into two periodontal defects, that had been surgically created in the buccal cortex in rat's molar. In the first defect a cementum/PDL-like complex characterized by a layer of aligned cementum-like tissue and associated PDL-like tissues was generated. In the second defect, 6–8 weeks after transplantation a PDL-like tissue was observed, with PDLSCs associated with the alveolar bone. This may suggest a potential functional role in periodontal tissue regeneration [12, 48]. A recently study demonstrate an osteogenic capability when the collagen membrane is used in conjunction with human PDLSCs to repair a calvaria defect of a rat [51]. In a retrospective pilot study, three male patients between 25 and 42 years with periodontal disease were selected for transplantation of PDLSCs. The researchers found a decrease in probing depth during post-operatory controls with a follow-up of 72 months [52].

1.5 Stem cells from the apical papilla

In 2006, a research team led by Dr. Wataru Sonoyama found apical papilla tissue on the exterior of the root foramen area, contained a population of stem cells identified them as Stem Cells from the Apical Papilla (SCAP). The team generated single-cells suspension from third molars of 18–20 years old adult. They proved that a transplant of SCAP and PDLSCs could form a root/periodontal complex in a mini-pig model [53]. A Further study revealed, that this tissue contains less cellular and vascular components than dental pulp, although there is a cell-rich zone between the apical papilla and the dental pulp [54]. These cells proliferate faster than DPSCs, and can differentiate into odontoblast, adipocytes and hepatocyte-like cells. They express biomarkers, such as CD13, CD44, CD73, CD90, CD105 and CD146 (MSCs), DSPP and osteocalcin (dentinogenic), Nestin and neurofilament M (neurogenic) or FGFR-1 (Fibroblast growth factor receptor – 1) and TGF-β-RI (Transforming growth factor beta isotype, receptor 1) (**Table 2**).

The presence of the mesenchymal marker STRO-1 is in doubt, sources exposed that it is present in a portion of these stem cells, meanwhile other claims that it is not expressed. SCAP could form hard tissue *in vitro* and *in vivo* after subcutaneous transplantation of a SCAP/Hydroxyapatite biocomplex into immunocompromised mice, although the precise characteristics of this hard tissue could not be determined [55]. Another approach of SCAP on regenerative therapies was conducted by Bellamy *et al.* [55], when a bioactive chitosan-based scaffold with a sustained TGF-β-releasing nanoparticles system was prepared, to evaluate if it would promote migration and enhances differentiation of SCAP. The study showed that the scaffold was releasing TGF-β in a sustained manner thus facilitating delivery of a critical concentration of this molecule at the opportune time, demonstrating properties conducting to cellular activities and a bioactive time of up to 4 weeks. SCAP showed greater viability, migration and biomineralization when it is compared with the control group.

SCAP displays a promising battery of characteristics, that are useful for regenerative engineering purposes, but for stem cell population, there is a substantial lack of clinical studies that needs to be experienced sooner than later [56].

1.6 Tooth-germ progenitor cells

The tooth germ, is an aggregation of progenitor cells that forms a tooth, consisting of the dental papilla, the dental follicle, and the enamel organ [12]. It has been determined that a novel population of stem cells can be isolated from a third molar, called: tooth-germ progenitor cells (TGPCs). These cells have notorious proliferative and a multipotent nature, which could be explained due to the fact that tooth germ of third molars are reported to develop after the age of 6 years, but remain undifferentiated until this time. TGPCs are able to differentiate into osteoblasts, neural cells, adipocytes, chondrocytes and hepatocytes [57, 58]. This capacity, raises interesting possibilities, as it has been proven that these cells can engraft successfully in carbon tetrachloride (CCl4)-treated liver injured rats and help them to restore the liver function after 4 weeks [57]. TGPCs express the MSCs biomarkers CD29, CD73, CD90, CD105, CD166 and STRO-1 (at least in parts of their total population), along with CD31, VEGFR2, VE-Cadherin and vWF (endothelial cell markers) and Cytokeratin-17, Cytokeratin-19, Epithelial cell adhesion molecule and vimentin (epithelial cell markers). TGPCs respond well with different materials scaffolds, (Poly ε-caprolactone, poly L-lactide and a mix of both) (**Table 2**) [59]. TGPCs and TGPCs transfected with Venus (a variant of green fluorescent protein) were implanted with HA into immunocompromised rats. New bone formation in the presence of osteocytes was observed in the newly formed bone matrix and an active osteoblast lining on the matrix surface [57]. As it can be noted, TGPCs display characteristics that make them a suitable option to be used for regenerative therapies, but it is clear that more studies are needed, before their use on patients.

1.7 Gingiva-derived stem cells

The gingiva is an oral tissue overlaying the alveolar ridge and retromolar region that is recognized as a biological barrier and a fundamental component of the oral mucosal immunity [12]. The gingival tissue is constantly subjected to thermal, chemical, mechanical and bacterial aggression. However, it has the capacity to restore itself completely, if the destruction of its collagen network occurs. This unique healing capacity indicates that this tissue should have a significant amount of stem cells [60]. The isolation and characterizations of a subpopulation of gingival fibroblasts that possess stem cells characteristics, called Gingiva-derived Mesenchymal Stem cells or Gingiva-derived Stem cells (GMSCs), was described by many different research groups [60–63]. GMSCs are a multipotent type MSCs, that can differentiate into adipogenic, chondrogenic and osteogenic lines, expressing markers such as CD29, CD44, CD73, CD90 and CD105; (**Table 3**) Subpopulations of these cells can express the markers CD146 and STRO-1, that are widely present by other oro-dental derived MSCs [60, 62–64].

It is important to notice the immuno-modulatory capacity displayed by GMSCs. These cells are capable to: elicit a potent inhibitory effect on T-cell proliferation [12], generate distinct immune tolerance [61, 65], elicit M2 polarization of macrophages through cytokine modulation and an increase of the expression of a mannose receptor [66], and alleviate the sensitization and elicitation of contact hypersensitivity [67], displaying many other immuno-modulatory capabilities as well [12]. There have been different in vitro studies that evaluate the potential of GMSCs related to tissue generation. Zhang and colleagues [60] demonstrated that a GMSCs-HA/TCP biocomplex incubated in osteogenic supplemented with collagen gel, could raise bone-related proteins such as osteocalcin, osteopontin and collagen [61].

Name	Niche	Biomarkers expressed	Biomarkers not expressed	Differentiation *in vitro*	Tissue Formation *in vivo*	Clinical Trials *human*
GMSCs	Gingival tissue overlaying the alveolar ridges and retromolar region	CD29, CD44, CD73, CD90 and CD105. CD146 and STRO-1 are expressed by fractions of their population	CD11b, CD19, CD34, CD45, CD117, CD200, CD271 and HLA-DR	Adipogenic, chondrogenic, neurogenic, entothelial and osteogenic lines.	A GMSCs-HA/TCP biocomplex incubated in osteogenic medium and supplemented with collagen gel raised the levels of bone-related proteins when transplanted subcutaneously into immunocompromised mice, suggesting new bone formation. This can also be observed after subcutaneous transplantation of a GMSCs/collagen gel biomatrix in the dorsal surface of immunocompromised mice.	N/A
					Newly formed bone with well-mineralized trabecular structure and an increase of bone-related proteins expression were found at the inner site of mandibular defects of Sprague Dawley rats after transplantation of a GMSCs/collagen gel biomatrix.	
					New bone formation and an increase of bone-related proteins expression was found in critical-size calvarial defects in rat model after transplantation of a GMSCs/collagen gel biomatrix.	
					Transplantation of a 3-D Poly-(lactide) scaffold enriched with GMSCs and GMSCs-CM on this same model showed a better osteogenic capacity compared to controls, repair of the calvarial defect, and upregulated genes involved in ossification and regulation of ossification.	

DOI: http://dx.doi.org/10.5772/intechopen.95090

Name	Niche	Biomarkers expressed	Biomarkers not expressed	Differentiation *in vitro*	Tissue Formation *in vivo*	Clinical Trials *human*
aBMMSCs	Bone marrow of the alveolar process	CD29, CD44, CD73, CD90, CD105 and CD146. A fraction of the population express STRO-1	CD11b, CD14, CD19, CD34, CD45, CD79α nor HLA-DR	Osteogenic, chondrogenic and adipogenic lines.	New bone formation along with cuboidal osteoblasts lining the surface of its margin was observed after transplantation of aBMMSCs mixed with HA/TCP ceramic powder into mice.	N/A
					Adipocityc fatty marrow support originated from aBMMSCs could also be observed around the site of the transplant.	
					Substantial new bone and osteocyte formation was found after transplantation of aBMMSCs mixed with matrixes with different ratio of HA/TCP into immunocompromised mice.	
					Newly formed cellular mixed fiber cementum, woven/lamellar bone and periodontal ligament was observed after transplantation of a biocomplex comprising aBMMSCs seeded into a chitosan/anorganic bovine bone (C/ABB) scaffold into beagle dogs.	

Abbreviations: aBMMSCs: *Alveolar Bone Marrow Mesenchymal Stem Cells;* ***GMSCs:*** *Gingiva-derived Mesenchymal Stem Cells;* ***N/A:*** *not applicable or determined.*

Table 3.
Principal characteristics of Oro-dental-derived MSCs: GMSCs and aBMMSCs.

GMSCs can generate tissues from neural crest cells, during embryonic development [65]. This data is supported on a study in which GMSCs were injected (subcutaneously) in four different immunodeficient Rag2 mice. Results showed no signs of tumors, into different organs after 6 months [64]. In another investigation, GMSCs were mixed with collagen gel matrix and transplanted (subcutaneously), into the dorsal surface of immunocompromised mice model. The results showed higher levels of osteopontin and collagen when it was compared with the control group, (supporting the findings of Zhang and colleagues in 2009). Also, this investigation proved a newly bone formation with mineralized trabecular tissue, after performing the transplantation of GMSCs, but this time into mandibular rat defects [68].

Another interesting capacity of GMSCs in regenerative therapies, is related to the use of the secretome (SM) in their cultures It has been proven, that implantation of a three-dimensional Poly- (lactide) scaffold enriched with GMSCs-SM on rat calvaria defect model, showed a better osteogenic capacity compared to group controls [69]. Although further studies are needed to prove that GMSCs can be useful in pre-clinical and clinical trials too, it is clear that these MSCs have great potential in orofacial tissue engineering, regeneration and repair.

1.8 Alveolar bone marrow mesenchymal stem cells

Bone Marrow Mesenchymal Stem Cells, are the predominant MSCs used in clinical studies for craniofacial tissue regeneration, with a high osteogenic ability [5]. Clinical trials regarding in the use of BMMSCs obtained from iliac bone, have shown promissory results, other evidence suggests that for craniofacial regeneration, it may be a better option to use craniofacial tissues as a cell source [70].

It has been shown that contrary to what happens with iliac bone marrow extraction, alveolar bone marrow MSCs (aBMMSCs) can be easily obtained from alveolar bone, during a dental surgery as: wisdom tooth extraction, crown lengthening surgery, and other examples. 0.5 cc of bone marrow are needed to predictably isolate these cells [71, 72], emerging as an interesting alternative in the craniofacial field.

BMMSCs and aBMMSCs have no significant differences on their osteogenic potential, as measured mRNA levels of osteocalcin, osteopontin, and bone sialoprotein are similar in both populations, but there are differences on their chondrogenic and adipogenic potentials. aBMMSCs are reported to differentiate with more difficulties toward these lines than BMMSCs [73]. aBMMSCs express the markers CD29, CD44, CD73, CD90, CD105 and CD146 while do not express the markers CD11b, CD14, CD19, CD34, CD45, CD79α nor HLA-DR, consistently showing the classic MSCs marker pattern (**Table 3**). A fraction of the cell population (approximately 3%) also expresses the marker STRO-1, a trend that can also be observed in other oro-dental derived MSCs [70, 74–76].

Several *in vitro* and *in vivo* studies have been performed with these stem cells. aBMMSCs mixed with HA/TCP ceramic powder were transplanted into immunodeficient mice. 8 weeks after transplantation a significant new bone formation could be observed around the material, and cuboidal osteoblasts were seen lining the surface of the margin of formed bone. In a different experience, aBMMSCs were transplanted into the left and right dorsal surfaces of 24 immunocompromised mice. The experimental groups consisted in: aBMMSCs mixed with a 60%HA/40%TCP (MBCP) matrix, aBMMSCs mixed with a 20% HA/80% TCP (MBCP plus) matrix and aBMMSCs mixed with deproteinized sterilized bovine bone (Bio-Oss). Substantial new bone and osteocyte formation as noted in the first two groups, while in the third case the new bone formation was poor. Similarly, positive immunostaining for alkaline-phosphatase, RUNX-2, osteocalcin and osteopontin was evidenced in the first two groups but only limited expression was found on the third group. It is important to notice that although Bio-Oss gave rise to the lower quantity of new bone, it also was associated with low osteoclasts formation, while both MBCP and MBCP plus induced a higher formation of these cells, so Bio-Oss cannot be discarded as a potential material for bone regeneration [77].

The potential of this stem cells in the periodontal regeneration field, was explored by seeding them into a chitosan/anorganic bovine bone (C/ABB) scaffold, and transplanting this biocomplex into six male beagle dogs with one-wall critical size periodontal defects. The experimental group that had the C/ABB seeded with aBMMSCs exhibited newly formed cellular mixed cementum, woven/lamellar bone and periodontal ligament in higher levels than the different controls used in the experiment [71].

1.9 Salivary gland stem cells

The use of salivary gland stem cells (SGSCs) in regenerative therapy is widely inclined toward the restoration of the function of salivary glands. When their function is impaired and saliva production decreases, current therapies are limited to bring secretagogues and artificial saliva, to restore salivary gland function.

The search of stem cells that can restore the lost function, has come to the exploration of salivary gland stem cells (SGSCs) as a novel resource [78, 79]. SGSCs express the markers CD24, CD29, CD34, CD44, CD49f, CD73, CD81, CD90, CD105, CD133, CD146, CD166, STRO-1, Nestin and aldehyde dehydrogenase (ALDH) (**Table 4**). There is a controversy if they express CD117 marker or not, as it was reported that SGSCs that were isolated from minor salivary glands do not express this marker [78, 80, 81]. These cells are capable of differentiate toward the classic MSCs lines; osteogenic, adipogenic and chondrogenic, and into amylase-expressing cells [82].

A study demonstrates the ability of SGSCs to restore the function of a damage salivary gland in irradiated rats. After one day, SGSCs were transplanted to each gland through intra-glandular injection, measuring their body weight and saliva flow rate during 60 days. The body weight of the rats decreased the first week, but after that, consistently increased until day 60, with significant difference respecting to the control group. Furthermore, the acinar and duct structures were evaluated, along with the composition of their mucosubstances. The parenchyma of the salivary glands of un-treated rats were intact, as well the parenchyma of the damaged-rats that were treated with SGSCs, while the parenchyma of the radiated but un-treated group showed vacuoles and a disrupted acinar structure. One week after the treatment, apoptotic cells could be observed in the un-treated damaged-rats, while in the treated group they were not present [82]. In another study, with the same protocol but differences irradiated dose and transplantation time, the results showed that SGSCs can restore homeostasis of salivary glands by a combination of engraftment, proliferation, differentiation and potential stimulation of recipient cells [80].

It is apparent that SGSCs are a potential useful solution for patients with xerostomia, thus requiring further studies to prove if these promissory results are replicated in pre-clinical or clinical interventions.

1.10 Periosteum-derived mesenchymal stem cells

The periosteum is in direct contact with the bone surface and contains a mixed cell population that includes fibroblasts, osteoblasts, pericytes and a subpopulation of MSCs known as Periosteum-derived stem cells (PDSCs) [83]. PDSCs (**Table 4**) express the biomarkers CD9, CD13, CD29, CD49e, CD44, CD54, CD73, CD 90, CD105, CD166 and HLA-ABC, while not expressing the markers CD14, CD31, CD33, CD34, CD38,

Name	Niche	Biomarkers expressed	Biomarkers not expressed	Differentiation *in vitro*	Tissue Formation *in vivo*	Clinical Trials *human*
SGSCs	Major, parotid, submandibular, sublingual and minor salivary glands	CD24, CD29, CD34, CD44, CD49f, CD73, CD81, CD90, CD105, CD133, CD146, CD166, STRO-1, Nestin and ALDH. CD117 expression is disputed	CD45 and CD271	Osteogenic, adipogenic, chondrogenic, and amylase-expressing cells.	In several different studies it has been shown that the transplantation of SGSCs toward previously irradiated salivary glands restore their function (measured by saliva flow rate), and promote a decrease of their degeneration by a combination of engraftment, proliferation, differentiation and potential stimulation of recipient cells. This suggests that they have potential to differentiate toward cell lines that conform the acinar and/or ductal structures of salivary glands.	N/A
PDSCs	Inner cell-rich cambium layer of the outer lining of long bones. Can be found on the upper vestibule, lower vestibule or hard palate	CD9, CD13, CD29, CD49e, CD44, CD54, CD73, CD 90, CD105, CD166 and HLA-ABC	CD14, CD31, CD33, CD34, CD38, CD45, CD106, CD117, CD133 and HLA-DR	Osteogenic, adipogenic and chondrogenic lines.	iPSCs (induced pluripotent stem cells) derived from PDSCs and un-differentiated PDSCs were transplanted under the kidney capsules of diabetic mice. Hyperglycemia and glucose tolerance improved, and human insulin was detected on their serum and kidney sections for both groups. These results suggest that these stem cells could engraft, proliferate and differentiate when subjected to these conditions.	N/A
					Autologous PDSCs in a Collagen I/Collagen II matrix were transplanted to Beagle dogs. Bone fill within the limits of implant threads and bone-implant contact was observed after transplantation. These results were not statistically similar that the ones yielded with the transplantation of BMMSCs using the same methodology.	

Name	Niche	Biomarkers expressed	Biomarkers not expressed	Differentiation *in vitro*	Tissue Formation *in vivo*	Clinical Trials *human*
OESCs	Basal layer of the oral mucosal epithelium	CD29, CD44, CD73 and CD90. Subsets of their population are positives for CD105, CD146 and STRO-1	CD34 and CD45	Osteogenic, chondrogenic, adipogenic and neurogenic lines.	in vivo differentiation potential toward corneal tissues has been thoroughly researched. Cultivated oral mucosal epithelial cell sheets (COMECS) have shown that OESCs can differentiate into stratified epithelial cells upon transplantation into rabbit corneal surface using this methodology, being well-attached to the host corneal stroma and able to survive up to two weeks after transplantation.	The integrity of the ocular surface of eyes with total bilateral limbal stem cell deficiency was restored for at least 2 years after transplantation of OESCs cultured with human amniotic membrane as biological substrate.
IPAPCs	Inflamed peri-apical tissues after endodontic infection	CD73, CD90 and CD105	CD45	Adipogenic and osteogenic lines.	Mineralized tissue was observed 8 weeks after transplantation of a IPAPCs-HA/TCP biocomplex into mice.	N/A
*LESCs**	Second and third layer of the epithelium cell layer at the base of the inter-papillary pit	Bmi-1	N/A	Keratinized epithelial cells.	N/A	N/A

Abbreviations: SGSCs: *Salivary Gland Stem Cells;* ***PDSCs:*** *Periosteum-derived Mesenchymal Stem Cells;* ***OESCs:*** *Oral Epithelial Stem Cells;* ***IPAPCs:*** *Inflamed Periapical Progenitory Cells;* ***LESCs:*** *Lingual Epithelial Stem Cells;* ***N/A:*** *not applicable or determined; *status as MSCs not yet conclusive.*

Table 4.
Principal characteristics of Oro-dental-derived MSCs: SGSCs, PDSCs, OESCs, IPAPCs and LESCs.

CD45, CD106, CD117, CD133 and HLA-DR. PDSCs can differentiate toward to: osteogenic, adipogenic and chondrogenic line [84]. It has been proven that PDSCs express clonogenical and proliferative activity independent of the age and the donor site [85].

In 2015, a three-dimensional culture system designed for mass production of PDSCs. The cells formed spheres by spontaneous aggregation, thus passing from a two-dimensional culture to a three-dimensional system. The spheres retained their viability and proliferation ability, even when the culture was scaled-up to 125 mL Erlenmeyer flasks. These results open up the possibility of developing a secure, fast and economic method to achieve high MSCs biomass for future clinical applications [86]. In another study, PDSCs were isolated, and then subjected to a three-step differentiation process to become: Induced Pluripotent Stem Cells (iPSCs; pluripotent stem cells generated artificially via genetic manipulation of somatic cells). Insulin release by iPSCs was confirmed in the immunocytochemical analysis. Hyperglycaemia and glucose tolerance of these mice were improved and human insulin was detected on their serum and kidney sections. Transplantation of undifferentiated PDSCs also improved blood glucose levels and increased serum human insulin levels [87]. In another interesting study PDSCs and BMMSCs were harvested from seven Beagle dogs. After this, the animals were subjected to teeth extraction, and after three months, implants were mixed with a Collagen I/Collagen II sponge as a scaffold and transplanted to a bone dehiscence created for this purpose. Both stem cells populations showed osteogenic potential *in vitro* evidenced by mineral nodule formation and expression of bone markers, and after transplantation both had similar bone fill within the limits of implant threads and bone-implant contact. There was no significant difference between both MSCs, thus presenting a similar potential for bone reconstruction [88].

1.11 Oral epithelial stem cells

The oral mucosal epithelium (OME) is a stratified tissue that posse tight junction proteins in its supra-basal layer and hemidesmosomes in its basal layer. These characteristics, which are similar to the characteristics of corneal epithelium, define OME as a potential source of material for cross-therapies in the reparation of damaged corneal surfaces [89]. Furthermore, the cultivated oral mucosal epithelial transplantation (COMET), a technique that uses OME to repair other tissues, has been used to repair intraoral mucosal defects and esophageal mucosa during endoscopic mucosal resection procedures, thus suggesting a wide variety of potential applications [90, 91]. The potential for regenerative therapies displayed by OME is related to the presence of a cell population with stemness potential, called Oral epithelial stem cells (OESCs), located in the basal layer of the OME [92].

OESCs are undifferentiated cells, ultra-structurally and biochemically, that retain a high capacity of long-term self-renewal and proliferative potential, that response to injury and certain growth stimuli [93]. These stem cells are capable to differentiate toward osteogenic, chondrogenic, adipogenic and neurogenic lines [94]. Regarding their surface markers, there are positive for CD105, CD146 and STRO-1, while they are consistently positive for CD29, CD44, CD73 and CD90 and negative for CD34 and CD45 (**Table 4**) [95]. Furthermore, the p75-positive subset of the population displayed higher *in vitro* proliferative capacity and clonal growth potential [96].

The use of COMECS for ocular transplantation has given good results, as this tissue has showed to be able to survive two weeks after being attached to rabbit corneal surfaces, being well-attached to the host corneal stroma, and involving differentiated stratified epithelial cells [95]. Nonetheless, alternative treatments that do not rely on cell sheets have also been studied. A clinical grade fibrin gel for the culture of OESCs was prepared utilizing fibrinogen and thrombin that served as base for the culture of OESCs previously harvested from oral mucosa. Tranexamic acid was used to prevent the digestion of the fibrin gel during the culture. A clinical trial was conducted to prove if cultivated oral mucosa epithelium expanded, without depending of cell sheets, could achieve improvement in two patients with histologically confirmed bilateral total limbal stem cell deficiency (LSCD). The use of OESCs for the regeneration of other tissues should be explored further, but these stem cells definitely have the potential to cause an impact regarding regeneration of damaged tissues.

1.12 Inflamed periapical progenitory cells and lingual epithelial stem cells

Inflammation of the periapical progenitory cells (IPAPCs), are MSCs that can be found in inflamed periapical tissues. It was explored that these cells can differentiate into adipogenic and osteogenic lines. Also, they proved that after mixing an IPAPCs culture with an HA/TCP matrix resulted in the appearance of mineralized tissue [97]. Regarding their surface marker expression, IPAPCs are positive for the classical MSCs markers CD73, CD90 and CD105, but only 66.3% of their population co-expressed the three of them at the same time (**Table 4**). Nevertheless, IPAPCs are consistently negative for CD45 [98]. Even though IPAPCs are difficult to harvest than the previously described MSCs, because they inhabit exclusively on inflamed periapical tissue, while the majority of the aforementioned oro-dental derived MSCs can be harvested from healthy patients, more studies should be conducted to definitely assess their characteristics and potential use on regenerative therapies.

The surface of the tongue is covered with stratified squamous cell layers, and the lingual epithelium is continuously replaced throughout the life of mammals, which suggest the presence of stem cells [99].

Lingual epithelial stem cells (LESCs), are located in the basal layer of the lingual epithelium. A population of cells that were harvested from the second and third layer of the epithelium cell layer at the base of the interpapillary pit, and are positive for the marker Bmi-1 (B cell-specific Moloney murine leukemia virus integration site 1), that has a role in cell cycle, self-renewal and maintenance of hemopoietic and neural stem cells [100].

The Bmi-1 stem cells, replace keratinized epithelial cells but no the taste bud cells. Studies have shown the presence of two types of stem cells (slow-cycling, long term stem cells and rapidly proliferating, short term stem cells), with different role in tissue maintenance and regeneration. There still unidentified the specific biomarkers for short term stem cells, this put in doubt if the mechanism of maintenance exists [100].

2. Combinatorial technology: nano-based stem cell therapy

For example, when dental pulpitis is diagnosed, the indicated treatment is to remove the pulp by an endodontic treatment. One of the most promising/emerging treatment approach is to regenerate this lost tissue. A study tried to replicate vital pulp tissue, with seeding SC from the dental tissue, with promising result. It is yet to be developed, an ideal cell-seeding system, due to the nature of the root and root canal system [101].

There is a need of regenerative therapies, capable to recover the function of the lost tissue due to diseases or trauma. To be a possible option, three elements are needed: cells, scaffolds / extracellular matrix and growing factors.

Tissue engineering it is bringing significant changes in clinical results. Nano-materials were first explored/used in 2002, for dental reconstruction. The income of new membranes in the guided tissue regeneration was the beginning of techniques considering three principal elements: SC, scaffolds and molecules signals. The combination of stem cells with nano-structured materials and scaffolds is a promising research area [102, 103].

2.1 Growth factors

These proteins generate a stimulus that induce cell growth (regulate, proliferation and migration) and the receptors binding in cell membrane. In tissue engineering the most proteins used includes: Hedgehog proteins (HHS), morphogenetic proteins (BMPs), interleukins, fibroblast growth factor (FGF) vascular endothelial growth factor (VEGF) and tumor necrosis factor (TNF) [104].

BPM have been studied and extensively applied for dental regeneration. These proteins can divide into four families (BMP-2/BMP-4, BMP-3/BMP-3B, BMP-5/BMP-6/BMP-7/BMP-8 and GDF-5/GDF-6/GDF-7), that shows an important function in the differentiation of dental biological cells (odontoblast and ameloblast) [104].

2.2 Scaffolds

Scaffolds are biomaterials that provide an optimal environment to cells allowing to: migrate, proliferate and differentiate. Biocompatibility is the main characteristic (among others as: mechanical strength, surface, pore size, biodegradable), that prevents cytotoxicity and inflammatory reactions, allowing an optimal regenerative functioning of the biomaterial. Materials with these properties are challenge in the tissue engineering field (**Figure 3**) [102–105].

Hydrogels are highly hydrophilic (due to the presence of carboxyl, amide, amino, hydroxyl groups) polymers commonly used as scaffolds, with the ability to support cell proliferation, migration and differentiation, letting a correct transport if oxygen and nutrient (**Figure 3**). Their preparation depends on the designed and the application, including physical, chemical, irradiation crosslink and free radical polymerization. In addition, chitosan and alginate-based hydrogels, demonstrate desirable biocompatibility [105, 106].

A common approach to developed a tissue, involves isolation of tissue-specific cells, from the patient and harvested in vitro. Cells are expanded and seeded into a scaffold of the targeted tissue then, the cell-loaded scaffold is transplanted into the patient, by a direct injection or trough implantation of the fabricated tissue at the desired site [106].

Porosity (total surface of the structure for incoming cells) is the key to provide space for cell migrate and vascularization of the tissue. The minimum pore size required is 100 μm, due to the cell size, transport and migration conditions. The degradation rate is intimately related to the porosity, high porosity can reduce the accumulation of acidic products.

These scaffolds can mimic the extracellular matrices, providing an integral structure and giving an optimal guidance to cellular organization. A successful approach to improve the cellular attachment, is the combination of a peptide sequence; Arginine-glycine-aspartic acid (RGD). This incorporation has shown a better binding between cells-RGD hydrogel scaffolds on different cells (fibroblast, osteoblast, muscle cells) [107]. Naturally polymer materials (collagen, fibrin, glycosaminoglycans, chitosan, alginates, starch, agarose, silk fibroin), are biocompatible, low cytotoxicity and inflammatory response. Collagen is a widely natural polymers, that provide mechanical support to the connective tissue [103].

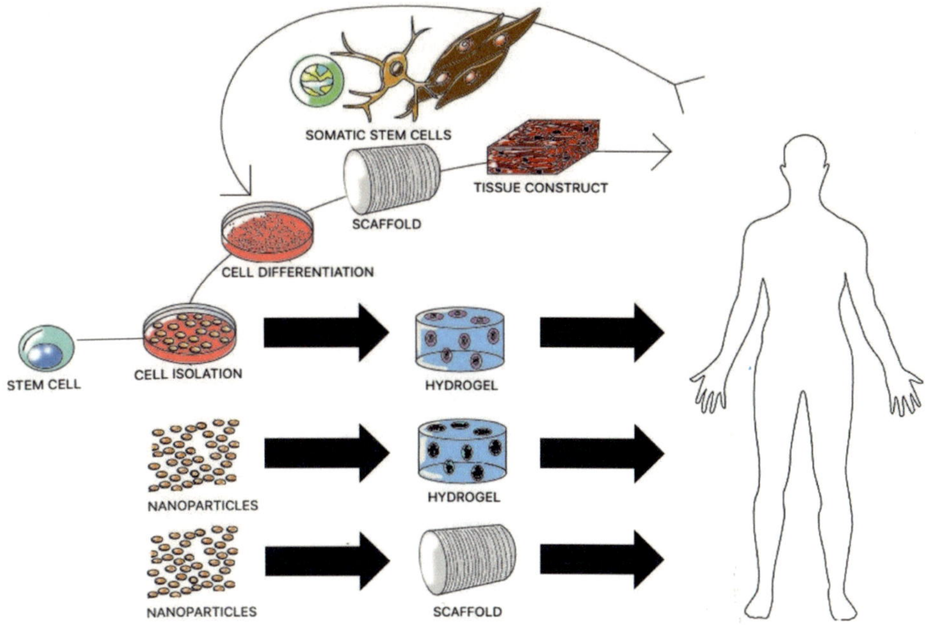

Figure 3.
Dental stem cells and their potential clinical applications in regenerative medicine.

Synthetic Polymer (poly-lactic acid, poly-glycolic acid, copolymers, poly-e-caprolacton, polyurethanes, poly-ortho ester, poly-anhydrides), are used because their high versatility, properties and reproducibility. A disadvantage of this polymers, is the less biocompatibility and not bioactive. The most used scaffold is poly-glycolic & poly-lactic acid [104].

Different techniques to fabricate scaffolds have been used to produce random structures with different pore size and reduced pore interconnections that facilitate cell support, adhesion, proliferation and differentiation. Among these techniques, we can find: solvent casting, phase inversion, freeze drying, melt-based technology, fiber bonding and high pressure-based. Lately, electrospinning has been studied for engineering applications [108].

3. Nanotechnology

The nanotechnology is the use of atoms, molecules or supra molecules structures for diverse purpose. Nanomaterials are made up of units of a size between 1 and 100 nm. Nanoparticles with sizes from 10 to 1000 nm, can provide high control of scaffolds properties, such as mechanical strength, improve biodegradability, corrosion rates, and a control of release bioactive agents [102], additionally, low solubility, short circulation life of bioactive molecules (growing factors and cytokines) [103–105].

The preparation methods, are based in the rupture of the material block (top-down), or the fabrication through the addition of components (atoms or molecules).

The objective of encapsulate the substance, is to preserve the function, and the possibility to have a controlled rate, of the substance.

Nanoparticles include nanospheres and nanocapsules, which vary in their morphology and architecture. Nanospheres are composed by a polymeric matrix, with the ability of a substance could join to its surface or disperses on it. On the other hand, nanocapsules are vesicular structures, made of synthetic or natural polymeric membrane, with the drug inside [101–103]. These substances are released by diffusion or degradation of the polymer. Nanoparticles, can be created from different types of materials (ceramic, metals, polymers).

3.1 Metallic nanoparticles

3.1.1 Gold nanoparticles

Using as a drug delivery, and in different size (20-50 nm), these metallic nanoparticles have antifungal action, in candida species, performing an interaction with cell membrane, that leads to the lysis of the cell. Golden nanoparticles offer antibacterial action over, gram-positive and gram-negative, due to the alteration in the biological process (ribosome for t-RNA binding) [109]. The increase surface to volume ratio, enhance the antibacterial and antifungal properties Additionally it changes the membrane potential and disrupt the ATP synthase, decreasing the metabolism of the microorganism.

In tissue engineering, has promising results, in new bone formation, when is used in a photocurable and biodegradable gelatin hydrogel. Also, can enhance osteogenic differentiation of stem cells, when is used coated over TiO2 surfaces and even as an injectable hydrogel scaffold. The objective of adding these nanoparticles, is to increase scaffolds structures and to guide cell behavior.

Gold nanoparticles, also can be applied for enhance MSCs properties. Used with VEGF, enhance cell migration on the scaffold of FN-Au nanoparticles.

3.1.2 Silver nanoparticles

Described as a colloid, this widely used metal, has antimicrobials properties. These particles can be formed by chemical or physical process. The physical methods used are, evaporation-condensation process, laser ablation of metallic bulk material, gamma irradiation or ultrasonic irradiation. The chemical methods consist in the use of sodium borohydrine or polyol as reducing agents. The size of the nanoparticles, could be controlled with the use of surfactants, this also depends on the obtention method and the reducing agents [105].

Silver ions, have been used for their antimicrobial effects, due to the possibility to block the respiratory system, and precipitate bacterial cellular protein. Depends on the size of the particles (1 to 10 nm), could have different potential against gram-negatives [110].

The particles also have been studied in tissue engineering. These particles have been incorporated into scaffolds, with diverse materials (gelatin, chitosan-alginate and cellulose acetate) with promising results on the antimicrobial activity with accelerated healing, in diabetic wound treatments. This result could be better with the use of a hydrogel, producing a contraction of the injury, due to the water content. In the same field, silver nanoparticles, have been employed to create chitin/nanosilver antimicrobial composite scaffold. This results in a better blood clotting, due to the effect of the silver to affect the coagulation path, by denaturing the anticoagulant proteins [111]. It is important to mention that in a porous chitosan-alginate, with biosynthesized silver particles, shown cytotoxic results in breast cancer cells [112].

3.2 Ceramic nanoparticles

Inorganics combinations, also metals, metal sulfides and oxides, used in the fabrication of materials with different porosity, shapes and forms. These nanoparticles, are classified as inert, bioactive or resorbable ceramics [103].

3.2.1 Bioactive nanoceramics

Bioglasses are materials, formed from different elements (sodium, silicone, magnesium, oxygen), that can be absorbed by the cells. These are promising materials due to the possibility to control con stimulate new tissue formation. There are different techniques to generate nanoscale bioactive glasses as: laser spinning, sol–gel (most common), micro-emulsion or gas-phase synthesis [113]. These nanoceramics, can bring a faster ion release, when compared with the bulk bioactive glasses, due to their better specific surface area, boosting the bioactivity and the protein adsorption. Bioactive glass nanoparticles, have interesting anti-bacterial and angiogenic properties. The use of boron in a cellulose construct, can bring promising results on dental tissue regeneration, that could increase cellular viability [114].

Bioactive glass nanoparticles, are also attractive for bone tissue engineering. In vivo experiments have exhibited new bone formation, in chitosan-gelatin hydrogels with 5% bioactive glass nanoparticles, after 8 weeks, compared to control groups.

3.2.2 Bioinert nanoceramics

As their positive interaction on the body tissue, bioinert nanoceramics, are used for different medical applications. Titanium dioxide, are commonly used, because of their exceptional biocompatibility (due to the oxide layer formed, on the surface). Their mechanical stability, corrosion resistance, high biocompatibility, are considered as highly recommended materials for biomedical applications. As one of the most utilized materials. These nanoparticles can be synthesized by hydrothermal, solvothermal, sol–gel and emulsion precipitation methods [115]. Nowadays, these nanostructured materials have been useful as bone scaffolds, bringing acceleration to the rate of apatite construction and increase the osteoblast adhesion, proliferation and differentiation [113]. The roughness of the dental implant, enhanced the adhesion and proliferation of osteoblast [114].

3.3 Polymeric nanoparticles

Compounds, containing predominantly carbon, hydrogen, oxygen and nitrogen in a monomeric chemical structure. With a size of 40–400 nm, and produced from synthetically polymers as poly- D,L.lactic-co-glycolic acid (PLGA) and from biopolymers (chitosan, alginate), these nanoparticles are attractive for drug delivery [115]. Using PLGA, has become interesting due to the biodegradation, biocompatibility, formulation techniques, on dental and periodontal treatments. The use of PLGA nanoparticles include effect on the oral biofilm, disrupting the plaque structure and direct impact on antibiotic resistance [116].

Classification of these nanoparticles, could be based on diverse measures such as: structure, structure and manufacturing method. Design, dimension, peripheral chemistry, porosity, mechanical strength, solubility, degradation rate, can be modified for dentistry purpose. Polymeric nanoparticles can be created, in different forms as: nanospheres, polymersomes, polymeric micelles, nanogels or even nanocapsules. For preparing these nanoparticles there are, diverse systems of emulsifications, supercritical fluid, nanoprecipitation, self-assembly [115].

Nowadays to enhanced the delivery of bioactive agents, nanoparticles changed from a simple delivery to multifunctional responsive systems, even the possibility to has a controlled release.

3.4 Iron oxide, zirconia and silver

The superparamagnetic iron oxide nanoparticles, with a controllable size and nontoxicity, are used as antimicrobial agent. With the use of an external magnetic field, these nanoparticles can be guided to the local infection [117].

Nano zirconia-alumina materials, are new implants materials, that avoid the biofilm formation. Also, they can be used as polish substance [118].

Silver nanoparticles have interesting properties as biocompatibility, low toxicity, low bacterial resistance, and antimicrobial. These particles can infiltrate and disrupts the bacteria wall and interact with de DNA. The tooth discoloration is a disadvantage to consider, thinking about esthetics treatments [108–118].

A collagen scaffold/silver nanoparticles/BMP-2 composite, presented antimicrobial activity and no adverse effects over adherence and proliferation of BMMSCs after preparation [108]. On other study, an injectable chitosan-based thermosensible hydrogel scaffold loaded with BMP-2-plasmid DNA-charged nanoparticles yielded good results on bony defects regeneration, in rat and dog models [106].

Nanostructured biomaterials have a modifiable nature, as they can be personalized by engineering their structure, shape, size, and surface properties in order to be applied in precise anatomical sites, allowing them to be used on many different contexts. Nanoparticles can be used to overcome some of the limitations of scaffold materials in bone regeneration, such as insufficient mechanical strength, issues related to cell growth and differentiation [108].

Nanotechnology has come, to revolutionize the biomedical field, with a reformed on the traditional approaches on tissue engineering and regenerative medicine. Using different types of nanoparticles (ceramics, metals, synthetic or natural polymeric), for various applications, including: bioactive agent delivery, tissue targeting and imaging, modulated scaffolds [118].

3.5 Nanotechnology and dental caries

The key to prevent dental caries is the remineralization of the enamel surface and to avoid the production of acid substance from the dental plaque. Unfortunately, saliva function, makes preventive products (toothpaste, mouthwash, fluor varnish), decrease their effectiveness due to the salivary flow rate (unstimulated: 0.3–0.4 mL/min, stimulated: 1–3 mL/min in adults) [119]. The creation of nanoparticles to enhance the fluoride concentration on dental surface, would allow increase effectiveness in the prevention of dental caries. The hydroxyapatite nanoceramic particles, have a promising future. A structure comparable to tooth and bone structure, biocompatible, and a stable form of phosphate salts, have been applied as bone substitutes. These particles, can join to dental tube and even seal them, reducing the sensibility [120, 121]. Various techniques have been established for the fabrication of hydroxyapatite nanoparticles with particular control over the nanostructure [120].

3.6 Nanotechnology and periodontal diseases

The loss of the surrounded structures of the tooth is a consequence of a disequilibrium of the oral microbiota, triggering a periodontal disease. The treatment objective consists in localized therapeutic substance. The inefficiency to reach an adequate penetration (periodontal pocket) and the inadequate period of contact of the substance, are points to consider for an alternative treatment [29–48].

Numerous nanoparticles into dental composites and adhesives, (zinc oxide, and silver), are used to impede the bacterial progression. Due to the large surface-to volume ratio, they are effective in the lysis of the bacterial membrane. Also, they are efficient obstructing the sugar metabolism, producing reactive oxygen species [122].

Tetracycline nanoparticles in calcium sulfate, are used in periodontal treatment as a matrix, in which drugs are dissolved. Because of their size, these particles could enter more deeper, in the infectivity pocket. Polymersomes are amphiphilic vesicles, that could enclose a substance. This vehicle, is used has a vehicle for antimicrobials (metronidazole), as an alternative to periodontal treatments [119].

3.7 Innovation in nano-based stem cell therapeutic systems

Stem cells with nanocarriers, has increasing as an interesting field, with favorable results. These mesenchymal stem cells could act as a reservoir for delivering nanoparticles [123, 124].

Innovative nanostructured materials could be useful in manipulating stem cells. DPSCs and Human umbilical vein endothelial cells (HUVECs) combined with an injectable, self-assembling peptide hydrogel scaffold exhibited vascularized pulp-like tissue with patches of osteodentin after transplantation [108]. The use of carbon nanomaterial's, such as carbon nanotubes, carbon nanohorns and/or graphene on bone tissue engineering, shows that these biocompatible materials can promote new bone formation and could even make possible the enhancement of their biocompatibility or induce new characteristics [118]. These examples test the capability of nanomaterials to offer versatile and relatively simple solutions to classical tissue engineering problems.

3.8 Perspective

There are promising results with the use of nanoparticles in tissue engineering, regeneration and repair; enhancing mechanical and biological characteristics, and/or even involving an anti-microbial effect. Though, there are still challenges ahead, to develop and advance in the wide medical and dental fields. Risk assessments (including data requirements and testing strategies) would be useful for better knowledge accumulation and technology advancement. While some nanomaterials might enjoy potential applications in the engineering area, additional research is needed to establish their therapeutic efficacy and safety [52].

Currently there is an emerging field, based on the dental delivery systems that could bring promising results in the therapeutic dental diseases. But there is insufficient knowledge, to let the expansion for such technologies in dental field [24–125].

New challenges will continue to emerge after more research is conducted regarding the possibilities of mixing nanotechnology with oral MSCs, but the promising results already obtained, and the extraordinary potential of both of them, mark this union as an important and interesting target for more investigation, research and innovation.

4. Conclusions

Tissue engineering is a promising and rapidly-evolving field in the clinical dental practice. Stem cells demonstrated the capability to produce dental tissues, bringing solutions to the healthcare services. Ongoing research efforts continue to establish their therapeutic efficacy and replication. Nanomaterials are essential, for the proper or "ïdeal" innovation, development and introduction (clinical translation) of novel, safe, non-invasive and effective therapies, in oro-dental tissue repair and beyond.

Funding and acknowledgments

This work was supported by generous funding and operating grants provided to the BioMAT'X R&D&I Group, part of CiiB (Centro de Investigación e Innovación Biomédica at UAndes), through the Faculty of Dentistry and Fondo de Ayuda a la Investigacion FAI - No. **INV-IN-2015-101 (2015–2019)**, Department for Research, Development and Innovation, Universidad de los Andes, Santiago de Chile. The corresponding author wishes to acknowledge supplementary funding provided under the awarded national grants from CORFO-CTecnológicos para la Innovación **#18COTE-89695** (the bioFLOSS project; 2018–2021) and CONICYT-FONDEF Chile **#ID16I10366** (the maxSALIVA project; 2016/17–2020).

Conflict of interest

The authors declare that the research was conducted in the absence of any commercial or financial relationships that could be construed as a potential conflict of interest.

Author details

Sebastián E. Pérez and Ziyad S. Haidar*
BioMAT'X R&D&I,Faculties of Dentistry and Medicine, Centro de Investigación e Innovación Biomédica (CiiB), Universidad de los Andes, Santiago de Chile, Chile

*Address all correspondence to: zhaidar@uandes.cl

References

[1] Shenghui HE, Nakada D, & Morrison SJ. Mechanisms of stem cell self-renewal. Annu Rev Cell Dev Biol. 2009; 25: 377-406.

[2] Ulloa-Montoya F, Verfaillie CM, & Hu WS. Culture systems for pluripotent stem cells. J Biosci Bioeng. 2005; 100,1: 12-27.

[3] Lewis P, Silajdžić E, Brison DR, Kimber SJ. Embryonic Stem Cells. Series in Biomedical Engineering. Springer; 2018; 1-51

[4] Pittenger MF, Mackay AM, Beck SC, Jaiswal RK, Douglas R, Mosca JD, Marshak DR. Multilineage potential of adult human mesenchymal stem cells. Science. 1999; 5411: 143-147

[5] White AC, & Lowry WE. Refining the role for adult stem cells as cancer cells of origin. Trends Cell Biol. 2015; 25: 11-20.

[6] Caplan AI. Mesenchymal stem cells. J Orthop Res. 1991; 9: 641-650.

[7] Dominici MLBK, Le Blanc K, Mueller I, Slaper-Cortenbach I, Marini, FC, Krause, DS & Horwitz EM. Minimal criteria for defining multipotent mesenchymal stromal cells. The International Society for Cellular Therapy position statement. Cytotherapy. 2006; 8: 315-317.

[8] Ullah I, Subbarao RB, & Rho GJ. Human mesenchymal stem cells-current trends and future prospective. Biosci Rep. 2015; 35: 2.

[9] Martinez-Saez D, Sasaki RT, Neves A da C, da Silva MCP. Stem Cells from Human Exfoliated Deciduous Teeth: A Growing Literature. Cells Tissues Organs. 2016; 202:269-280.

[10] Shakoori P, Zhang Q, Le A. Applications of Mesenchymal Stem Cells in Oral and Craniofacial Regeneration. Oral Maxillofacial Surg Clin N Am 2017; 29: 19-25

[11] Liu J, Yu F, Sun Y, Jiang B, Zhang W, Yang J, ... & Liu S. Concise reviews: Characteristics and potential applications of human dental tissue-derived mesenchymal stem cells. Stem cells. 2015; 33: 627-638

[12] Wang H, Zhong Q, Yang T, Qi Y, Fu M, Yang X, Zhao Y. Comparative characterization of SHED and DPSCs during extended cultivation in vitro. Mol Med Rep. 2018; 17: 6551-6559.

[13] Martens W, Sanen K, Georgiou M, Struys T, Bronckaers A, Ameloot M, Lambrichts I. Human dental pulp stem cells can differentiate into Schwann cells and promote and guide neurite outgrowth in an aligned tissue-engineered collagen construct in vitro. FASEB J. 2014; 28: 1634-1643.

[14] Pierdomenico L, Bonsi L, Calvitti M, Rondelli D, Arpinati M, Chirumbolo G, Staffolani N. Multipotent mesenchymal stem cells with immunosuppressive activity can be easily isolated from dental pulp. Transplantation. 2005; 80: 836-842.

[15] Wada N, Menicanin D, Shi S, Bartold PM, & Gronthos S. Immunomodulatory properties of human periodontal ligament stem cells. J Cell Physiol. 2009; 219: 667-676.

[16] Zhao Y, Wang L, Jin Y, Shi S. Fas ligand regulates the immunomodulatory properties of dental pulp stem cells. J Dent Res. 2012 91: 948-954.

[17] Daltoe FP, Mendonca PP, Mantesso A, Deboni, MCZ. Can SHED or DPSCs be used to repair/regenerate non-dental tissues? A systematic review of in vivo studies. Braz Oral Res. 2014; 28: 1-7.

[18] Nakashima M, Iohara K, Murakami M, Nakamura H, Sato Y,

Ariji Y, Matsushita K. Pulp regeneration by transplantation of dental pulp stem cells in pulpitis: a pilot clinical study. Stem Cell Res Ther. 2017; 8: 61.

[19] Li Y, Zhao S, Nan X, Wei H, Shi J, Li A, Gou J. Repair of human periodontal bone defects by autologous grafting stem cells derived from inflammatory dental pulp tissues. Stem Cell ResTher. 2016; 7: 141.

[20] d'Aquino R, De Rosa A, Lanza V, Tirino V, Laino L, Graziano A, Papaccio, G. Human mandible bone defect repair by the grafting of dental pulp stem/ progenitor cells and collagen sponge biocomplexes. Eur Cell Mater. 2009; 18: 75-83.

[21] Kushnerev E, Shawcross SG, Sothirachagan S, Carley F, Brahma A, Yates JM, Hillarby MC. Regeneration of corneal epithelium with dental pulp stem cells using a contact lens delivery system. Invest Ophthalmol Vis Sci. 2016; 57: 5192-5199.

[22] de Mendonça Costa A, Bueno DF, Martins MT, Kerkis I, Kerkis A, Fanganiello RD, Passos-Bueno, MR. Reconstruction of large cranial defects in nonimmunosuppressed experimental design with human dental pulp stem cells. J Craniofac Surg. 2008; 19: 204-210.

[23] Király M, Kádár K, Horváthy DB, Nardai P, Rácz GZ, Lacza Z, et al. Integration of neuronally predifferentiated human dental pulp stem cells into rat brain in vivo. Neurochem Int. 2011; 59:371-381.

[24] Botelho J, Cavacas MA, Machado V, & Mendes JJ. Dental stem cells: recent progresses in tissue engineering and regenerative medicine. Ann Med. 2017; 49: 644-651.

[25] Honda MJ, Imaizumi M, Tsuchiya S, & Morsczeck C. Dental follicle stem cells and tissue engineering. J Oral Sci. 2010; 52: 541-552.

[26] Yildirim S, Zibandeh N, Genc D, Ozcan EM, Goker K, & Akkoc T. The comparison of the immunologic properties of stem cells isolated from human exfoliated deciduous teeth, dental pulp, and dental follicles. Stem Cells Int. 2016; 2: 1-15.

[27] Mori G, Ballini A, Carbone C, Oranger A, Brunetti G, Di Benedetto A, Grano M. Osteogenic differentiation of dental follicle stem cells. Int J Med Sci. 2012; 9: 480.

[28] Madiyal A, Babu S, Bhat S, Hegde P, Shetty A. Applications of stem cells in dentistry: A review. Gulhane Med J. 2018; 1: 60.

[29] Sowmya S, Chennazhi KP, Arzate H, Jayachandran P, Nair SV, Jayakumar R. Periodontal specific differentiation of dental follicle stem cells into osteoblast, fibroblast, and cementoblast. Tissue Eng Part C Methods. 2015; 21: 1044-1058.

[30] Patil R, Kumar BM, Lee WJ, Jeon RH, Jang SJ, Lee YM, Rho GJ. Multilineage potential and proteomic profiling of human dental stem cells derived from a single donor. Exp Cell Res. 2014; 320: 92-107.

[31] Yang B, Chen G, Li J, Zou Q, Xie D, Chen Y, Guo W. Tooth root regeneration using dental follicle cell sheets in combination with a dentin matrix-based scaffold. Biomaterials. 2012; 33: 2449-2461.

[32] Kang YH, Lee HJ, Jang SJ, Byun JH, Lee JS, Lee HC, Park BW. Immunomodulatory properties and in vivo osteogenesis of human dental stem cells from fresh and cryopreserved dental follicles. Differentiation. 2015; 90: 48-58.

[33] Miura M, Gronthos S, Zhao M, Lu B, Fisher LW, Robey PG, Shi S. SHED: stem cells from human exfoliated deciduous teeth. Proc Nat Acad Sci U.S.A. 2003 100: 5807-5812.

[34] Sakai VT, Zhang Z, Dong Z, Neiva KG, Machado MAAM, Shi S, Nör J E. SHED differentiate into functional odontoblasts and endothelium. J Dent Res. 2010; 89: 791-796.

[35] Zhang N, Chen B, Wang W, Chen C, Kang J, Deng SQ, Han F. Isolation, characterization and multi-lineage differentiation of stem cells from human exfoliated deciduous teeth. Mol Med Rep. 2016; 14: 95-102.

[36] Nakajima K, Kunimatsu R, Ando K, Ando T, Hayashi Y, Kihara T, Nikawa H. Comparison of the bone regeneration ability between stem cells from human exfoliated deciduous teeth, human dental pulp stem cells and human bone marrow mesenchymal stem cells. Biochem Biophys Res Commun. 2018; 497: 876-882.

[37] Taraslia V, Lymperi S, Pantazopoulou V, Anagnostopoulos AK, Papassideri IS, Basdra EK, Anastasiadou E. A High-Resolution Proteomic Landscaping of Primary Human Dental Stem Cells: Identification of SHED-and PDLSC-Specific Biomarkers. Int J Mol Sci. 2018; 19: 158.

[38] Chen K, Xiong H, Xu N, Shen Y, Huang Y, Liu C. Chondrogenic potential of stem cells from human exfoliated deciduous teeth in vitro and in vivo. Acta Odontol Scand . 2014; 72: 664-672.

[39] Su WT, Chen XW. Stem cells from human exfoliated deciduous teeth differentiate into functional hepatocyte-like cells by herbal medicine. Biomed Mater Eng. 2014; 24: 2243-2247

[40] Lee HS, Jeon MJ, Kim SO, Kim SH, Lee JH, Ahn SJ, Song JS. Characteristics of stem cells from human exfoliated deciduous teeth (SHED) from intact cryopreserved deciduous teeth. Cryobiology. 2015; 71: 374-383.

[41] Seo BM, Sonoyama W, Yamaza T, Coppe C, Kikuiri T, Akiyama K, Shi S. SHED repair critical-size calvarial defects in mice. Oral Dis. 2008 14: 428-434.

[42] Zheng Y, Liu Y, Zhang CM, Zhang HY, Li WH, Shi S, Wang SL. Stem cells from deciduous tooth repair mandibular defect in swine. J Dent Res. 2009; 88: 249-254.

[43] Khoroushi M, Foroughi MR, Karbasi S, Hashemibeni B, Khademi AA. Effect of Polyhydroxybutyrate/Chitosan/Bioglass nanofiber scaffold on proliferation and differentiation of stem cells from human exfoliated deciduous teeth into odontoblast-like cells. Mater Sci Eng C. 2018; 89: 128-139.

[44] Jin Yan. Revitalization of Immature Permanent Teeth with Necrotic Pulps Using SHED Cells [Internet]. 2018. Available at: https://clinicaltrials.gov/ct2/show/NCT01814436

[45] Açil Y, Yang F, Gulses A, Ayna M, Wiltfang J, Gierloff M. Isolation, characterization and investigation of differentiation potential of human periodontal ligament cells and dental follicle progenitor cells and their response to BMP-7 in vitro. Odontology. 2016; 104: 123-135.

[46] Prateeptongkum E, Klingelhöffer C, Müller S, Ettl T, Morsczeck C. Characterization of progenitor cells and stem cells from the periodontal ligament tissue derived from a single person. J Periodontal Res. 2016; 51: 265-272.

[47] Seo BM, Miura M, Gronthos S, Bartold PM, Batouli S, Brahim J, Shi S. Investigation of multipotent postnatal stem cells from human periodontal ligament. Lancet. 2004; 364: 149-155.

[48] Ng TK, Yung JS, Choy KW, Cao D, Leung CK, Cheung HS, Pang CP. Transdifferentiation of periodontal ligament-derived stem cells into retinal ganglion-like cells and its microRNA signature. Sci Rep. 2015; 5: 16429.

[49] Collado-González M, García-Bernal D, Oñate-Sánchez RE, Ortolani-SeltenerichPS,LozanoA,FornerL, Rodríguez-Lozano FJ. Biocompatibility of three new calcium silicate-based endodontic sealers on human periodontal ligament stem cells. Int Endod J. 2017 50: 875-884.

[50] Diomede F, D'Aurora M, Gugliandolo A, Merciaro I, Orsini T, Gatta V, Mazzon E. Biofunctionalized Scaffold in Bone Tissue Repair. Int J Mol Sci. 2018; 19: 1022.

[51] Feng F, Akiyama K, Liu Y, Yamaza T, Wang TM, Chen JH, Shi S. Utility of PDL progenitors for in vivo tissue regeneration: a report of 3 cases. Oral Dis. 2010; 16: 20-28.

[52] Sonoyama W, Liu Y, Fang D, Yamaza T, Seo BM, Zhang C, Wang S. Mesenchymal stem cell-mediated functional tooth regeneration in swine. PloS one. 2006; 1: 79.

[53] Sonoyama W, Liu Y, Yamaza T, Tuan RS, Wang S, Shi S, Huang GTJ. Characterization of the apical papilla and its residing stem cells from human immature permanent teeth: a pilot study. J Endod. 2008; 34: 166-171.

[54] Yagyuu T, Ikeda E, Ohgushi H, Tadokoro M, Hirose M, Maeda M, Kirita T. Hard tissue-forming potential of stem/progenitor cells in human dental follicle and dental papilla. Arch Oral Biol. 2010; 55: 68-76.

[55] Bellamy C, Shrestha S, Torneck C, & Kishen A. Effects of a Bioactive Scaffold Containing a Sustained Transforming Growth Factor-β1–releasing Nanoparticle System on the Migration and Differentiation of Stem Cells from the Apical Papilla. J Endod. 2016; 42: 1385-1392.

[56] Ikeda E, Yagi K, Kojima M, Yagyuu T, Ohshima A, Sobajima S, Kawase M. Multipotent cells from the human third molar: feasibility of cell-based therapy for liver disease. Differentiation. 2008; 76: 495-505.

[57] Doğan A, Yalvaç ME, Şahin F, Kabanov AV, Palotás A, Rizvanov AA. Differentiation of human stem cells is promoted by amphiphilic pluronic block copolymers. Int J Nanomed. 2012; 7: 4849.

[58] Calikoglu Koyuncu AC, Gurel Pekozer G, Ramazanoglu M, Torun Kose G, Hasirci V. Cartilage tissue engineering on macroporous scaffolds using human tooth germ stem cells. J Tissue Eng Regen Med. 2017;11: 765-777.

[59] Fournier BP, Ferre FC, Couty, L, Lataillade JJ, Gourven M, Naveau A, Gogly B. Multipotent progenitor cells in gingival connective tissue. Tissue Eng Part A. 2010; 16: 2891-2899.

[60] Zhang Q, Shi S, Liu Y, Uyanne J, Shi Y, Shi S, Le AD. Mesenchymal stem cells derived from human gingiva are capable of immunomodulatory functions and ameliorate inflammation-related tissue destruction in experimental colitis. J Immunol. 2009; 183: 7787-7798.

[61] Zhang Q, Nguyen AL, Shi S, Hill C, Wilder-Smith P, Krasieva TB, Le AD. Three-dimensional spheroid culture of human gingiva-derived mesenchymal stem cells enhances mitigation of chemotherapy-induced oral mucositis. Stem Cells Dev. 2011 21: 937-947

[62] El-Sayed KMF, Paris S, Graetz C, Kassem N, Mekhemar M, Ungefroren H, Dörfer C. Isolation and characterisation of human gingival margin-derived STRO-1/MACS+ and MACS− cell populations. Int J Oral Sci. 2015; 7: 80.

[63] Santamaría S, Sanchez N, Sanz M, Garcia-Sanz JA. Comparison of periodontal ligament and gingiva-derived mesenchymal stem cells for regenerative therapies. Clin Oral Investig. 2017; 21: 1095-1102.

[64] Tang L, Li N, Xie H, & Jin, Y. Characterization of mesenchymal stem cells from human normal and hyperplastic gingiva. J Cell Physiol. 2011; 226: 832-842.

[65] Zhang QZ, Su WR, Shi SH, Wilder-Smith P, Xiang AP, Wong A, Le AD. Human gingiva-derived mesenchymal stem cells elicit polarization of m2 macrophages and enhance cutaneous wound healing. Stem Cells. 2010; 28: 1856-1868.

[66] Su WR, Zhang QZ, Shi SH, Nguyen AL, Le AD. Human gingiva-derived mesenchymal stromal cells attenuate contact hypersensitivity via prostaglandin E2-dependent mechanisms. Stem Cells. 2011: 29: 1849-1860.

[67] Wang F, Yu M, Yan X, Wen Y, Zeng Q, Yue W, Pei X. Gingiva-derived mesenchymal stem cell-mediated therapeutic approach for bone tissue regeneration. Stem Cells Dev. 2011; 20: 2093-2102.

[68] Diomede F, Gugliandolo A, Scionti D, Merciaro I, Cavalcanti MF, Mazzon E, Trubiani O. Biotherapeutic effect of gingival stem cells conditioned medium in bone tissue restoration. Int J Mol Sci. 2018; 19: 329.

[69] Mason S, Tarle SA, Osibin W, Kinfu Y, Kaigler D. Standardization and safety of Alveolar bone–derived stem cell Isolation. J Dent Res. 2014; 93: 55-61.

[70] Zang S, Jin L, Kang S, Hu X, Wang M, Wang J, Wang Q. Periodontal Wound Healing by Transplantation of Jaw Bone Marrow-Derived Mesenchymal Stem Cells in Chitosan/ Anorganic Bovine Bone Carrier into One-Wall Infrabony Defects in Beagles. J Periodontol. 2016; 87: 971-981.

[71] Matsubara T, Suardita K, Ishii M, Sugiyama M, Igarashi A, Oda R, Miyazaki K. Alveolar bone marrow as a cell source for regenerative medicine: differences between alveolar and iliac bone marrow stromal cells. J Bone Miner Res. 2005; 20: 399-409.

[72] Park, JC, Kim JC, Kim YT, Choi SH, Cho KS, Im GI, Kim CS. Acquisition of human alveolar bone-derived stromal cells using minimally irrigated implant osteotomy: in vitro and in vivo evaluations. J Clin Periodontol. 2012; 39: 495-505.

[73] Pekovits K, Kröpfl JM, Stelzer I, Payer M, Hutter H, Dohr G. Human mesenchymal progenitor cells derived from alveolar bone and human bone marrow stromal cells: a comparative study. Histochem Cell Biol. 2013; 140: 611-621.

[74] El-Sayed KMF, Boeckler J, Dörfer CE. TLR expression profile of human alveolar bone proper-derived stem/progenitor cells and osteoblasts. J Craniomaxillofac Surg. 2017; 45: 2054-2060

[75] Park, JC, Oh SY, Lee JS, Park SY, Choi, EY, Cho KS, Kim CS. In vivo bone formation by human alveolar-bone-derived mesenchymal stem cells obtained during implant osteotomy using biphasic calcium phosphate ceramics or B io-O ss as carriers. J Biomed Mater Res B Appl Biomater. 2016; 104: 515-524.

[76] Andreadis D, Bakopoulou A, Leyhausen G, Epivatianos A, Volk J, Markopoulos A, Geurtsen W. Minor salivary glands of the lips: a novel, easily accessible source of potential stem/ progenitor cells. Clin Oral Investig. 2014; 18: 847-856.

[77] Emmerson E, Knox SM. Salivary gland stem cells: A review of development, regeneration and cancer. Genesis. 2018; 56: e23211.

[78] Pringle S, Maimets M, van der Zwaag M, Stokman MA, van Gosliga D, Zwart E, Coppes RP. Human salivary gland stem cells functionally restore

radiation damaged salivary glands. Stem Cells. 2016; 34: 640-652.

[79] Wang SQ, Wang YX, Hua H. Characteristics of Labial Gland Mesenchymal Stem Cells of Healthy Individuals and Patients with Sjögren's Syndrome: A Preliminary Study. Stem Cells Dev. 2017; 26: 1171-1185.

[80] Jeong J, Baek H, Kim YJ, Choi Y, Lee H, Lee E, Kwon H. Human salivary gland stem cells ameliorate hyposalivation of radiation-damaged rat salivary glands. Exp Mol Med. 2013; 45: e58.

[81] Wang YL, Hong A, Yen TH, Hong HH. Isolation of Mesenchymal Stem Cells from Human Alveolar Periosteum and Effects of Vitamin D on Osteogenic Activity of Periosteum-derived Cells. J Vis Exp. 2018; 135: e57166.

[82] Choi YS, Noh SE, Lim SM, Lee CW, Kim CS, Im MW, Kim DI. Multipotency and growth characteristic of periosteum-derived progenitor cells for chondrogenic, osteogenic, and adipogenic differentiation. Biotechnol Lett. 2008; 30: 593-601.

[83] Ceccarelli G, Graziano A, Benedetti L, Imbriani M, Romano F, Ferrarotti F, Cusella De Angelis GM. Osteogenic Potential of Human Oral-Periosteal Cells (PCs) Isolated from Different Oral Origin: An In vitro Study. J Cell Physiol. 2016; 231: 607-612.

[84] Cha HM, Kim SM, Choi YS, Kim DI. Scaffold-free three-dimensional culture systems for mass production of periosteum-derived progenitor cells. J Biosci Bioeng. 2015; 120: 218-222.

[85] Dao LT, Park EY, Lim SM, Choi YS, Jung HS, Jun HS. Transplantation of insulin-producing cells differentiated from human periosteum-derived progenitor cells ameliorate hyperglycemia in diabetic mice. Transplantation. 2014; 98: 1040-1047.

[86] Ribeiro FV, Suaid FF, Ruiz KG, Salmon CR, Paparotto T, Nociti Jr FH, Casati, MZ. Periosteum-derived cells as an alternative to bone marrow cells for bone tissue engineering around dental implants. A histomorphometric study in beagle dogs. J Periodontol. 2010; 81: 907-916.

[87] Hsueh YJ, Huang SF, Lai JY, Ma SC, Chen HC, Wu SE, Lai CH. Preservation of epithelial progenitor cells from collagenase-digested oral mucosa during ex vivo cultivation. Sci Rep. 2016; 6: 36266.

[88] Takagi R, Yamato M, Kanai N, Murakami D, Kondo M, Ishii T, Okano T. Cell sheet technology for regeneration of esophageal mucosa. World J Gastroenterol. 2012; 18: 5145

[89] Amemiya T, Nakamura T, Yamamoto T, Kinoshita S, Kanamura N. Autologous transplantation of oral mucosal epithelial cell sheets cultured on an amniotic membrane substrate for intraoral mucosal defects. PloS one. 2015; 10: e0125391.

[90] Papagerakis S, Pannone G, Zheng L, About I, Taqi N, Nguyen NP, Prince ME. Oral epithelial stem cells—implications in normal development and cancer metastasis. Exp Cell Res. 2014; 325: 111-129.

[91] Nakamura T, Endo KI, Kinoshita S. Identification of human oral keratinocyte stem/progenitor cells by neurotrophin receptor p75 and the role of neurotrophin/p75 signaling. Stem Cells. 2007; 25: 628-638.

[92] Locke M, Davies LC, Stephens P. Oral mucosal progenitor cell clones resist in vitro myogenic differentiation. Arch Oral Biol. 2016; 70: 100-110.

[93] Zhang QZ, Nguyen AL, Yu WH, Le AD. Human oral mucosa and gingiva: a unique reservoir for mesenchymal stem cells. J Dent Res. 2012; 91: 1011-1018

[94] Nakamura T, Yokoo S, Bentley AJ, Nagata M, Fullwood NJ, Inatomi T, Kinoshita S. Development of functional human oral mucosal epithelial stem/progenitor cell sheets using a feeder-free and serum-free culture system for ocular surface reconstruction. Sci Rep. 2016; 6: 37173.

[95] Sheth R, Neale MH, Shortt AJ, Massie I, Vernon AJ, Daniels JT. Culture and characterization of oral mucosal epithelial cells on a fibrin gel for ocular surface reconstruction. Curr Eye Res. 2005; 40: 1077-1087.

[96] Kolli S, Ahmad S, Mudhar HS, Meeny A, Lako M, Figueiredo FC. Successful application of ex vivo expanded human autologous oral mucosal epithelium for the treatment of total bilateral limbal stem cell deficiency. Stem Cells. 2014; 32: 2135-2146.

[97] Liao J, Al Shahrani M, Al-Habib M, Tanaka T, Huang GTJ. Cells isolated from inflamed periapical tissue express mesenchymal stem cell markers and are highly osteogenic. J Endod. 2011; 37: 1217-1224.

[98] Chrepa V, Pitcher B, Henry MA, Diogenes A. Survival of the apical papilla and its resident stem cells in a case of advanced pulpal necrosis and apical periodontitis. J Endod. 2017; 43: 561-567.

[99] Hume WJ. Kinetics of cell replacement in the stratum granulosum of mouse tongue epithelium. Cell Tissue Kin. 1986; 19: 195-203.

[100] Hisha H, Tanaka T, Ueno H. Lingual Epithelial Stem Cells and Organoid Culture of Them. Int J Mol Sci. 2016; 17: 168.

[101] Na S, Zhang H, Huang F, Wang W, Ding Y, Li D, Jin Y. Regeneration of dental pulp/dentine complex with a three-dimensional and scaffold-free stem-cell sheet-derived pellet. J Tissue Eng Regen Med. 2013; 10: 261-270.

[102] Li G, Zhou T, Lin S, Shi S, Lin Y. Nanomaterials for craniofacial and dental tissue engineering. J Dent Res. 2017; 96: 725-732.

[103] Mitsiadis TA Orsini G. Regenerative Dentistry Using Stem Cells and Nanotechnology. Nanoscience and Nanotechnology for Human Health. Wiley. 2017; 263-292.

[104] Moro JS, Barcelos RCS, Terra TG, Danesi CC. l. Tissue engineering perspectives in dentistry: review of the literature. RGO, Rev Gaúch Odontol. 2018;66: 361-367

[105] Sun CY, Che YJ, Lu SJ. Preparation and application of collagen scaffold-encapsulated silver nanoparticles and bone morphogenetic protein 2 for enhancing the repair of infected bone. Biotechnol Lett. 2015; 37: 467-473.

[106] El-Sherbiny IM, Yacoub MH. Hydrogel scaffolds for tissue engineering: Progress and challenges, Global Cardiology Science and Practice 2013; 3: 316-342.

[107] Carletti E, Motta A, Migliaresi C. Scaffolds for tissue engineering and 3D cell culture. Methods Mol Biol. 2011; 695: 17-39. doi: 10.1007/978-1-60761-984-0_2. PMID: 21042963.

[108] Dissanayaka WL, Hargreaves KM, Jin L, Samaranayake LP, Zhang C. The interplay of dental pulp stem cells and endothelial cells in an injectable peptide hydrogel on angiogenesis and pulp regeneration in vivo. Tissue Eng Part A. 2014; 21: 550-563.

[109] Ibrahim Khan, Khalid Saeed, Idrees Khan,Nanoparticles: Properties, applications and toxicities,Arabian Journal of Chemistry, Volume 12. 2019: 908-931.

[110] Morones, J. R., Elechiguerra, J. L., Camacho, A., Holt, K., Kouri, J. B., Ramírez, J. T. The bactericidal effect of

silver nanoparticles. Nanotechnology. 2005; 16: 2346-2653.

[111] Madhumathi, K., Kumar, P. S., Abhilash, S., Sreeja, V., Tamura, H., Manzoor, K., et al. Development of novel chitin/nanosilver composite scaffolds for wound dressing applications. J. Mater. Sci. Mater. Med. 2010; 21: 807-813.

[112] Venkatesan, J., Lee, J.-Y., Kang, D. S., Anil, S., Kim, S.-K., Shim, M. S. Antimicrobial and anticancer activities of porous chitosanalginate biosynthesized silver nanoparticles. Int. J. Biol.Macromol. 2017; 98: 515-525.

[113] James Zhijian Shen, Jenny Fäldt. Requirements of Bioactive Ceramics for Dental Implants and Scaffolds, Advanced Ceramics for Dentistry. Butterworth-Heinemann,2014: 279-300,

[114] Zheng, K., Wu, J., Li, W., Dippold, D., Wan, Y., and Boccaccini, A. R. Incorporation of Cu-containing bioactive glass nanoparticles in gelatin-coated scaffolds enhances bioactivity and osteogenic activity. ACS Biomater. Sci. *2018;* 4: 1546-1557.

[115] J R JONES, Bioactive ceramics and glasses,In Woodhead Publishing Series in Biomaterials, Tissue Engineering Using Ceramics and Polymers, Woodhead Publishing. 2007; 52-71,

[116] Qian, J., Xu, W., Yong, X., Jin, X., and Zhang, W. Fabrication and *in vitro* biocompatibility of biomorphic PLGA/nHA composite scaffolds for bone tissue engineering. Mater. Sci. Eng.*2014;* 36: 95-101.

[117] Subhashree Priyadarsini, Sumit Mukherjee, Monalisa Mishra, Nanoparticles used in dentistry: A review, Journal of Oral Biology and Craniofacial Research,.2018: 8: 58-67.

[118] Danielle S. W. Benoit, Kenneth R. Sims, and David Fraser. Nanoparticles for Oral Biofilm Treatments. ACS Nano. 2019: 13: 4869-4875.

[119] Olusegun A, Makun HA, Ogara IM, et al. Dietary Factors, Salivary Parameters, and Dental Caries. Intech. 2012; 1:38.

[120] Evans, A., Leishman, S.J., Walsh, L.J. Inhibitory effects of children's toothpastes on *Streptococcus mutans*, *Streptococcus sanguinis* and *Lactobacillus acidophilus*. Eur Arch Paediatr Dent. *2015;* 16: 219-226.

[121] C. de Melo Alencar, *et al.* Clinical efficacy of nano-hydroxyapatite in dentin hypersensitivity: a systematic review and meta-analysis.J. Dent. 2019; 82: 11-21.

[122] Mercado N, Bhatt P, Sutariya V, Florez FLE, Pathak Y V. Application of Nanoparticles in Treating Periodontitis: Preclinical and Clinical Overview. In: Pathak Y V, ed. *Surface Modification of Nanoparticles for Targeted Drug Delivery*. Springer International Publishing; 2019:467-480.

[123] Accomasso L, Gallina C, Turinetto V, Giachino C. Stem Cell Tracking with Nanoparticles for Regenerative Medicine Purposes: An Overview. Jendelova P, ed. *Stem Cells Int*. 2016; 7920358

[124] Maman P, Nagpal M, Gilhotra RM, Aggarwal G. Nano Era of Dentistry-An Update. Curr Drug Deliv. 2018; 15:186-204

[125] Maryam Koopaie,Nanoparticulate systems for dental drug delivery, In Woodhead Publishing Series in Biomaterials,Nanoengineered Biomaterials for Advanced Drug Delivery, Elsevier.2020; 525-559.

Chapter 5

Non-integrating Methods to Produce Induced Pluripotent Stem Cells for Regenerative Medicine: An Overview

Immacolata Belviso, Veronica Romano, Daria Nurzynska, Clotilde Castaldo and Franca Di Meglio

Abstract

Induced Pluripotent Stem cells (iPSC) are adult somatic cells genetically reprogrammed to an embryonic stem cell-like state. Due to their autologous origin from adult somatic cells, iPSCs are considered a tremendously valuable tool for regenerative medicine, disease modeling, drug discovery and testing. iPSCs were first obtained by introducing specific transcription factors through retroviral transfection. However, cell reprogramming obtained by integrating methods prevent clinical application of iPSC because of potential risk for infection, teratomas and genomic instability. Therefore, several integration-free alternate methods have been developed and tested thus far to overcome safety issues. The present chapter provides an overview and a critical analysis of advantages and disadvantages of non-integrating methods used to generate iPSCs.

Keywords: induced pluripotent stem cells (iPSCs), cell reprogramming, dermal fibroblasts, integration-free methods, regenerative medicine

1. Introduction

The entrance of induced Pluripotent Stem Cells (iPSCs) in the stem cell scene represents a novel approach for studying human diseases and a promising tool for regenerative medicine [1].

The compelling need to overcome ethical and technical issues related to the production and utilization of Embryonic Stem Cells (ESCs) has prompted to search for a method to induce the pluripotency in terminally differentiated cells pushing them to an embryonic-like state.

Several studies, therefore, have been focused on characterizing and isolating unique transcriptional factors expressed by ESCs, presuming that their expression was sufficient to confer to adult cells the peculiar features of pluripotent cells [2]. The hypothesis that genome is not irreversibly modified during the differentiation and that some factors residing in ESCs can confer pluripotency to terminally differentiated nuclei has given a boost to bypass both the practical and ethical concerns related to the use of ESCs and has paved the way for the development of cutting-edge approaches for tissue regeneration, like cellular reprogramming by artificially inducing the pluripotency [3].

Cell reprogramming consists in converting adult somatic cells in undifferentiated cells defined by an acquired pluripotency, typically showed by ESCs. Many techniques have been developed to achieve the goal since in 2006 Yamanaka and colleagues succeeded in the undertaking challenge of identifying four specific transcription factors (Oct4, SOX2, c-Myc, and KLF4) capable of reprogramming murine or human fibroblasts to embryonic-like cells, and termed them "induced pluripotent stem cells" [4]. The four factors recognized by Yamanaka are involved in multiple mechanisms and are pivotal for the pluripotency of embryonic stem cells, for embryonic development and to determine cell fate [5].

The great potential residing in iPSCs was soon noticeable, primarily for the possibility to obtain stem cell lineages customized for each patient, able to give rise to the needed cell type, then, for the chance to overcome organ shortage difficulties and to avoid invasive medical procedures to treat degenerative diseases [6].

Additionally, iPSCs share several features with ESCs showing similarities for morphology and culturing conditions: they both grow arranging in dome-shaped colonies (**Figure 1**) and need to be cultured in presence of a layer of feeder cells and/or specific cytokines [7]. Furthermore, iPSCs express equal stemness markers showed by ESCs, a common proliferation potential, the capability to self-renew and differentiate into the three fundamental germ layers [8].

It is considerably relevant that iPSCs can also provide effective disease models to investigate cellular and molecular mechanisms involved in the development of pathologies and a platform for toxicological and pharmacological screening [9].

Until the sprawl of cell reprogramming, ESCs were considered the most promising and innovative tool for the research and clinical application in the field of regenerative medicine. Due to their ability to grow indefinitely and to differentiate into cells of the three germ layers while maintaining the pluripotency, ESCs rapidly gained the attention of the scientific community [10]. Despite the tremendous potential they hold for tissue and organ regeneration, at now, the clinical application of ESCs is limited and still faces many obstacles. The use of ESCs, in fact, raises several controversies and the studies focused on the understanding of their biology are strictly regulated or even forbidden in many countries. The reason of such restraint primarily resides in their origin and isolation techniques, as ESCs derive from the inner cell mass of mammalian blastula, the early stage of embryonic development, and common methods for their isolation require the destruction of the embryo, triggering ethical concerns [11].

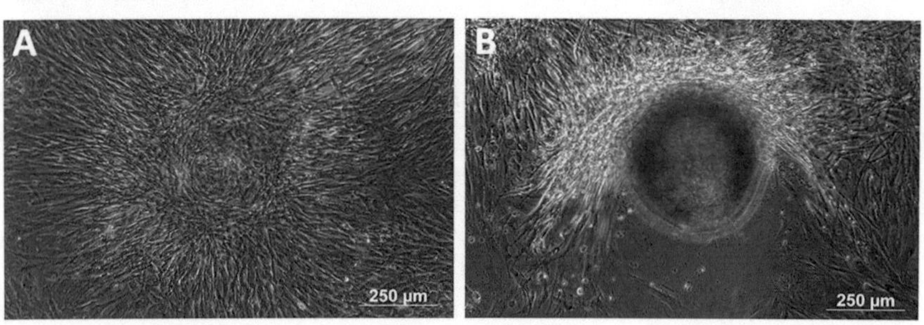

Figure 1.
Skin fibroblast reprogrammed by mRNAs codifying for Oct4, SOX2, c-Myc, KLF4, Nanog, LIN28. Representative images of iPSCs arranging after 24 hours to form a colony (A) that appeared clearly visible ten days later (B). Scale bar is 250 µm.

Beside the ethical issue, several other hurdles limit the concrete employment of ESCs, such as the risk of rejection related to their immunogenicity, the challenging conditions to culture and expand ESC lines and then to maintain the undifferentiated state ensuring their stability [12–14]. Additionally, there is a risk for tumor formation if ESCs are not fully addressed into a specific differentiated cell type prior to implantation [15]. Finally, about the therapeutic application of ESCs in human studies, another major concern is the use of non-human and xenogenic materials such as fetal bovine serum for cell culture [16].

However, the pluripotency makes ESCs unique, and this astonishing differentiation capability renders them very attractive to research studies, to the extent that a big effort has been put recently into the search for methods to artificially reproduce their pluripotency (**Figure 2**).

Nonetheless, the efficiency of cell reprogramming remains low, hence, the reprogramming techniques are under intense investigation so as to generate induced pluripotent stem cells ameliorating the efficiency of the process, the quality and safety of the derived cells [17]. The improvement generally targets several aspects of the reprogramming methods: primarily the source of somatic cells, as many studies suggest that some cells are more prone than others to be reprogrammed into certain cell types; [18] reprogramming factor cocktail; [19] the conditions to culture and maintain the iPSCs and, above all, the technique to introduce the reprogramming factors [20].

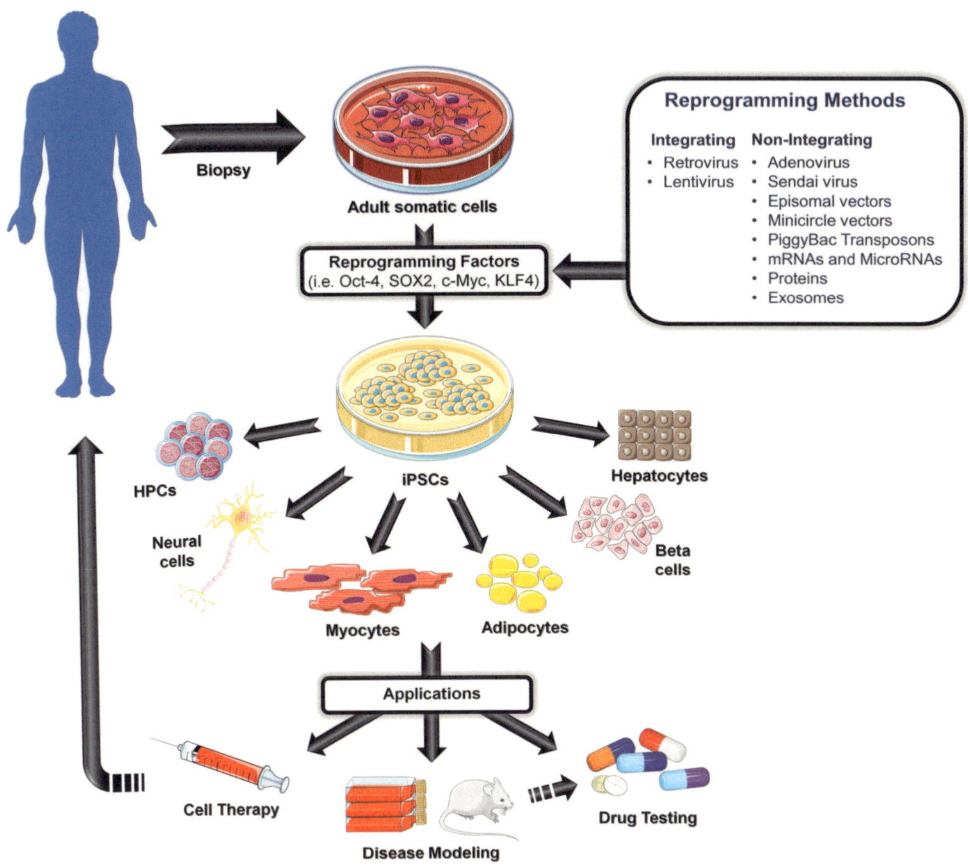

Figure 2.
Human iPSC technology allows, through the introduction of reprogramming factors into adult somatic cells, to obtain pluripotent cells capable of differentiating towards several mature cells which can be used for providing cells for regenerative medicine, for in vitro or in vivo disease modeling, and for screening and developing new drugs. (The figure was prepared with the support of Servier Smart Medical Art, https://smart.servier.com/).

A major issue related to the production of iPSCs, in fact, is the use of retroviruses to obtain a permanent integration of the reprogramming factors in the host cell genome, leading to teratoma formation due to the residual expression of oncogenes like c-Myc and KLF4 [21].

Different methods are known, at the present, to induce the expression of the reprogramming factors, classified in two major categories: non-viral and viral vector-based methods [22]. Viral-based methods include integrating viruses like Retrovirus and Lentivirus and non-integrating viruses, such as Adenovirus, Sendai virus [23].

According to several studies, all these methods provide good results in terms of effectiveness of cell reprogramming, hence, the choice of the suitable method strictly depends on the cell type used and on the subsequent applications of the iPSCs obtained [24].

Since from the first studies on reprogramming programs the most common method to generate iPSCs included the employment of retroviruses or lentiviruses to deliver Yamanaka factors [25–27]. Retroviruses integrate into host's genome allowing a satisfying expression of reprogramming factors. The first retrovirus used to deliver specific transcription factors into mouse and human fibroblasts was the Moloney Murine Leukemia Virus (MMLV), capable to infect only actively dividing cells and silent in immature cells such as ESCs [22, 28].

Conversely, the most common lentivirus used as a delivery vector derives from HIV. Usually lentiviruses have higher cloning capacities and infection efficiency than retroviruses. Unlike MMLV based retroviruses, lentiviruses could replicate both in dividing and non-dividing cells. Lentiviruses, with the respect to retroviruses have two safety advantages, the lack of integration near the transcription site of start and the capacity to deliver simultaneously different reprogramming factors in a single construct [29].

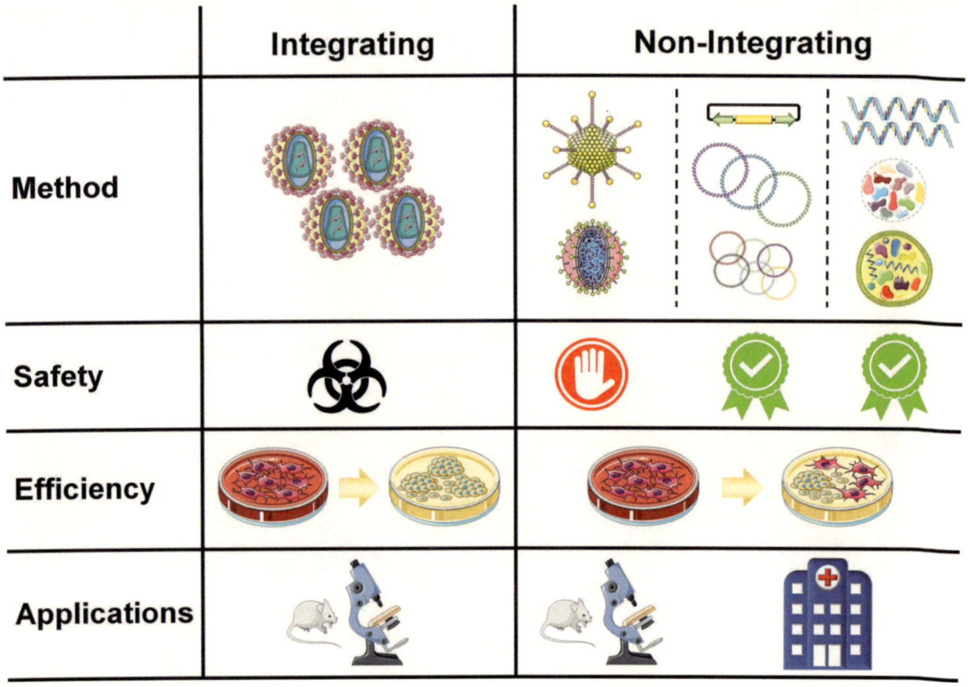

Figure 3.
The scheme summarizes the major advantages and disadvantages of integrating vs non-integrating methods currently employed for adult somatic cells reprogramming. (The figure was prepared with the support of Servier Smart Medical Art, https://smart.servier.com/).

However both vectors made of retrovirus and lentivirus carry significant risk of insertion mutagenesis during transfection related to their genomic integration; [26] therefore, even if they are properly silenced, viral transgenes can eventually be reactivated during differentiation or during the maturation of iPSCs, with high risk for tumorigenicity [6].

Therefore, while they represent a valuable research tools, they cannot be safely employed in the clinical application (**Figure 3**).

2. Introducing non-integrating methods

The efficiency and safety of generating and using iPSCs show a negative balance, and thus clinical employment of iPSC technology is still waiting for an effective protocol better poising these two fundamental features [30].

Even though the integration of reprogramming factors in iPSCs generated using viral methods offers high efficiency and a good yield, it is risky and represents a strong limitation for further clinical applications. Indeed, the residual expression of Yamanaka factors in the derived cells, such as the oncogene c-Myc, causes several genetic and epigenetic mutations, along with transcriptional abnormalities, despite the silencing of these genes during reprogramming. The integration of the reprogramming factors, in fact, is responsible for disruption of coding regions, promoters, and enhancers/repressors causing the instability of the gene network of the iPSCs obtained. Genetic aberrations are strongly related to cancer onset, hence, the maintenance of genomic stability of iPSCs without dragging integrating viral vectors sequences is highly desirable (**Figure 3**). To overcome all these relevant safety issues newer protocols are currently under development for deriving iPSCs without any integration while addressing the low efficiency showed by earlier reprogramming methods [31].

3. Non-integrating viral-based methods: advantages and disadvantages

In order to fulfill the above-mentioned requirements several integration-free methods have been developed, many of them employing viruses. It is important to underline that, even if all these methods are classified as "non-integrating", avoiding even a partial and negligible integration of viral genome into the host cells is not possible (**Figures 2** and **3**).

3.1 Adenovirus

Adenovirus is DNA virus that can reprogram cellular metabolism in a variety of ways, like increasing glucose uptake in cells and stimulating the synthesis of lactate, and produce many other metabolic changes related to cancer. Several studies have shown the effectiveness of the adenovirus as a vector to deliver specific differentiation factors to generate iPSCs without integration into host's genome.

The use of Adenovirus as a delivering method for reprogramming factors shows a certain effectiveness, allowing, at the same time, the production of quite safe and integration-free iPSCs. As a matter of fact, Stadtfeld and colleagues have demonstrated that human iPSCs generated from adenovirus are pluripotent and can be differentiated into all three germ layers in vitro and in vivo [32]. Zhou and Freed produced iPSCs from human embryonic fibroblasts using adenoviral vectors expressing c-Myc, KLF4, Oct4, and SOX2, and the iPSCs obtained expressed ESCs specific markers, showed a great differentiation potential and were free of any viral or transgene integration [33]. However, despite the employment of the adenovirus method eliminate the risk for malignant transformation associated with retrovirus or lentivirus, it shows disadvantages, such as the lower efficiency and the shorter expression kinetics requiring repeated transductions to maintain an adequate level of transgene expression [33].

Additionally, not all the cell types are capable to generate iPSCs with this method alone as shown by Okita and colleagues in their studies they were unable to obtain murine hepatocyte iPSCs clones introducing the four reprogramming factors in the adenoviral vector alone, but the entire process required additional transfections of Oct3/4 and KLF4 or Oct3/4 and SOX2 by retrovirus [34].

3.2 Sendai virus

Sendai virus is an RNA virus that can infect a wide range of cell types either proliferating or quiescent and does not enter the nucleus of host cells. RNA virus-derived vectors are considered an attractive tool to vehicle Yamanaka factors, as they show a low risk of genomic insertion and are commonly used to reprogram neonatal and adult fibroblasts, and blood cells. The virus, while replicating, remains in the cytoplasm after infection and can be washed out of the host cells by several passages. Sendai virus shows a high transduction efficiency as confirmed by the expression of transgenes delivered yet detectable within a few hours after transduction, with a maximum expression after 24 hours after transduction. Sendai virus vectors have been largely studied and have emerged for their capability of successfully produce iPSCs with a non- detectable presence of viral RNA reprogramming adult human fibroblasts and circulating T cells [35].

As Sendai virus is an RNA virus it holds the great advantage that does not enter the nucleus of the host cells and allows a highly efficient reprogramming [36]. Further, Sendai virus-based vectors are replication deficient, and their copies became diluted during cell divisions, and eventually virus-free iPSCs are available after about 10 passages. Thus, this reprogramming technique works to obtain iPSCs without introducing changes to genome. However, their relatively short expression strongly limits their use in biological and research application that require long-term manipulation for somatic cell reprogramming.

4. Non-viral-based reprogramming methods

Due to the highlighted safety issues, it is necessary to develop efficient non-viral reprogramming methods. To generate iPSCs completely free from any viral contamination, researchers have modified and used DNA-based vectors, such as plasmids, episomal vectors, minicircle vectors, piggyBac transposons and non-DNA-based methods to deliver Yamanaka factors as mRNAs, microRNAs and proteins, as well as the direct reprogramming by exosomes (**Figure 2**) [37].

The common denominator of these methods is a much lower reprogramming efficiency as compared to lentiviral vectors-based reprogramming (**Figure 3**).

4.1 DNA-based methods

They require the use of elements composed of DNA to induce the expression of the reprogramming factors into the target cells. The most used elements include circular DNA vectors of different sizes (episomal vectors and minicircles) and mobile DNA sequences able to move and integrate to different locations within the genome by a cut and paste mechanism (PiggyBac).

4.1.1 Episomal vectors

One of the first integration-free techniques used for cell reprogramming includes the employment of non-replicating or replicating episomal vectors. This method is a quite simple technique not requiring special skills by the operators performing the experiments. Beside these advantage, reprogramming by the means of episomal vectors produces iPSCs still containing fragments of plasmidic DNA, due to the low transfection power that requires multiple transfections to obtain an appropriate expression level of the desired genes in the derived cells. Due to such a low transfection efficacy, the possibility of DNA fragments integration is highly increased, and it is crucial to improve the technique focusing on the reduction of transfection frequency and genetic fragments integration. Reprogramming by episomes is an excellent choice if employing blood cells but needs modification of standard culture conditions to reprogram fibroblasts into iPSCs [34].

4.1.2 Minicircle vectors

Minicircle vectors were first developed as smaller alternates to episomal vectors with a higher efficiency of transfection. They are circular, non-viral DNA elements that have been freed from a prokaryotic vector containing sequences of interest i.e. Oct3/4, SOX2, Nanog, LIN28, Green Fluorescent Protein (GFP). Expression of minicircle-coded genes occurs in both dividing and non-dividing cells with high efficiency, and typically yield higher expression levels of desired proteins, as they are less likely to be inactivated and silenced by cellular mechanisms targeting foreign nucleic acids [38, 39].

4.1.3 PiggyBac transposons

In PiggyBac transposon reprogramming, transgene sequence can be removed from integration site without changing host's DNA. It requires only the inverted terminal repeats, flanking a transgene and transient expression of the transposase to catalyze insertion or excision events [40]. All the mentioned methods show disadvantages, for example, the Sendai virus is effective on all cell types, but requires a lot of passages to obtain iPSCs. The PiggyBac method could represent an attractive alternate but studies in human cells are still limited and weak [40].

4.2 Non-DNA-based methods

Most common reprogramming strategies are based on the use of DNA. All these techniques are effective in achieving a successful reprogramming of the somatic cell, but they are considered less safe as some fragments of the DNA employed can integrate into the host cells genome due to the repeated treatments required to obtain the appropriate expression level of the desired genes. To avoid this safety issues, several groups focused on the development of protocols including non-DNA based methods for reprogramming, such as the use of mRNAs, microRNAs, or recombinant proteins (**Figures 2** and **3**).

Beside reprogramming, and subsequent differentiation into desired cell type, several authors have recently reported the possibility of trans-differentiation, or conversion of one cell type to another one, while bypassing the iPSC-state. An example is the direct conversion of myocardial scar fibroblasts (MSFs) to cardiomyocytes by infection of human MSFs with a lentivirus vector encoding the potent cardiogenic transcription factor myocardin [41].

The direct reprogramming, in fact, is a procedure by which a mature, fully differentiated cell is converted into another cell type, completely or partially bypassing an intermediate pluripotent state. The direct reprogramming is an interesting new approach of regenerative medicine allowing to overcome the numerous problems related to the use of stem cells. Additionally, it has a low risk for genetic alterations and tumor development, as the reprogramming by this technique avoids risky genetic manipulation and the use of viruses or other strategies causing the residual integration of exogenous genetic material.

4.2.1 mRNAs

High-efficiency, synthetic mRNA-based reprogramming was recently described [42]. Synthetic mRNAs codifying for Yamanaka factors are modified to overcome innate antiviral responses. Since mRNA is translated to protein in the cytoplasm, it does not enter the nucleus, minimizing chance of unwanted modifications of hosts DNA. This method appears to work fast and efficiently, but the major disadvantage is that mRNA is degraded in few days. As such, repeated transfection is required for successful reprogramming [42, 43].

The direct delivery of synthetic mRNAs for the conversion of adult mature cells into iPSCs is an example of direct reprogramming. An effective protocol including the employment of this method was proposed by Warren et al. The idea of delivering mRNA directly raised from the possibility of random DNA fragment integration when DNA is used to derive iPSCs. This procedure is based on the in vitro transcription by the means of templates previously amplified by molecular biology techniques to encode the four Yamanaka reprogramming factors. A strong limitation related to the employment of this procedure is due to the multiple administrations required to gain an adequate protein expression levels, therefore the entire reprogramming process consists in a daily mRNA transfection and the derivation of iPSCs can take up to 18 days. Nonetheless, the transfection of human dermal fibroblast with Yamanaka's reprogramming factors combined with Nanog and LIN28, from Thomson's approach, have been reported as inducing the arrangement of cells in colonies as early as 24 h after the first transfection (**Figure 1**) [18, 19]. To increase the efficiency of the technique, the delivery of mRNAs is combined with hypoxic culture conditions that seem to double the efficiency of reprogramming. However, direct cell reprogramming mediated by mRNA is risky, as the numerous and repeated administrations of them to ensure a high expression level of proteins of interest can eventually trigger the activation of c-Myc, with a high risk for tumor development. A pivotal improvement for this procedure could target the frequency of mRNAs administration and the activation of the oncogene c-Myc.

4.2.2 MicroRNAs

MicroRNAs are small molecules of non-coding RNA primarily involved in gene expression regulation at both transcriptional and post-transcriptional level; in particular, they are responsible for gene silencing. Several studies have reported that including microRNAs in the traditional procedures employed for reprogramming can positively impact the efficiency of the process. Equally to other procedures not requiring DNA, reprogramming by microRNAs produces iPSCs free from exogenous DNA integration, but the needing of multiple administrations makes the procedure complicated and time consuming [44].

4.2.3 Recombinant proteins

To overcome the issue related to the introduction of exogenous DNA into derived iPSCs, another approach consists in the employment of recombinant proteins as reprogramming factors. Protein-based reprogramming carries the advantage that it does not cause any genetic changes. As already mentioned, current methods of protein-based reprogramming are less efficient that lentiviral delivery of Yamanaka factors [42, 45]. Typically, synthesized in bacteria, Yamanaka factors are modified so that they express basic amino acids or other transport peptides enabling to cross the cell membrane [4].

Some studies have led to the development of different methods to isolate, purify, and then deliver reprogramming factors in form of recombinant proteins [33, 45].

The reprogramming mediated by recombinant proteins is challenging and need several improvements. The synthesis of a consistent amount of proteins is quite hard and requires specific skills that make the technique ineffective for a number of laboratories.

4.2.4 Exosomes

The modern trend for cell reprogramming consists in the direct conversion of a cell into another by the means of exosomes containing a cocktail of reprogramming factors for a specific purpose, named reprosomes. With the respect to the iPSCs, reprogramming cells by exosomes seems to be more likely for clinical applications, as it requires easier procedures and the risk for tumor formation and mutations is low [46].

Exosomes are nanovesicles with a size ranging between 30 and 200 nm. They are secreted by all cell types and circulate in many body fluids, from where they can be easily isolated. After the discovery that exosomes are able to transfer molecules of biological relevance, like mRNA, miRNA and proteins to one cell to another eliciting phenotypical changes, several studies are ongoing to define their potential as an integration-free method for cellular reprogramming. Despite several advantages offered by the use of exosomes, like the easy extraction method, the reduction of immunological host response and the possibility to reprogram cells without genetical manipulation, their effective employment is still under investigation and the procedures for their isolation and characterization are still limited by a low efficiency and a poor specificity [47, 48].

5. Conclusions

The improvement of non-integrating methods is now the target for cell reprogramming to derive iPSCs. In fact, these methods do not require the incorporation of viral genome into the host cells, avoiding the risk of tumor development. The safety of these methods, that makes the derived cells more appealing for clinical applications, is a common strong point, although beside the above-mentioned specific issues related to each method, the common major weakness is represented by a general low efficiency respect to the traditional integrating approaches. The original protocol proposed by Yamanaka for generating iPSCs from adult somatic cells was based on the insertion of only four factors: octamer-binding transcription factor-3/4 (OCT3/4), SRY-related high-mobility group (HMG)-box protein-2 (SOX2), Myc, and Kruppel-like factor-4 (KLF4), or Nanog and LIN28 instead of Myc and KLF4 [4]. A major obstacle in cellular reprogramming, beside the risk of tumor formation due to the integrating methods, is the very low efficiency of the reprogramming procedure, strictly related to several factors, such as the type of cell to be reprogrammed, the method of delivering the reprogramming factors and culture conditions. Although the non-integrating methods offer a safer way to produce iPSCs for further clinical application, it is crucial to focus on the enhancement of the efficiency of the existing and ongoing protocols. In this respect, several strategies have been developed, such as the employment of promoters or enhancers boosting the reprogramming of somatic cells have being developed. Regulatory genes involved in proliferation and cell cycle modulators represent a valid example among the approaches proposed, although if on one side they allow a better yield, on the other they have the disadvantage of being potentially tumorigenic [49, 50].

Additional candidates investigated for their ability to increase up to 100 folds the efficiency of reprogramming, due to their capability of remodeling chromatin, are small molecules and inhibitor factors, such as valproic acid (VPA) and histone deacetylase (HDAC) inhibitor. Further, the use of VPA together with hypoxic conditions greatly boosts the efficiency of reprogramming [51–53]. The remodeling of chromatin induces a dynamic modification of chromatin architecture that allows the access to the condensed DNA by proteins involved in transcriptional regulation mechanism and responsible for the modulation of the gene expression in the cells [54].

Other factors heavily impacting on the efficiency of reprogramming are culture conditions, the possible employment of supporting feeder cells, and the composition of culture medium [55, 56]. It is well documented that reprogramming under hypoxic conditions of 5% O2 instead of the atmospheric 21% O2 increases the reprogramming efficiency of mouse embryonic fibroblasts (MEFs) and human dermal fibroblasts. The presence of a layer of feeder cells is extremely important to support cells during the reprogramming procedures, as feeder cells are responsible for the secretion of growth factors essential for cell survival. Usually, mouse feeder cells are used to support the growth and culture of iPSCs, but they must be removed before the use in clinical applications. Basically, feeder cells consist in a layer of growth-arrested cells unable to divide, which provides extracellular secretions to help other cells to proliferate. However, the use of animal derived feeder cells rises safety issues for the clinical applications due to the contamination of pathogens cross-transfer. To overcome this limitation, the use of Matrigel, a mixture of extracellular matrix proteins such as laminin, collagen and fibronectin, and supplemented with a medium conditioned by feeder cells, as substitute supporting layer is widely popular to produce and support iPSCs [19, 57–58].

A successful reprogramming also depends on the choice of the proper cell type to reprogram. The original protocol proposed by Yamanaka included the use of fibroblasts, first from mouse, then from humans, and these cells still remain the favorite cell type, primarily for the easiness of harvesting by skin biopsy. However, even among the different types of fibroblasts several studies highlighted that they are not reprogrammable with the same efficiency [18]; hence, other cell sources need to be found. In fact, the specific promptness of cell to be reprogrammed is strictly related to the endogenous expression of some reprogramming factors and from the starting differentiation state. Currently, there are different strategies, which allow choosing the appropriate cell source, the delivery method, and the system to boost the efficiency of cell reprogramming to derive iPSCs in the safer manner. Nevertheless, all these techniques need to be strongly boosted in order to be considered useful for a clinical application of the derived iPSCs.:

Conflict of interest

The authors declare no conflict of interest.

Author details

Immacolata Belviso, Veronica Romano, Daria Nurzynska, Clotilde Castaldo*
and Franca Di Meglio
Department of Public Health, University of Naples Federico II, Naples, Italy

*Address all correspondence to: clotilde.castaldo@unina.it

References

[1] Inoue H, Nagata N, Kurokawa H, Yamanaka S. iPS cells: a game changer for future medicine. EMBO J. 2014;33(5):409-417. DOI: 10.1002/embj.201387098

[2] Thomson JA, Itskovitz-Eldor J, Shapiro SS, Waknitz MA, Swiergiel JJ, Marshall VS, Jones JM. Embryonic stem cell lines derived from human blastocysts. Science. 1998;282(5391):1145-1147. DOI: 10.1126/science.282.5391.1145

[3] Tada M, Takahama Y, Abe K, Nakatsuji N, Tada T. Nuclear reprogramming of somatic cells by in vitro hybridization with ES cells. Curr Biol. 2001;11(19):1553-1558. DOI: 10.1016/s0960-822(01)00459-6

[4] Takahashi K, Yamanaka S. Induction of pluripotent stem cells from mouse embryonic and adult fibroblast cultures by defined factors. Cell. 2006;126(4):663-676. DOI: 10.1016/j.cell.2006.07.024

[5] Cartwright P, McLean C, Sheppard A, Rivett D, Jones K, Dalton S. LIF/STAT3 controls ES cell self-renewal and pluripotency by a Myc-dependent mechanism. Development. 2005;132(5):885-896. DOI: 10.1242/dev.01670

[6] Yu J, Vodyanik MA, Smuga-Otto K, Antosiewicz-Bourget J, Frane JL, Tian S, Nie J, Jonsdottir GA, Ruotti V, Stewart R, Slukvin II, Thomson JA. Induced pluripotent stem cell lines derived from human somatic cells. Science. 2007;318(5858):1917-1920. DOI: 10.1126/science.1151526

[7] Puri MC, Nagy A. Concise review: Embryonic stem cells versus induced pluripotent stem cells: the game is on. Stem Cells. 2012;30(1):10-14. DOI: 10.1002/stem.788

[8] Kang L, Wang J, Zhang Y, Kou Z, Gao S. iPS cells can support full-term development of tetraploid blastocyst-complemented embryos. Cell Stem Cell. 2009;5(2):135-138. DOI: 10.1016/j.stem.2009.07.001

[9] Ye L, Swingen C, Zhang J. Induced pluripotent stem cells and their potential for basic and clinical sciences. Curr Cardiol Rev. 2013;9(1):63-72. DOI: 10.2174/15734031380507627811

[10] Moon SY, Park YB, Kim DS, Oh SK, Kim DW. Generation, culture, and differentiation of human embryonic stem cells for therapeutic applications. Mol Ther. 2006;13(1):5-14. DOI: 10.1016/j.ymthe.2005.09.008

[11] de Wert G, Mummery C. Human embryonic stem cells: research, ethics and policy. Hum Reprod. 2003;18(4):672-682. DOI: 10.1093/humrep/deg143

[12] Drukker M, Benvenisty N. The immunogenicity of human embryonic stem-derived cells. Trends Biotechnol. 2004;22(3):136-141. DOI: 10.1016/j.tibtech.2004.01.003

[13] Ludwig TE, Levenstein ME, Jones JM, Berggren WT, Mitchen ER, Frane JL, Crandall LJ, Daigh CA, Conard KR, Piekarczyk MS, Llanas RA, Thomson JA. Derivation of human embryonic stem cells in defined conditions. Nat Biotechnol. 2006;24(2):185-187. DOI: 10.1038/nbt1177

[14] Lu J, Hou R, Booth CJ, Yang SH, Snyder M. Defined culture conditions of human embryonic stem cells. Proc Natl Acad Sci U S A. 2006;103(15):5688-5693. DOI: 10.1073/pnas.0601383103

[15] Damdimopoulou P, Rodin S, Stenfelt S, Antonsson L, Tryggvason K, Hovatta O. Human embryonic stem cells. Best Pract Res Clin Obstet

Gynaecol. 2016;31:2-12. DOI: 10.1016/j.bpobgyn.2015.08.010

[16] Richards M, Fong CY, Chan WK, Wong PC, Bongso A. Human feeders support prolonged undifferentiated growth of human inner cell masses and embryonic stem cells. Nat Biotechnol. 2002;20(9):933-936. DOI: 10.1038/nbt726

[17] Yamanaka S. Strategies and new developments in the generation of patient-specific pluripotent stem cells. Cell Stem Cell. 2007;1(1):39-49. DOI: 10.1016/j.stem.2007.05.012

[18] Sacco AM, Belviso I, Romano V, Carfora A, Schonauer F, Nurzynska D, Montagnani S, Di Meglio F, Castaldo C. Diversity of dermal fibroblasts as major determinant of variability in cell reprogramming. J Cell Mol Med. 2019;23(6):4256-4268. DOI: 10.1111/jcmm.14316

[19] Belviso I, Sacco AM, Romano V, Schonauer F, Nurzynska D, Montagnani S, Di Meglio F, Castaldo C. Isolation of Adult Human Dermal Fibroblasts from Abdominal Skin and Generation of Induced Pluripotent Stem Cells Using a Non-Integrating Method. J Vis Exp. 2020;(155). DOI: 10.3791/60629

[20] Omole AE, Fakoya AOJ. Ten years of progress and promise of induced pluripotent stem cells: historical origins, characteristics, mechanisms, limitations, and potential applications. PeerJ. 2018;6:e4370. DOI: 10.7717/peerj.4370

[21] Okita K, Ichisaka T, Yamanaka S. Generation of germline-competent induced pluripotent stem cells. Nature. 2007;448:313-317. DOI: 10.1038/nature05934

[22] Han JW, Yoon YS. Induced pluripotent stem cells: emerging techniques for nuclear reprogramming. Antioxid Redox Signal. 2011;15(7):1799-1820. DOI: 10.1089/ars.2010.3814

[23] Malik N, Rao MS. A review of the methods for human iPSC derivation. Methods Mol Biol. 2013;997:23-33. DOI: 10.1007/978-1-62703-348-0_3

[24] Park IH, Zhao R, West JA, Yabuuchi A, Huo H, Ince TA, Lerou PH, Lensch MW, Daley GQ. Reprogramming of human somatic cells to pluripotency with defined factors. Nature. 2008;451(7175):141-146. DOI: 10.1038/nature06534

[25] Brambrink T, Foreman R, Welstead GG, Lengner CJ, Wernig M, Suh H, Jaenisch R. Sequential expression of pluripotency markers during direct reprogramming of mouse somatic cells. Cell Stem Cell. 2008;2(2):151-159. DOI: 10.1016/j.stem.2008.01.004

[26] Stadtfeld M, Brennand K, Hochedlinger K. Reprogramming of pancreatic beta cells into induced pluripotent stem cells. Curr Biol. 2008;18(12):890-894. DOI: 10.1016/j.cub.2008.05.010

[27] Kitamura T, Koshino Y, Shibata F, Oki T, Nakajima H, Nosaka T, Kumagai H. Retrovirus-mediated gene transfer and expression cloning: powerful tools in functional genomics. Exp Hematol. 2003;31(11):1007-1014. PMID: 14585362

[28] Hotta A, Ellis J. Retroviral vector silencing during iPS cell induction: an epigenetic beacon that signals distinct pluripotent states. J Cell Biochem. 2008;105(4):940-948. DOI: 10.1002/jcb.21912

[29] Wernig M, Lengner CJ, Hanna J, Lodato MA, Steine E, Foreman R, Staerk J, Markoulaki S, Jaenisch R. A drug-inducible transgenic system for

direct reprogramming of multiple somatic cell types. Nat Biotechnol. 2008;26(8):916-924. DOI: 10.1038/nbt1483

[30] Wernig M, Meissner A, Foreman R, Brambrink T, Ku M, Hochedlinger K, Bernstein BE, Jaenisch R. In vitro reprogramming of fibroblasts into a pluripotent ES-cell-like state. Nature. 2007;448(7151):318-324. DOI: 10.1038/nature05944

[31] Domínguez O, Martínez D, Manzanares M, Ortega S, Serrano M. Reprogramming in vivo produces teratomas and iPS cells with totipotency features. Nature. 2013;502(7471):340-345. DOI: 10.1038/nature12586

[32] Stadtfeld M, Nagaya M, Utikal J, Weir G, Hochedlinger K. Induced pluripotent stem cells generated without viral integration. Science. 2008;322(5903):945-949. DOI: 10.1126/science

[33] Zhou W, Freed CR. Adenoviral gene delivery can reprogram human fibroblasts to induced pluripotent stem cells. Stem Cells. 2009;27(11):2667-2674. DOI: 10.1002/stem.201

[34] Okita K, Nakagawa M, Hyenjong H, Ichisaka T, Yamanaka S. Generation of mouse induced pluripotent stem cells without viral vectors. Science. 2008;322(5903):949-953. DOI: 10.1126/science.1164270

[35] Fusaki N, Ban H, Nishiyama A, Saeki K, Hasegawa M. Efficient induction of transgene-free human pluripotent stem cells using a vector based on Sendai virus, an RNA virus that does not integrate into the host genome. Proc Jpn Acad Ser B Phys Biol Sci. 2009;85(8):348-362. DOI: 10.2183/pjab.85.348

[36] Nakanishi M, Otsu M. Development of Sendai virus vectors and their potential applications in gene therapy and regenerative medicine. Curr Gene Ther. 2012;12(5):410-416. DOI: 10.2174/156652312802762518

[37] Deng XY, Wang H, Wang T, Fang XT, Zou LL, Li ZY, Liu CB. Non-viral methods for generating integration-free, induced pluripotent stem cells. Curr Stem Cell Res Ther. 2015;10(2):153-158. DOI: 10.2174/1574888x09666140923101914

[38] Jia F, Wilson KD, Sun N, Gupta DM, Huang M, Li Z, Panetta NJ, Chen ZY, Robbins RC, Kay MA, Longaker MT, Wu JC. A nonviral minicircle vector for deriving human iPS cells. Nat Methods. 2010;7(3):197-199. DOI: 10.1038/nmeth.1426

[39] Narsinh KH, Jia F, Robbins RC, Kay MA, Longaker MT, Wu JC. Generation of adult human induced pluripotent stem cells using nonviral minicircle DNA vectors. Nat Protoc. 2011;6(1):78-88. DOI: 10.1038/nprot.2010.173

[40] Thibault ST, Singer MA, Miyazaki WY, Milash B, Dompe NA, Singh CM, Buchholz R, Demsky M, Fawcett R, Francis-Lang HL, Ryner L, Cheung LM, Chong A, Erickson C, Fisher WW, Greer K, Hartouni SR, Howie E, Jakkula L, Joo D, Killpack K, Laufer A, Mazzotta J, Smith RD, Stevens LM, Stuber C, Tan LR, Ventura R, Woo A, Zakrajsek I, Zhao L, Chen F, Swimmer C, Kopczynski C, Duyk G, Winberg ML, Margolis J. A complementary transposon tool kit for *Drosophila melanogaster* using P and piggyBac. Nat Genet. 2004;36(3):283-287. DOI: 10.1038/ng1314

[41] van Tuyn J, Pijnappels DA, de Vries AA, de Vries I, van der Velde-van Dijke I, Knaän-Shanzer S, van der Laarse A, Schalij MJ, Atsma DE. Fibroblasts from human postmyocardial infarction scars acquire properties of cardiomyocytes after transduction with a recombinant myocardin gene. FASEB

J. 2007;21(12):3369-3379. DOI: 10.1096/fj.07-8211com

[42] Warren L, Manos PD, Ahfeldt T, Loh YH, Li H, Lau F, Ebina W, Mandal PK, Smith ZD, Meissner A, Daley GQ, Brack AS, Collins JJ, Cowan C, Schlaeger TM, Rossi DJ. Highly efficient reprogramming to pluripotency and directed differentiation of human cells with synthetic modified mRNA. Cell Stem Cell. 2010;7(5):618-630. DOI: 10.1016/j.stem.2010.08.012

[43] Plews JR, Li J, Jones M, Moore HD, Mason C, Andrews PW, Na J. Activation of pluripotency genes in human fibroblast cells by a novel mRNA based approach. PLoS One. 2010;5(12):e14397. DOI: 10.1371/journal.pone.0014397

[44] Miyoshi N, Ishii H, Nagano H, Haraguchi N, Dewi DL, Kano Y, Nishikawa S, Tanemura M, Mimori K, Tanaka F, Saito T, Nishimura J, Takemasa I, Mizushima T, Ikeda M, Yamamoto H, Sekimoto M, Doki Y, Mori M. Reprogramming of mouse and human cells to pluripotency using mature microRNAs. Cell Stem Cell. 2011;8(6):633-638. DOI: 10.1016/j.stem.2011.05.001

[45] Kim D, Kim CH, Moon JI, Chung YG, Chang MY, Han BS, Ko S, Yang E, Cha KY, Lanza R, Kim KS. Generation of human induced pluripotent stem cells by direct delivery of reprogramming proteins. Cell Stem Cell. 2009;4(6):472-476. DOI: 10.1016/j.stem.2009.05.005

[46] Saleem SN, Abdel-Mageed AB. Tumor-derived exosomes in oncogenic reprogramming and cancer progression. Cell Mol Life Sci. 2015;72(1):1-10. DOI: 10.1007/s00018-014-1710-4

[47] Zhang Y, Liu Y, Liu H, Tang WH. Exosomes: biogenesis, biologic function and clinical potential. Cell Biosci. 2019;9:19. DOI: 10.1186/s13578-019-0282-2

[48] Qadir F, Aziz MA, Sari CP, Ma H, Dai H, Wang X, Raithatha D, Da Silva LGL, Hussain M, Poorkasreiy SP, Hutchison IL, Waseem A, Teh MT. Transcriptome reprogramming by cancer exosomes: identification of novel molecular targets in matrix and immune modulation. Mol Cancer. 2018;17(1):97. DOI: 10.1186/s12943-018-0846-5

[49] Takenaka C, Nishishita N, Takada N, Jakt LM, Kawamata S. Effective generation of iPS cells from CD34+ cord blood cells by inhibition of p53. Exp Hematol. 2010;38(2):154-162. DOI: 10.1016/j.exphem.2009.11.003

[50] Hu X, Eastman AE, Guo S. Cell cycle dynamics in the reprogramming of cellular identity. FEBS Lett. 2019;593(20):2840-2852. DOI:10.1002/1873-3468.13625

[51] Yu J, Chau KF, Vodyanik MA, Jiang J, Jiang Y. Efficient feeder-free episomal reprogramming with small molecules. PLoS One. 2011;6(3):e17557. DOI: 10.1371/journal.pone.0017557

[52] Hou P, Li Y, Zhang X, Liu C, Guan J, Li H, Zhao T, Ye J, Yang W, Liu K, Ge J, Xu J, Zhang Q, Zhao Y, Deng H. Pluripotent stem cells induced from mouse somatic cells by small-molecule compounds. Science. 2013;341(6146):651-654. DOI: 10.1126/science.1239278

[53] Doering L, Khatri R, Petry SF, Sauer H, Howaldt HP, Linn T. Regulation of somatostatin expression by vitamin D3 and valproic acid in human adipose-derived mesenchymal stem cells. Stem Cell Res Ther. 2019;10(1):240. DOI: 10.1186/s13287-019-1330-x

[54] Apostolou E, Ferrari F, Walsh RM, Bar-Nur O, Stadtfeld M, Cheloufi S, Stuart HT, Polo JM, Ohsumi TK, Borowsky ML, Kharchenko PV, Park PJ, Hochedlinger K. Genome-wide chromatin interactions of the Nanog

locus in pluripotency, differentiation, and reprogramming. Cell Stem Cell. 2013;12(6):699-712. DOI: 10.1016/j.stem.2013.04.013

[55] Lu HF, Chai C, Lim TC, Leong MF, Lim JK, Gao S, Lim KL, Wan AC. A defined xeno-free and feeder-free culture system for the derivation, expansion and direct differentiation of transgene-free patient-specific induced pluripotent stem cells. Biomaterials. 2014;35(9):2816-2826. DOI: 10.1016/j.biomaterials.2013.12.050

[56] Zhang Y, Wei C, Zhang P, Li X, Liu T, Pu Y, Li Y, Cao Z, Cao H, Liu Y, Zhang X, Zhang Y. Efficient reprogramming of naïve-like induced pluripotent stem cells from porcine adipose-derived stem cells with a feeder-independent and serum-free system. PLoS One. 2014;9(1):e85089. DOI: 10.1371/journal.pone.0085089

[57] Ghasemi-Dehkordi P, Allahbakhshian-Farsani M, Abdian N, Mirzaeian A, Saffari-Chaleshtori J, Heybati F, Mardani G, Karimi-Taghanaki A, Doosti A, Jami MS, Abolhasani M, Hashemzadeh-Chaleshtori M. Comparison between the cultures of human induced pluripotent stem cells (hiPSCs) on feeder-and serum-free system (Matrigel matrix), MEF and HDF feeder cell lines. J Cell Commun Signal. 2015;9(3):233-246. DOI: 10.1007/s12079-015-0289-3

[58] Groß B, Sgodda M, Rasche M, Schambach A, Göhring G, Schlegelberger B, Greber B, Linden T, Reinhardt D, Cantz T, Klusmann JH. Improved generation of patient-specific induced pluripotent stem cells using a chemically-defined and matrigel-based approach. Curr Mol Med. 2013;13(5):765-776. DOI: 10.2174/1566524011313050008

Chapter 6

The Use of Ferritin as a Carrier of Peptides and Its Application for Hepcidin

Mohamed Boumaiza, Samia Rourou, Paolo Arosio and Mohamed Nejib Marzouki

Abstract

Hepcidin a 25-amino-acid and highly disulfide bonded hormone, is the central regulator of iron homeostasis. In this chapter we propose ferritin as a peptide carrier to promote the association of the hybrid hepcidin/ferritin nanoparticle with a particular cell or tissue for therapeutic or diagnostic use. Indeed, human ferritin H-chain fused directly (on its 5'end) with camel mature hepcidin was cloned into the pASK-43 plus vector and expressed using BL21 (DE3) pLys *E. coli* strain. The transformed *E.coli* produced efficiently hepcidin-ferritin construct (hepcH), consisting of 213 amino acids with a molecular weight of 24 KDa. The recovered product is a ferritin exposing hepcidin on outer surface. The hepcH monomer was characterized by immunoblotting using a monoclonal antibody specific for human ferritin and a polyclonal antibody specific for hepcidin-25. The results were also confirmed by MALDI-TOF mass spectrometry. The recombinant native human ferritin and the commercial human hepcidin-25 were used as controls in this experiment. The assembly of hepcH, as an heteropolymer molecule, was performed in presence of denatured human ferritin-H and -L chains. After cysteine oxidation of the recombinant nanoparticles, cellular binding assays were performed on mammalian cells such as mouse monocyte–macrophage cell line J774, HepG2 and COS7.

Keywords: camel hepcidin, chimeric nanoparticle, *engineered recombinant E. coli*, human ferritin, *protein folding*

1. Introduction

The combination of chemistry, biology, and nanotechnology is expected to make significant contributions to the field of medical diagnosis and therapeutics. In this framework, the use of nanoparticles in vaccine formulations allows not only improved antigen stability and immunogenicity, but also targeted delivery and slow release. Protein cage architectures such as virus capsids and ferritins are versatile nanoscale platforms willing to both genetic and chemical modifications. The incorporation of multiple functionalities within these nanometer-sized protein architectures reveals their potential to serve as functional nanomaterials with applications in medical imaging and therapy. For example, RGD-4C, a cell specific targeting peptide, which binds $\alpha v\beta 3$ integrins upregulated on tumor vasculature, was genetically incorporated on the exterior surface of a human H-chain ferritin nanoparticle [1]. Interestingly, this modified protein cage binds specifically cancer cells in vitro. Thus, the use of ferritin cage architecture is an exciting and promising strategy to serve as a multifunctional platform for the biomimetic synthesis of magnetic nanoparticles. It can be engineered for cell-specific targeting.

Ferritin is probably the most used protein in bio-nanotechnology. This is due to its well-known structural features, high stability, capability to mineralize metals in its cavity, self-assembly and possibility to redesign its interior and exterior by protein engineering. It has been used to encapsulate molecules, for the synthesis of inorganic cores, for functional nanostructured composite material, for magnetic nanoparticles for MRI applications and for carrying various epitopes. Most published studies used the human H or L ferritin chains, which are able to self-assemble in different proportions to produce a variety of heteropolymers. This allows the possibility to adorn ferritin surface with multiple functionalities through genetic and chemical modifications to achieve desired properties for therapeutic and/or diagnostic purposes. In particular, it can be used as a peptide carrier to target specific receptors. Unfortunately, there are no data published concerning functional biological peptides genetically fused to ferritin are missing.

In this chapter, we plan to exploit this approach by fusing hepcidin to the ferritin molecule. In fact, ferritin and hepcidin are central molecules implicated in the regulation of iron homeostasis and the fusion of the two can carry several advantages. For example, the injection of iron-loaded ferritin in a ten days wild mouse induces the expression of *BMP6* and *Hamp1* at dose-dependent manner. Such result cannot be obtained through an injection of FAC (ferric ammonium citrate) or holo-transferrin. However, the injection of uncharged ferritin has no effect on the expression of *BMP6* or *Hamp1*.

We also proposed to use ferritin to carry hepcidin, another key protein of iron metabolism. It is a small hormone peptide that control systemic iron homeostasis (ferritin is a major controller of cellular iron homeostasis). The production of chimeric ferritin complexes that expose on the surface of limited number of functional hepcidin is of interest. It is a tool that allows deep studies in relation to the mechanism of interaction between hepcidin and ferroportin and how the complex is degraded. It might indicate alternative approaches to control hepcidin activity and systemic iron homeostasis. Ferritin is composed of 24 subunits. Once defined the conditions to insert a novel function and to co-assemble different subunits in a highly stable molecule that carries are defined, it is possible to produce molecules with many more functions and it can be applied to other peptides and hormones.

The aim of this chapter is to describe an efficient strategy to fuse the full-length hepcidin to the N-terminus of ferritin-H chain (which in the assembled protein is exposed on the surface). The produced chimeric protein will be tested:

1. As iron regulatory hormone (by studying the hepcidin-ferroportin interaction) which can be useful for patients with iron disorders.

2. As drug-delivery agent.

2. Methods

2.1 Expression and solubilization of HepcH monomer

Human ferritin H-chain fused directly, on its 5'end, with camel mature hepcidin was cloned into the pASK-IBA 43 plus vector (**Table 1**) and expressed using *E. coli* BL21 (DE3) pLysS. Growth of the transformed *E. coli* was done in 1 L LB medium (10 g

Primers	Sequence 5′ to 3′	Using
NheI hFTH F	CAAATGGCTAGCACGACCGCGTCCA	Construction of pASK-IBA43 plus hFTH vector
BamHI hFTH R	TCGAGGGATCCCCGGGTTAGCTTTCATT	Construction of pASK-IBA43 plus hFTH vector
NheI H25 F	ATAGACGCTAGCATGGACACCCACTTCCCCATCTGC	Construction of pASK-IBA43 plus HepcD-hFTH vector
NheI H25 R	ATAGACGCTAGCGGTCTTGCAGCACATCCCAC	Construction of pASK-IBA43 plus HepcD-hFTH vector
pASK F	GAGTTATTTTACCACTCCCT	Sequencing
pASK R	CGCAGTAGCGGTAAACG	Sequencing

Table 1.
Sequences of the primes used in this study.

Tryptone, 5 g Yeast extract, 5 g NaCl), with100μg/ml AMP, at 37°C, for 1-2 h until OD = 0,5. Expression was induced by the addition of 200 μl anhydroteracycline (1 mg/ml), final concentration 200 μg/L, for 4 h. Cells were harvested by centrifugation at 7000 RPM for 10 min. The pallet was washed twice in Tris–HCl 20 mM pH 7,4 and sonicated, for cytoplasmic protein extraction, at the following conditions: 1 min: 30 sec, cycle5, power 72%. The sonicated pallet was centrifuged at 12000 RPM and washed twice in Tris 20 mM, 2 M Urea, 0,1% TritonX100, pH 7,4. The insoluble HepcH, precipitating with the inclusion bodies from the *E.coli* paste, was solubilized with a weight to volume ratio of 1:1 in 6 M Guanidine hydrochloride (GdnHCl) pH 4,7. The suspension was sonicated at the same conditions to homogenate the solution and incubated with stirring, for 18 h at 4°C.

2.2 Assembly and cysteine oxidation of HepcH-FTH heteropolymers

To enhance the assembling of HepcH as an heteropolymer molecule, it was mixed, with the molar ratio hepcidin/ferritin of 1:5, in presence of denatured FTH in 6 M GdnHCl pH 7. The mixture was then diluted at least 10-fold into 0,1 M sodium phosphate pH 7,4, in the presence of 5 mM beta-mercaptoethanol (3 mM DTT and 1 mM EDTA), and incubated with stirring for 18 h at 4°C, for the renaturation of the heteropolymer. The diluted solution was then clarified by centrifugation, at 4000RPM for 15 min, at least twice to separate the soluble fraction from the insoluble cellular debris. A 10-fold concentration was performed with a 100-KDa molecular weight cutoff membrane. The renatured HepcH-FTH heteropolymer was then purified using a gel filtration on a Sepharose 6B column and analyzed on native gel 8%. A slightly modified protocol of HepcH-FTH renaturation, using different molar ratios of hepcidin/ferritin, was described by Boumaiza et al. [2]. Both protocols showed to be efficient for the production of correctly assembled and functional HepcH-FTH heteropolymer. Cysteine oxidation for the final refolded HepcH-FTH renatured in the proportion hepcidin/ferritin = 1:5, was carried out using the glutathione redox system (GSH/GSSG) as described by Jordan et al. [3].

2.3 Cell culture

Mouse monocyte–macrophage cell line J774 (Lombardy and Emilia Romagna Experimental Zootechnic Institute) was cultured as previously described by

Delaby et al. [4]. Briefly, cells were grown in DMEM (PAA Laboratories GmbH), 10% endotoxin-free fetal bovine serum (Euroclone), 0.04 mg/mL gentamicin (Euroclone), 2 mM l-glutamine (PAA Laboratories GmbH), and maintained at 37°C in 5% CO2. They (200,000 cells/well) were seeded onto 12- well plates, and after 24 h were grown for 12 h in presence of 100 μM ferric ammonium citrate (FAC) to induce ferroportin expression. The day after, cells were incubated with HepcH-FTH at final concentrations of 0.5 μM and 0.2 μM. Controls were cells without ferric ammonium citrate (FAC) treatment and cells incubated with native FTH homopolymer. Experiments were performed at 37°C for 30 min and 2 h. After this time, the supernatant was discarded and the cells washed with cold PBS and lysed using cold buffer (200 mM Tris–HCl at pH 8, 100 mM NaCl, 1 mM EDTA, 0.5% NP-40, 10% glycerol, 1 mM sodium fluoride, 1 mM sodium orthovanadate, complete protease inhibitor cocktail; Roche). Protein content was determined by colorimetric BCA assay (bicinchoninic acid assay, Pierce), 30 μg of total proteins were separated by native and denatured polyacrylamide gel electrophoresis and Western blotting, for the detection of proteins bound and internalized by the J774 cells, as well as the mass spectroscopy analysis were performed as described previously [5].

3. Results and discussion

Ferritin is probably the most used protein in bionanotechnology. This is due to its well-known structural features, high stability, capability to mineralize metals in its cavity, self-assembly and possibility to redesign its interior and exterior by protein engineering [6, 7]. Hepcidin, a 25 amino acid peptide belonging to the β-defensins family, was isolated for the first time from plasma and human urine respectively by Krause *et al.* [8] and Park *et al.* [9]. It is a cysteine-rich cationic peptide, engaged with four disulfide bridges, which plays a major role in innate immunity and iron homeostasis [10]. It is induced by iron and inflammation and is suppressed by iron deficiency and hypoxia. It binds and inhibits ferroportin1, the only cellular iron exporter, thus, high hepcidin reduces while low hepcidin increases systemic iron availability. This hormone acts via its N-terminal part and more precisely the 7–9 amino acids including a single thiol cysteine, comprised the minimal structure that retained hepcidin activity [11] and can be refolded *in-vitro*. The 3D structure of human hepcidin is known [3]. Recombinant human and mouse hepcidins were expressed in *E. coli* in fusion with a Thioredoxin and treated by two sequential proteolytic enzymes to obtain functional hepcidin, in low yield <10% [12]. We used this procedure to clone and express camel hepcidin, in collaboration with Prof. Marie-Agnès Sari in the laboratory of Chemistry and Pharmacological and Toxicological Biochemistry (UMR 8601) at the University Paris Descartes. We showed that this hepcidin is functionally equivalent to human one in binding and inhibiting ferroportin using mouse monocyte–macrophage cell line J774 treated with Fe-nitrilotriacetate. Camel hepcidin differs from human hepcidin in 2 residues, which make it more stable [13]. Thus, we planned to use camel hepcidin to make hybrid molecules with ferritin. For this purpose, we have approached the laboratory of Prof. Paolo Arosio in Brescia that has a long experience in the production of recombinant proteins and is working on ferritin and hepcidin. The aim of this work was to fuse the full length hepcidin to the N-terminus of ferritin-H chain, which is exposed on the surface in the assembled protein. The chimeric subunit was assembled in the 24-mer shells together with various proportion of H or L chains to produce hybrid heteropolymers. These latter that can carry 1 to 24 hepcidin moieties and other functions that can be engineered and can include the electron dense iron core as tracer.

We cloned the gene encoding camel hepcidin in fusion with the 5′ of the cDNA for heavy chain of human ferritin into the pASK-IBA 43plus vector (**Figure 1A, B**) for high expression in *E. coli*. The clone was verified and expressed the chimeric peptide in high amount but it was insoluble and could not be easily refolded in a soluble and active 24-mer shell. Thus, we planned to carry out this project with different strategies:

The construct was expressed in the prokaryotic system *E.coli* BL21 (DE3) pLysS, and the peptides were initially characterized on polyacrylamide gel in denaturing conditions (**Figure 2A**), western blotting (**Figure 2B**) and MALDI-TOF mass spectrometry. Hepcidin carries 8 cysteines that form 4 disulfide bridges in the folded molecule, while FTH has three cysteines, which do not form bonds. Thus, the presence of free -SH groups was also quantified throughout all the purification and refolding processes. We planned to produce bicistronic constructs that express the chimeric hepcidin-FTH and the FTH-WT, with an approach that has been found successful for the production of insoluble ferritin mutants [14]. We obtained ferritin shells with low proportion of chimeric hepcidin (**Figure 1C, D**). In parallel, we have performed co-renaturation together with ferritin-H or L chains. We obtained molecules with various amounts of hepcidin. To this aim the *in-vitro* refolding of the fusion protein hepcH was done with different molar ratio of H and L chains, in order to optimize the assembly of the hybrid nanoparticles [2]. Purified fusion hepcidin–ferritin H subunit (**Figure 3D**) assembled together with H- or L-chains at a ratio of 1:5, produced a stable and functional 24-mer ferritin exposing about 4 hepcidin per shell (**Figure 1C, D**; **Figure 3C**). HepcH-FTH heteropolymer was purified and characterized by analysis on polyacrylamide gel in non-denaturing condition and by western blotting (**Figure 3E, F, G, H**). MALDI-TOF spectra of the final oxidized HepcH-FTH heteropolymer exhibited, average mass peaks at m/z 21135.97 and at 243775.51 (**Figure 4A**) which corresponds to the theoretical average mass [M + H] + of 21225.64 of FTH (183 amino acids), and of 24410.50 to HepcH (213 amino acids).

These procedures have produced ferritin shells that expose on the surface the hepcidin moiety. In order to control the correct folding, the cysteines of the

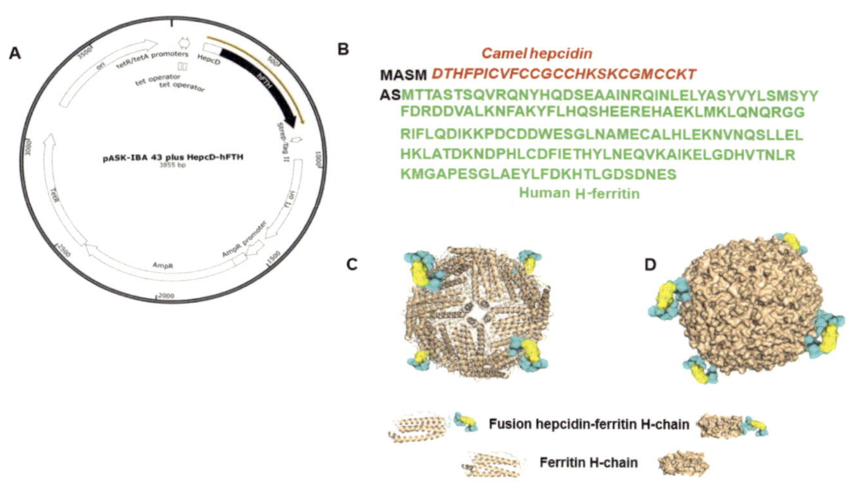

Figure 1.
(A) Construction of the recombinant HepcH pASK-IBA 43 plus vector. (B) Amino acid sequence of the fusion HepcH protein. In this recombinant protein, the coding sequence of camel hepcidin, in red and italic, was fused directly to the 5′ end of human H-ferritin, in green, and cloned into pASK-IBA43 plus vector. (C) Schematic representation (left) and space-filling diagram (right) of the assembled HepcH-FTH heteropolymer (with molar ratio hepcidin/ferritin = 1:5).

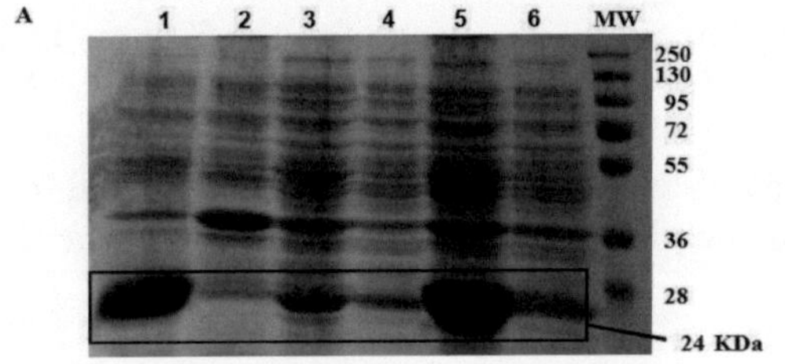

Figure 2.
(A) SDS-PAGE analysis of the induced and uninduced E.coli transformed by the recombinant HepcH-FTH pASK-IBA 43 plus vector. Lane 1 and 2, induced and uninduced pellet respectively (insoluble fraction). Lane 3 and 4, induced and uninduced supernatant (soluble fraction). Lane 5 and 6, induced and uninduced total sonicate (total protein). (B) Western blot analysis of the recombinant HepcH monomer (in denaturing conditions). Lane 1, rabbit hepcidin antibodies recognized the human hepcidin-25 (control). Lane2, rabbit hepcidin antibodies recognized the recombinant HepcH. Lane3, rHo2 antibodies recognized the recombinant HepcH. Lane4, rHo2 antibodies recognized the recombinant human H-ferritin (control).

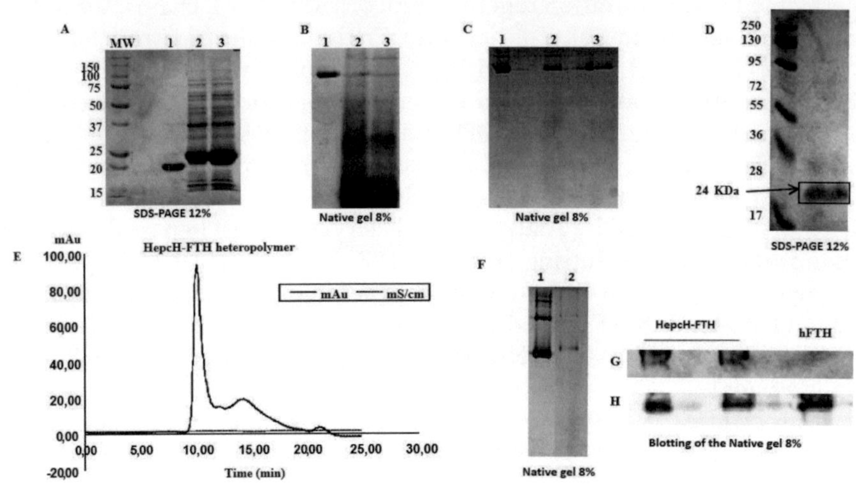

Figure 3.
Renaturation of the insoluble HepcH monomer in absence and in presence of FTH. (A) Purified FTH (line1) and solubilized HepcH monomer (line 2 and 3) analyzed on denaturing conditions. (B) FTH homopolymer (line1) and renatured HepcH, in absence of FTH, analyzed on non-denaturing conditions (line 2 and 3). (C) FTH homopolymer (line1) and renatured HepcH in presence of FTH with molar ratio of hepcidin/ ferritin = 1:5 (lane 2 and 3) analyzed on non-denaturing conditions. (D) SDS-PAGE analysis of the purified HepcH, from the insoluble fraction (IS), by gel filtration on a Sepharose 6B column (GE Healthcare, life sciences). (E) Fast protein liquid chromatography chromatogram showing the purification of HepcH-FTH heteropolymer using a gel filtration on a Sepharose 6B column and analyzer on non-denaturing conditions (F). (G) Western blot analysis of the purified HepcH-FTH heteropolymer using the anti-rabbit hepcidine-25 and the human ferritin-H antibodies, rHo2, as control (H).

molecule was reduced and then slowly oxidized under controlled conditions (to allow the formation of the correct four disulfide bridges constituting the hormone). In case the cysteine of the ferritin interferes with the process or its monitoring by spectroscopic techniques, they could be removed by site-directed mutagenesis.

The functionality of the assembled heteropolymer was analyzed by its capacity to bind with high affinity the ferroportin, which is the natural hepcidin receptor. To this goal, we used the macrophagic cell line J774 that expose evident ferroportin after treatment with iron. The cells were incubated with the hybrid molecules and the binding analyzed directly with traced anti-ferritin antibodies. Binding specificity was analyzed by adding ferritin and synthetic hepcidin. This process was repeated with the various heteropolymer types. Next, we studied the biological activity of the chimera,

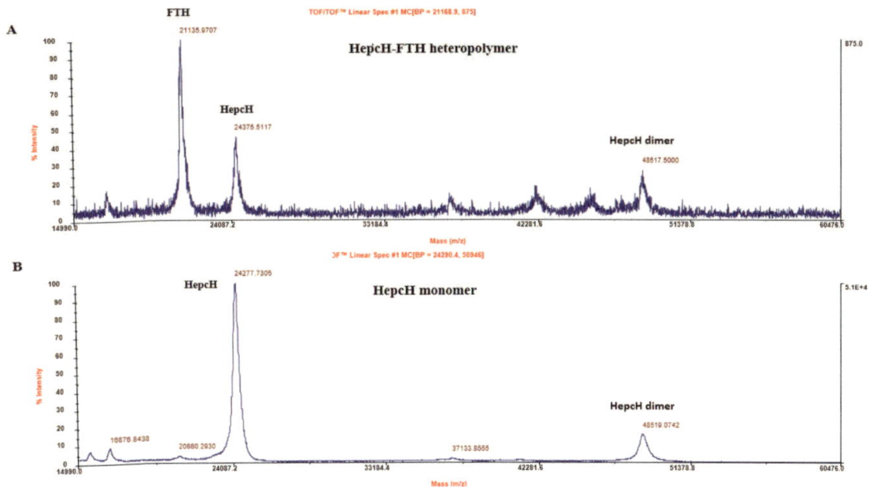

Figure 4.
(A) High-resolution MALDI-TOF/TOF mass analysis of the recombinant assembled HepcH-FTH heteropolymer and the recombinant human ferritin FTH homopolymer (B).

in particularly if it is taken up and degraded together with ferroportin, as it occurs with the hepcidin. Hybrid and native ferritin binding to murine J774 cells were monitored using monoclonal anti-human FTH antibody rH02 that does not cross-react with the mouse ferritins [15]. This was confirmed by treating J774 cells with mouse ferritin alone or together with HepcH-FTH. The obtained results (**Figure 5A**) showed that these antibodies are specific only to human H-ferritin. J774 cells treated with 100 μM FAC showed to be able to internalize HepcH-FTH heteropolymers after 30 min to 2 h of incubation at 37°C (**Figure 5B**). Hepcidin exerts it function by binding and then inducing ferroportin degradation, and in fact we observed that after 2 h incubation, with a final concentration of 0.2 μM, more efficiently than human hepcidin-25 used as control

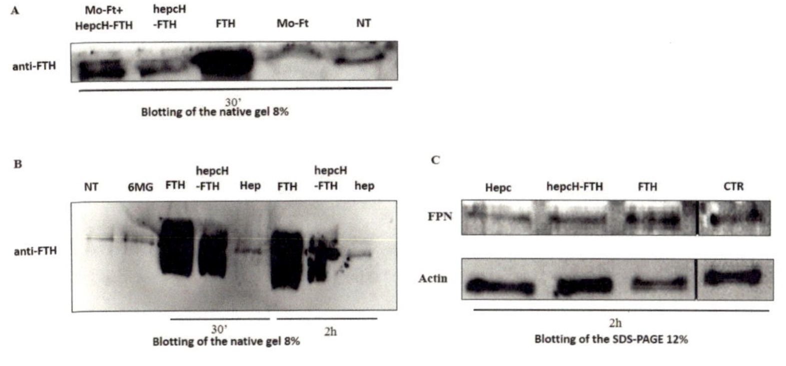

Figure 5.
(A) Western blot analysis of the J774 cells treated with mouse ferritin (Mo-Ft), FTH, human hepcidin-25 and HepcH-FTH heteropolymer using anti-FTH antibodies (rHo2). Lane 1, cells treatment with 0.5 μM Mo-Ft and HepcH-FTH; lane 2, cells treatment with 0.5 μM FTH; lane 3, cells treatment with 0.5 μM Mo-Ft; lane 4, untreated cells. (B) Western blot analysis of the J774 cells treated with 0.5 μM HepcH-FTH heteropolymer and FTH, using anti-FTH antibodies (rHo2). Lane 1, non-treated cells; lane2, cells treated with 6 M guanidine; lane 3, cells treated with 0.5 μM FTH for 30'; lane 4, cells treated with 0.5 μM HepcH-FTH for 30'; lane 5, cells treated with human hepcidin for 30 min; lane 6, cells treated with FTH for 2 h; lane 7, cells treated with HepcH-FTH for 2 h; lane 8, cells treated with human hepcidin for 2 h. (C) Western blotting analysis of the SDS-PAGE of cell lysates using polyclonal anti-rabbit ferroportin antibody. CTR: Untreated cells. FTH: Cells treatment with 0.5 μM native FTH for 2 h. HepcH-FTH: Cells treatment with 0.2 μM HepcH-FTH (with molar ration of 1:5) for 2 h. Hepc: Cells treatment with 0.5 μM synthetic human hepcidin-25 for 2 h. non-adjacent bands, from the same blot, were denoted by vertical black lines.

(**Figure 5C**). Indeed, the level of ferroportin in the J774 cells decreased, as it occurred in the cells treated with the synthetic hepcidin, while the incubation with FTH had no evident effect. This indicates that heteropolymer is biologically functional. Consequently, folded camel hepcidin activity against FPN1 could be enhanced thanks to its exposition, through its N-terminal part, at the H-ferritin surface nanocage [16]. This will probably offer a tool for a detailed study of the events after ferroportin binding the hepcidin. The heavy ferritin iron core and the fate of iron will facilitate the monitoring of the process.

As perspectives, the examination of the chronic effect of the purified heteropolymer injections on liver iron accumulation in a mouse model of hereditary hemochromatosis could be monitored. Indeed, hepcidin-1 knockout mice (hepc1$^{-/-}$) can be used, as a model, to eliminate any possibility of endogenous hepcidin contributing to the regulation of iron loading. This strategy can also be developed by producing ferritin subunits carrying other functionalities or epitopes, in order to have multifunctional complexes. Moreover, involving the approach can be applied for other peptides/hormones for the design of 'smart' molecular systems programmed to allow the transport in the body of potent anticancer agents in an innocuous manner toward safe tissues. Thus, these hybrid molecules will be useful for future therapeutic applications to improve health and life quality of a great number of patients with iron disorders or cancer diseases.

4. Conclusion

Ferritin is a well-known molecule with enormous potentiality in biotechnology. It has been already used to encapsulate molecules, as contrast in MRI and to carry epitopes. This chapter offers an original strategy to design a new bifunctional hybrid protein, which can be proposed as a stable iron regulatory molecule or a drug-delivery agent. The results could be exploited by scientists to produce ferritin subunits carrying other functionalities or epitopes, in order to have multifunctional complexes. It can be a new platform with utmost importance in the field of cell and gene therapies.

Acknowledgements

Special thanks to Fernando Carmona, Maura Poli, Michela Asparti and Paola Ruzzenenti, from the Molecular Biology Laboratory, and to Alessandra Gianoncelli and Michela Bertuzzi, from the Proteomics Platform, at the Department of Molecular and Translational Medicine, University of Brescia, Viale Europa 11, Brescia, Italy for their valuable contribution to this work since 2014. Great recognition to Institut Pasteur de Tunis, Université Tunis El Manar, 13, place Pasteur. BP. 74, Tunis, 1002, Tunisia for the payment of the publication fees of this chapter.

Conflict of interest

Authors declare that they have no conflict of interest.

Abbreviations

HepcH	fusion camel hepcidin-human ferritin H-chain subunit
FTH	human ferritin H
HepcH-FTH	24-mer heteropolymer comprising camel hepcidinhuman ferritin H assembled with FTH

Author details

Mohamed Boumaiza[1,2*], Samia Rourou[1], Paolo Arosio[3]
and Mohamed Nejib Marzouki[2]

1 Biotechnology Development Unit, Laboratory of Molecular Microbiology, Vaccinology and Biotechnology Development, Institut Pasteur de Tunis, Université Tunis El Manar, 13, Place Pasteur. BP. 74, Tunis, 1002, Tunisia

2 Laboratoire d'ingénierie des Protéines et des Molécules Bioactives, Institut National des Sciences Appliquées et de Technologie (I.N.S.A.T.) BP 676, Cedex1080, Tunis, Tunisie

3 Molecular Biology Laboratory, Department of Molecular and Translational Medicine, University of Brescia, Viale Europa 11, Brescia, Italy

*Address all correspondence to: mohamed12boumaiza@gmail.com

References

[1] Uchida M, Flenniken ML, Allen M, Willits DA, Crowley BE, Brumfield S, Willis AF, Jackiw L, Jutila M, Young MJ, Douglas T. Targeting of cancer cells with ferrimagnetic ferritin cage nanoparticles. J Am Chem Soc. 2006 Dec 27;128(51):16626-33. doi: 10.1021/ja0655690. PMID: 17177411.

[2] Boumaiza M, Carmona F, Poli M, Asperti M, Gianoncelli A, Bertuzzi M, Ruzzenenti P, Arosio P, Marzouki MN (2017). Production and characterization of functional recombinant hybrid heteropolymers of camel hepcidin and human ferritin H and L chains. Protein Engineering, Design and Selection. 30:77-84, https://doi.org/10.1093/protein/gzw066.

[3] Jordan JB, Poppe L, Haniu M, Arvedson T, Syed R, Li V, Kohno H, Kim H, Schnier PD, Harvey TS, Miranda LP, Cheetham J, Sasu BJ. (2009). Hepcidin revisited disulfide connectivity dynamics and structure.J. Biol. Chem. 284: 24155-24167.

[4] Delaby,C., Pilard,N., Gonçalves,A.S., Beaumont,C. and Canonne,H.F. (2005) Blood, 106, 3979-3984.

[5] Boumaiza M, Poli M, Carmona F, Asperti M, Gianoncelli A, Bertuzzi M, Arosio P, Marzouki MN (2019). Cellular binding analysis of recombinant hybrid heteropolymer of camel hepcidin and human ferritin H chain. The unexpected human H-ferritin binding to J774 murine macrophage cells. Molecular Biology Reports https://doi.org/10.1007/s11033-019-05234-3.

[6] Jutz G, van Rijn P, Santos Miranda B, Böker A. Ferritin: a versatile building block for bionanotechnology. Chem Rev. 2015 Feb 25;115(4):1653-701. doi: 10.1021/cr400011b. Epub 2015 Feb 16. PMID: 25683244.

[7] Jeon JO, Kim S., Choi E., Shin K., Cha K., So IS, Kim SJ, Jun E., Kim D., Ahn HJ, Lee BH, Lee SH and Kim IS (2013). Designed Nanocage Displaying Ligand-Specific Peptide Bunches for High Affinity and Biological Activity. ACS NANO 7: 7462-7471.

[8] Krause A., Neitz S., Magert H.J., Schulz A., Forssmann W.G., Schulz K.P., Adermann K. (2000). LEAP-1, a novel highly disulfide bonded human peptide, exhibits antimicrobial activity. FEBS let. 480: 147-50.

[9] Park C.H., Valore E.V., Waring A.J., Ganz T. (2001). Hepcidin, a urinary antimicrobial peptide synthesized in the liver. J. Biol. Chem. 276: 7806-7810.

[10] Falzacappa M.V.V., Muckenthaler M.U. (2005). Hepcidin: iron-hormone and antimicrobial peptide. Gene, 364: 37-44.

[11] Preza GC, Ruchala P, Pinon R, Ramos E, Qiao B, Peralta MA, Sharma S, Waring A, Ganz T and Nemeth E (2011). Minihepcidins are rationally designed small peptides that mimic hepcidin activity in mice and may be useful for the treatment of iron overload. J Clin Invest. 121: 4880-4888.

[12] Gagliardo B, Faye A, Jaouen M, Deschemin JC, Cannone-Hergaux JF, Vaulont S, Sari MA (2008). Production of biologically active forms of recombinant hepcidin, the iron regulating hormone. FEBS J. 275: 3793-3803.

[13] Boumaiza M, Abidi S (2019). Chapter One - Hepcidin CDNA Evolution in Vertebrates. In Vitamins and Hormones; Litwack, G., Ed.; Iron Metabolism: Hepcidin; Academic Press, 2019; Vol. 110, pp 1-16. https://doi.org/10.1016/bs.vh.2019.01.001.

[14] Luscieti S, Santambrogio P, Langlois d'Estaintot B, Granier T,

Cozzi A, Poli M, Gallois B, Finazzi D, Cattaneo A, Levi S, Arosio P. Mutant ferritin L-chains that cause neurodegeneration act in a dominant-negative manner to reduce ferritin iron incorporation. J Biol Chem. 2010 Apr 16;285(16):11948-57. doi: 10.1074/jbc.M109.096404. Epub 2010 Feb 16. PMID: 20159981; PMCID: PMC2852932.

[15] Arosio P, Cozzi A, Ingrassia R, Levi S, Luzzago A, Ruggeri G, Iacobello C, Santambrogio P, Albertini A (1990) A mutational analysis of the epitopes of recombinant human H-ferritin. Biochim Biophys Acta 1039:197-203

[16] Kanekiyo M, Wei C-J, Yassine HM, McTamney PM, Boyington JC, Whittle JRR, Rao SS, Kong W-P, Wang L, Nabel GJ (2013) Self-assembling influenza nanoparticle vaccines elicit broadly neutralizing H1N1 antibodies. Nature 499:102-106.

Chapter 7

A Purpose-Built System for Culturing Cells as *In Vivo* Mimetic 3D Structures

Krzysztof Wrzesinski, Søren Alnøe, Hans H. Jochumsen, Karoline Mikkelsen, Torsten D. Bryld, Julie S. Vistisen, Peter Willems Alnøe and Stephen J. Fey

Abstract

Culturing cells in 3D is often considered to be significantly more difficult than culturing them in 2D. In practice, this is not the case: the situation is that equipment needed for 3D cell culture has not been optimised as much as equipment for 2D. Here we present a few key features which must be considered when designing 3D cell culture equipment. These include diffusion gradients, shear stress and time. Diffusion gradients are unavoidably introduced when cells are cultured as clusters. Perhaps the most important consequence of this is that the resulting hypoxia is a major driving force in the metabolic reprogramming. Most cells in tissues do not experience liquid shear stress and it should therefore be minimised. Time is the factor that is most often overlooked. Cells, irrespective of their origin, are damaged when cultures are initiated: they need time to recover. All of these features can be readily combined into a clinostat incubator and bioreactor. Surprisingly, growing cells in a clinostat system do not require specialised media, scaffolds, ECM substitutes or growth factors. This considerably facilitates the transition to 3D. Most importantly, cells growing this way mirror cells growing *in vivo* and are thus valuable for biomedical research.

Keywords: clinostat, functionality, hypoxia, spheroids and organoids, *in vivo* mimetic, culture time, minimisation of infections, direct observation, media change

1. Introduction

Cells are pre-programmed to carry out certain functions – this represents their potential. At the same time, they are sensitive to physical or biological changes in their surrounding environment and will modify their function accordingly – and this becomes their constantly changing actuality. Cells *in vivo* are surrounded by an extracellular matrix (ECM) and are actively communicating with other cells. This forms part of an active environment which modifies and integrates their activities.

In the early days of cell culture in the 1950's the focus was to get cells to propagate rapidly and reliably in flasks, facilitated by the destruction of their ECM. With the realisation that cells grown in 3D conditions are more mimetic of human cell biology, the focus has changed away from getting the cells to propagate to getting the cells to function (physiologically). These two conditions mark the extremes in a spectrum of cellular activity [1].

Bearing this in mind, there are a number of factors that should be considered when changing this focus and transitioning from the classical 2D cell culture to 3D cell culture. These factors not only indicate which 3D culture systems could be expected to be advantageous over others but also indicate which should generate data that is more representative of the *in vivo* performance of such cells.

Perhaps, the most significant difference between 2D and 3D culture is the establishment of longer diffusion gradients for the majority of cells and thus the cells will experience significantly different levels of oxygen, CO_2, nutrients and waste products.

Related to the diffusion gradients is the amounts of various compounds in the environment around cells: cells in 2D are typically exposed to levels of for example O_2 and glucose which are not seen in the intact, healthy organism.

Another very significant difference will be the establishment of channels of communication between cells that are not only juxtapositioned but also further away. In 2D, immortal cells are typically passaged roughly every week (and shorter for faster growing cells). At the end of this cycle, cells are usually treated with enzymes or cocktails (containing trypsin, collagenases or other compounds) that damage proteins protruding from the plasma membrane and which dissolve or fragment the ECM. Similar cocktails may be used to produce cell suspensions from tissue biopsies, or these biopsies may be pressed through a mesh to 'liberate' cells. All these treatments release proapoptotic factors, damage cells and have a significant impact on gene expression. Cells will attempt to repair this damage and recover, but need time to do so. So, the final factor to consider is time.

While there are numerous publications illustrating that 3D cell culture can mimic functionalities of human tissues, perhaps one of the most graphic is shown in **Figure 1** where a freshly extirpated human liver biopsy and 29 day old C3A spheroids have been biosynthetically labelled with $[^{35}S]$-methionine and their proteins extracted and run on high resolution two-dimensional gels (IPG-SDS). Notice that, not only are the proteins expressed in very similar amounts, but also that their post-translationally modifications are very similar.

For many purposes in medical research, what is needed is a model system that accurately reflects what happens in the living organism - more often than not a human being – to shed light on many different processes, whether normal physiology or what goes wrong in disease, or infections by microorganisms, or the effects of compounds during treatment or poisoning.

3D cell culture promises to offer what is needed, but the field is still relatively new and many of the products used are small modifications of existing products that have been available for many years and as such, many have not been ideally suited to the purpose.

2. A purpose-built system for culturing cells

For these reasons, when we started to design some equipment specifically designed to support 3D cell culture. In doing so, we used four aims to guide the process. These were:

1. Use *in vivo* functionality as a yardstick

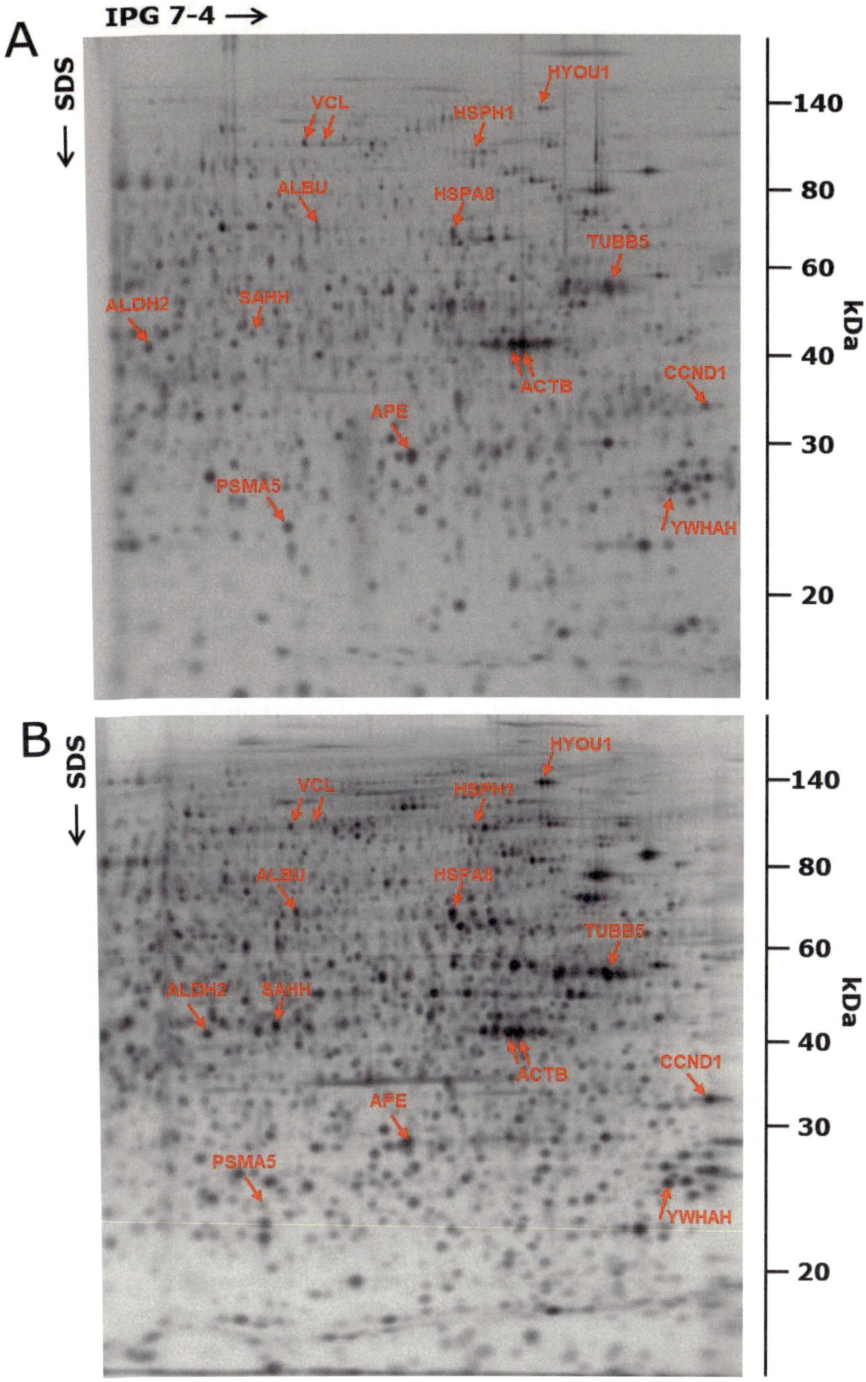

Figure 1.
Human biopsy tissue (ca. 0.5 mm^3) and spheroids (29 day-old, ca. 1 mm^3) were biosynthetically labelled for 20 hrs with [^{35}S]-methionine. Some of the proteins are named for reference: ACTB, Actin beta; ALBU, Albumin; ALDH2, Aldehyde dehydrogenase 2; APE, Apolipoprotein E; CCND1, Cyclin D; HSPA8, Heat shock protein 8; HSPH1, Heat shock protein H1; HYOU1, Hypoxia up-regulated protein 1; PSMA5, Proteasome subunit alpha type-5; SAHH, S-adenosyl-L-homocysteine hydrolase; TUBB5, Tubulin beta chain 5; VCL, Vinculin; YWHAH, 14–3-3 protein eta. The tissue was homogenised, freeze dried, redissolved in lysis buffer and analysed by 2DGE according to [2]. Images were collected using AGFA phosphorimager plates and reader. [^{35}S]-methionine labelled (A) human liver and (B) C3A spheroids.

2. Allow the cells to do what they want. Do not provide unnecessary compounds and do not stress them in any unphysiological way.

3. Keep the culture conditions as close to that seen *in vivo* as is practical.

4. Keep it simple (both for the cells and the user).

The main requirements that we addressed were: diffusion gradients, shear stress and time.

2.1 Diffusion gradients

Atmospheric oxygen (21%) provides a partial pressure (pO_2) of about 145 mm Hg (ca. 190 μM) to cells grown in 2D cultures. This is considerably more than the partial pressure of oxygen measured in tissues (11% to 0.1%) which should be considered as normoxic for cell culture [3]. Thus, cells grown in 2D cultures are exposed to unphysiological, hyperoxic conditions.

In the human body cells are usually located within 200 μm of a capillary [4] (corresponding to only 10 to 40 cell layers thick). Because cells are actively consuming oxygen, there will be a diffusion gradient into the cell. This is not problematic in 2D because the cultures are typically only one cell layer thick, but it becomes a challenge in 3D because there the spheroids can become tens or hundreds of cell layers thick. Despite that there may be a preferential transport of oxygen through cells and tissues by hydrophobic channelling within membranes, suggesting that oxygen diffusion within cells and tissues may be faster than through water, there will clearly be a limit [5].

In seminal work, Sutherlands group clearly demonstrated that the pO_2 in the centre of a spheroid fell to 0% when the radius was greater than 250 μm, corresponding quite well with the *in vivo* measurements [6]. The oxygen diffusion gradient started considerably outside of spheroids (ca. 100–200 μM) and continued to fall to the centre of the spheroid. They showed that this was an oxygen diffusion-depletion zone surrounding the spheroid and that in it the partial oxygen pressure fell by one third.

A flow of media past a spheroid significantly reduced this zone and had a very significant effect on the oxygenation of the spheroid. This allowed the spheroids to become larger before their cores reached anoxia. The beneficial effect of flow was almost completely negated if the spheroid was resting on a gas impermeable surface (e.g. glass or a gas-impermeable membrane) [6]. Spheroids appear to have a large capacity to adapt and significantly reduce their consumption when the supply of either O_2 or glucose or both is restricted [7–9].

Interestingly, hepatocytes, (which express haemoglobin *in vivo*), when grown as spheroids, massively overexpress (x30) haemoglobin, presumably to assist with oxygen transport into the oxygen depleted core [1]. Based on the changes in protein expression seen as cells recover their tissue mimetic metabolic equilibrium, it has been proposed that one of the strongest forces driving this recovery process which re-establishes the *in vivo* phenotype is hypoxia (affecting proteins like HIF 1 alpha (the main hypoxia sensor) and HYOU1 (a stress-responsive protein - see **Figure 1**)) [9]. The oxygen gradient formed has also been shown to have a marked effect on the formation of hepatic zonation during the differentiation of human embryonic stem cells and thus there will be a gradient of differences in metabolic enzymes into the spheroid [10].

Exactly the same arguments apply to CO_2: it has been demonstrated that CO_2 (as HCO_3^-) diffuses through spheroids of many cell types essentially as if the cells are not there [11]. Cells in clusters increase their aerobic respiration and decrease

DOI: http://dx.doi.org/10.5772/intechopen.96091

oxidative phosphorylation as they reprogram to a more anabolic based metabolism. This reduces their need for O_2 and their production of CO_2. Although this was first noted by Warburg in relation to cancer [12], it probably more strongly reflects the effects of 'mis-culture' of tumour cells in 2D rather than a metabolic style reflective of tumours *in vivo*.

Interestingly the rate of glucose diffusivity through spheroids of different cell types has been shown to differ by a factor of up to 4. The diffusion into a spheroid is quite rapid and an equilibrium is established after about 1 hour (single cells reach this equilibrium within a minute) [13]. These differences may be correlated to how tightly connected the cells become. C3A spheroids have been shown to rapidly deplete normoglycaemic media (5.5 mM) of glucose within 8 hours, converting much of it to glycogen. The cells were then able to reconvert the glycogen to glucose and survive for the next 40 (or 64 hrs) hrs until the next media exchange [9].

Diffusion gradients will also apply to nutrients and waste products. For example, NH_3 is produced by transamination followed by deamination, from biogenic amines and purine and pyrimidine bases. NH_3 (as NH_4OH) is a smaller and less lipophilic molecule and thus its diffusivity five times slower than CO_2 through cells than through pure water at 37 °C making it more difficult to 'escape' [11].

The conclusions are clear for 3D cell culture: without a vasculature, cell clusters should not be too big in order to avoid anoxia (and ensuing necrosis) and should be irrigated on all sides to diminish the depletion zone and accelerate gas, substrate and metabolite exchange.

2.2 Shear stress

There is a growing appreciation that the mechanical properties and cell mechanics, play an important role in gene expression and cell development. The concept that is emerging is that cell types which experience shear stress *in vivo*, (usually fluid movement induced) actually need the stress to differentiate correctly (and retain their differentiation) and that shear stress is detrimental to cells that are not naturally exposed *in vivo* [14].

Thus, in some cases shear stress is positive: see-saw shaking of induced pluripotent stem cell (iPSC) constructs for 17 days promoted cell aggregation, and induced significantly higher expression of chondrogenic-related marker genes than observed in static cultures [15]. A platform rocking at 7 ° with a 3 second cycle results in an average shear stress of about 0.01 Pascal [16]. These shear forces are however distributed unevenly – both spatially and temporally during the motion of the container (bag, or flask) [17]. A similar, ultra-low shear stress is also seen in clinostat cultures. In this case though, the shear stress is distributed essentially homogeneously spatially and temporarily throughout the culture [9].

Fluid-induced shear stress (ca. 0.02–0.06 Pa) in microfluidic devices *in vitro* increased the mechanical properties of neocartilage [18] and have been shown to be beneficial for several epithelial or endothelial cell layers (as seen in ducts, blood vessels and the kidney) [19, 20].

Stirred tank suspension bioreactors and orbital shakers are used widely [21–23] but both result in significantly higher shear forces (0.3–0.66 Pa and 0.6–1.6 Pa respectively) and are considered to be in the critical/lethal range for mammalian cells [24].

Since most cells are found in tissues which experience very little shear stress, equipment that is designed to cultivate cells from these tissues should expose cell clusters to as little shear stress as possible. It is easier to reintroduce shear stress if needed, than to struggle to remove it from a system not designed to be shear stress free.

2.3 Time

As mentioned above, enzymatic treatment of tissues or cells in 2D damages both the ECM and surface located proteins (including their modifications). This raises a number of questions.

The first is as to whether this damage can be repaired, i.e. can the 3D cultures recover the metabolic or physiological properties that they exhibited *in vivo* in the living organism. *In vivo* performance thus becomes an important benchmark – even though it may be very difficult to measure.

If the damage cannot be repaired, then the question raised is whether this failure is due to a limitation of the cells used, whether several cell types are needed, whether the procedures used prevent the recovery, or whether it is a true limitation that the performance cannot be replicated *in vitro*. Answering this question could therefore require a great deal of research. Fortunately, it appears that often the damage can be repaired.

If it can, the next question is how long do cells need to repair this damage?

A final question is that if the damage can be repaired, then once the cells have recovered, how stable is the 3D culture, i.e. for how long can the 3D culture be used?

The answer to these questions depends very much on the origin of the cells. For immortal cells, there are now numerous publications suggesting that these cells need to grow as spheroids for at least 2 weeks to recover their *in vivo* functionality [25–27]. Stem cells, including induced pluripotent stem cells appear to need a wide variety of times – some need only a few days while others never fully recover *in vivo* functionality [27, 28]. As a general rule primary cells seem to retain (most of) their functionality but use some of their mortal time to re-establish partial tissue organisation [29–31].

One observation that appears to be true for the majority of cells, irrespective of their origin, is that they grow considerably much slower as spheroids or organoids as they do in 2D cultures. Thus, doubling times in 3D may be as long as every 50 or 100 days rather than the 1 to 2 days seen in 2D [32, 33]. This makes sense: tissues and tumours *in vivo* do not double in volume every day or even every week. In other words, cells grown in 2D *in vitro* do not represent either their parental tissue or the tumour from which they were isolated. For example, the HepG2 cell line has a doubling time of 1.4 days [8] compared to 135 days for an average hepatocellular carcinoma [34] and approximately 327 days for liver hepatocytes [35].

Starting with isolated cells in culture, it is necessary therefore to anticipate that the cells need to re-adapt to being in clusters once again. There is a lot that needs to occur in such a readaptation process: for example, isolated cells do not have tight junctions and so their import and export pumps will have mixed: and need to be 're-deployed' to different regions of the plasma membrane once tight junction has been re-established [36]. While this is critically important for most cells, the specialisation of pumps in the liver cells is exquisite and intricate [37]. Redeployment of pumps might not be an active process – the cell after all was not designed to work in 2D cultures. Hence, the cell may have to rely on protein turnover to degrade the misplaced pumps and on membrane delivery processes to establish the pumps on the correct sides of the tight junctions. And there are innumerable other redeployments (changes to the cytoskeleton [1], organelle organisation, gene and protein expression, epigenetic marking [38], post-translational modifications and metabolic reprogramming [8, 9]) to complete.

The take home message here is that researchers have to be much more patient and expect that they will need to maintain 3D cultures for extended periods of time (weeks or months). With this in mind, these extended periods will place a premium on cultures that are highly reproducible and preferably also high yield. Cultures that reach and maintain a dynamic equilibrium for weeks or months will be advantageous in that they will mimic the homeostasis seen in tissues and will provide a large window of utility. Within this window, it will be possible to for example collect multiple samples from the same culture (like collecting biopsies from the same animal at different times) or perform repeated treatment studies [39]. These samples could be used for the same assay at different times or multiple different assays at the same time, or both if there is sufficient biomass available. But the stability of the biological process needs to be documented throughout this window before perturbation experiments can be initiated [32, 40].

Maintaining cultures for extended times greatly increases the risk of infections, and thus requires great care. This can be facilitated if all aspects of a 3D culture system have to be considered so that the culture is well protected from external contamination.

3. A clinostat incubator

So – what does a cell culture system that addresses all of these issues look like?

First it is a CO_2 incubator. The incubator constructed can maintain a steady temperature both over time and within its volume. The inclusion of a powerful fan to mix the air within the incubator ensures no differences in temperature or gas partial pressures (and speed temperature recovery after the door has been opened). Measurements show that the difference in temperature between the top of the chamber and the bottom are less than 0.2 °C.

Figure 2 illustrates that the incubator quickly reaches running conditions after about 15 minutes when it is first switched on and that it can maintain a steady temperature and CO_2 % (in the figure, over 12 hrs).

When the door is opened, the controlling software switches off the fan, heaters and the UV-C lamp (if active) and closes the CO_2 valve. Closing the door reactivates these functions. **Figure 3** illustrates the effect of opening the door wide open (90 °) for respectively either 30 seconds or two minutes showing that running conditions are re-established by about 4 or 6 minutes.

Note that the internal temperature in the culture vessel falls by a maximum of only 0.1 °C while the door is open illustrating that the cultures are not exposed to any cold shock which would affect their gene expression.

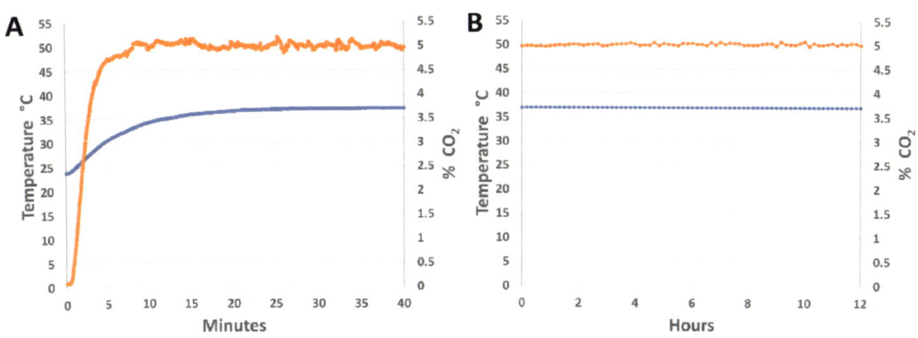

Figure 2.
% CO_2 ● and temperature ● levels at (A) initial start up and (B) during a 12 hour period. Measurements were collected using the internal sensors.

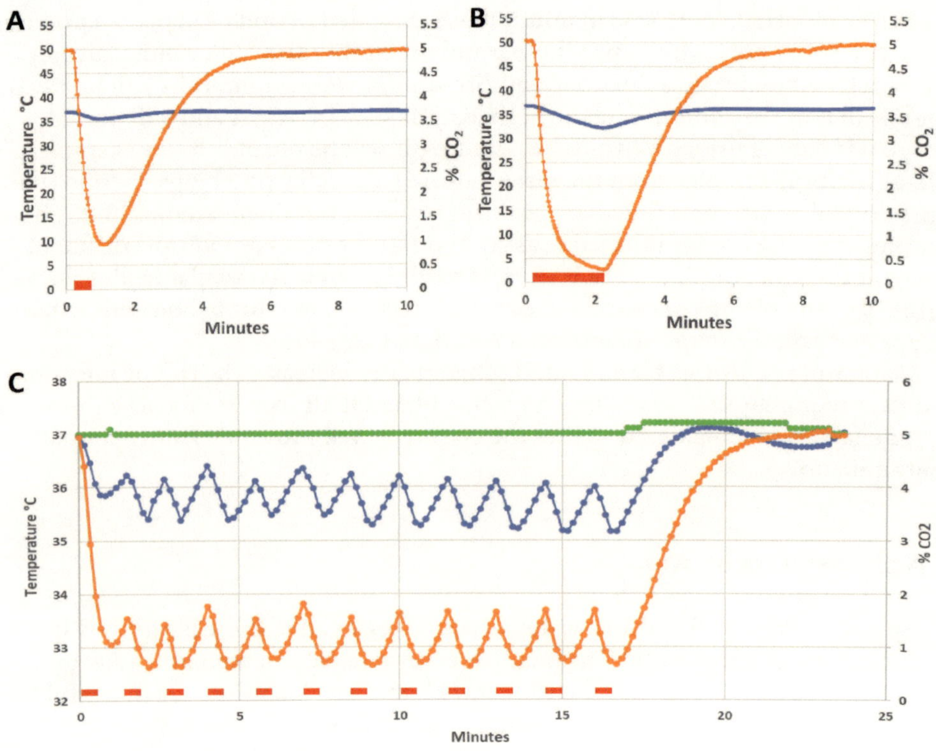

Figure 3.
The effect on CO_2 % ● and temperature ● levels of opening the door to 90 ° for either 30 seconds or 2 minutes (as indicated by the red bars). C) Illustrates the effect on the temperature inside a culture vessel ● of changing the media in the 6 cultures (open door for 30 seconds to take out the culture vessel, 1 minute to change the media, 30 seconds to return the vessel, 1 minute to prepare the sterile bench for the next vessel – All repeated 6 times) Measurements were collected using the internal sensors and an external thermocouple inside a culture vessel.

4. Clinostat technology

In order to reduce the diffusion depleted zone to a minimum, we have adopted the clinostat technology. Introduced for cell culture more than 20 years ago, this technology has been used to culture hundreds of different types of cells and tissues (cell lines, stem cells, primary cells) as well as bacteria and viruses and produced some excellent research. The major limitation of the initial equipment was that it was difficult to use (for example the culture chamber could not be opened but had to be accessed via luer lock ports).

Basically, a clinostat keeps cell clusters in suspension by rotating the culture vessel in a vertical direction (like a wheel). At the right speed, the uplift caused by the effect of liquid viscosity between the vessel and the clusters is balanced by the effect of gravity (these systems are often referred to as 'simulated microgravity' because the clusters appear to float or be maintained in a 'stationary orbit' (relative to the culture vessel)). Thus, the incubator that has been built has been equipped with clinostat motors. These have to run very smoothly so that there is no vibration (which would otherwise shake the clusters apart). **Figure 4** A) would reveal 50/60 Hz mains 'noise' effects while B) would reveal high frequency noise.

To retain 'continuity' with previously published data, we have maintained the basic geometry of the culture chamber.

The next requirement is to be able to open the culture vessel easily for the purpose of introducing or removing cell clusters, for changing the media, or adding compounds or collecting samples.

Figure 5 illustrates a culture vessel with a top access port for media exchange, a front access port for collecting individual cell clusters, and front window that can be removed to reveal a petri-dish like 10 mL culture chamber.

Changing the growth media is illustrated in the video (https://bit.ly/2PkiE9m). The culture chamber is removed from the incubator and the spheroids are allowed to sink to the bottom. The top port plug is removed and 90–95% of the media is sucked away using a sterile syringe and long needle. Fresh media is introduced in the same way, making sure to overfill the growth chamber so that any bubbles are driven into the 'drip-cup' around the top port. The plug is then replaced, the drip cup emptied,

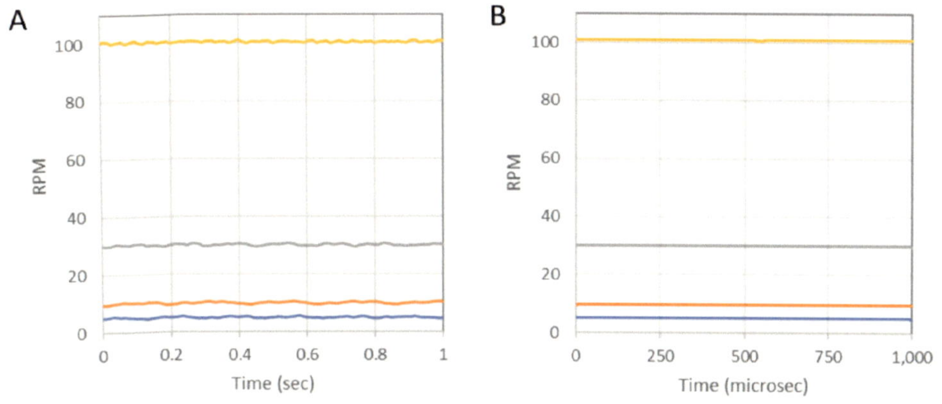

Figure 4.
Variations in the rotational speed of a clinostat motor. (A) Long term variations during 1 second: RPM (± STD) 5.03 ± 0.210; 10.03 ± 0.277; 30.21 ± 0.278; 100.38 ± 0.224. (B) Sort term variations during one thousandth of a second. RPM (± STD) 5.12 ± 0.002; 9.82 ± 0.004; 30.13 ± 0.008; 100.66 ± 0.007. The Permanent Magnet Synchronous Motor (PMSM) used for the clinostat was loaded with a dummy inertia block to mimic the weight of the full culture vessel and run with an Odrive V3.6 motor drive and controller software with anticogging feature. A TLE5012B encoder and digital oscilloscope (Picoscope 2200) was used to measure rpm, Measurements were made each microsecond.

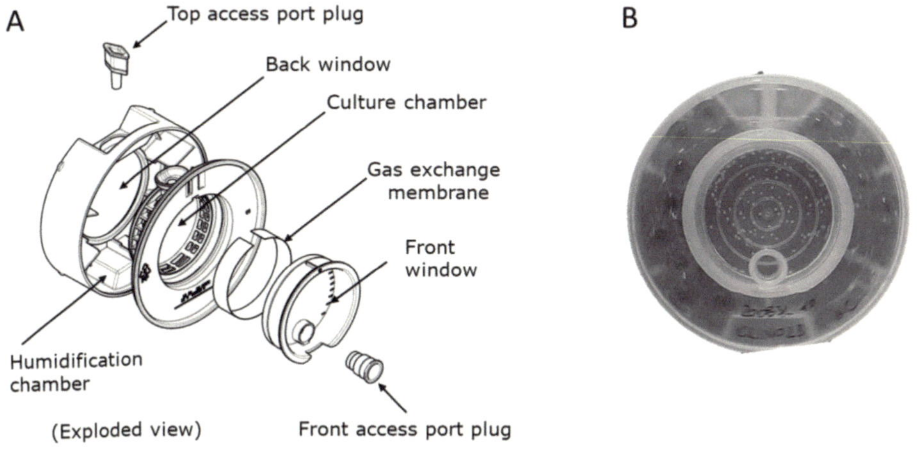

Figure 5.
A culture vessel designed to provide easy access to the culture chamber. (A) Exploded view of parts. (B) Front view showing spheroids in the culture chamber (white spots).

washed with 70% ethanol for sterility and the culture vessel replaced in the clinostat incubator. The whole procedure takes less than 40 seconds, resulting in minimal stress for the cell clusters (a video of this can be seen on CelVivo's website). Small samples of the media can be collected at any time using the same approach.

In this design (**Figure 5**), the gas exchange membrane has been moved from its 'cylinder end' position to a circumferential 'side' position whilst still retaining essentially the same area to allow rapid gas exchange between the culture chamber and the humidification chamber. Relocating the gas exchange membrane allows the culture chamber to be illuminated from the back and observed from the front (using the cameras), facilitating inspection of the clusters without disturbing the culture, or even opening the incubator door. This also helps to minimise infection risks.

5. Humidification

Most incubators are humidified with water trays or tanks, which usually increase the relative humidity close to 100% to prevent cultures from losing water and concentrating the media. This is fortunate because CO_2 normally does not transverse dry membranes very readily. By hydrating the atmosphere, CO_2 can dissolve into the water vapour (giving H_2CO_3) and then diffuse easily across the membrane [41].

Unfortunately, the combination of high humidity and the warm temperatures inside an incubator are strongly conducive to infections and so regular thorough cleaning is necessary to prevent contamination of the cultures.

Microbial infection can be mitigated if the humidification of the incubator chamber can be reduced. For that reason, a culture vessel has been designed that can humidified itself. This permits the incubator to be run in a 'dry state' (i.e. with only ambient humidity). Assuming that the air around the incubator contains 40% relative humidity, (at 20 °C and normal pressure), then when this air enters the incubator and is warmed up to 37 °C, its relative humidity will fall to 13.9% making microorganism growth more difficult.

The culture vessel is humidified by placing water beads in a circumferential chamber around the gas exchange membrane and allowing air exchange into this

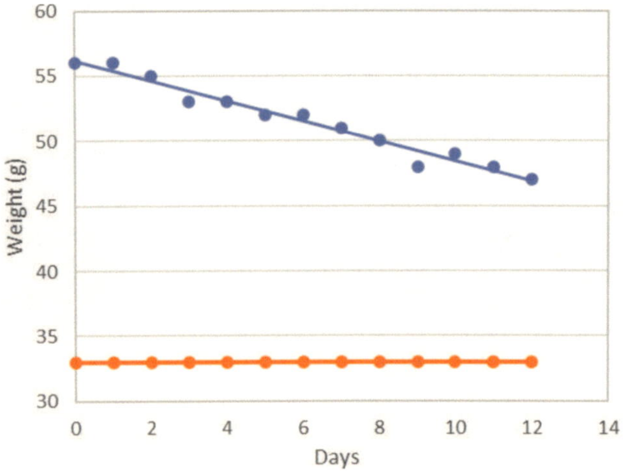

Figure 6.
Loss of water from water beads in a culture vessel in a clinostat incubator at 37 °C. Two culture vessels, one containing hydrated water beads (blue line) and the other containing unhydrated beads (orange line) were rotated at 20 rpm in a clinostat incubator at 37 °C and weighed on a daily basis.

chamber. In use, the hydrated beads release water linearly with time to the atmosphere (1 mL water gives about 1.67 L water vapour) and maintain a very high humidity close to the membrane and facilitating gas exchange (**Figure 6**).

6. Illumination and visualisation

The circumferential position of the gas exchange membrane facilitates another feature of the culture chamber. Because there is nothing on either planar side of the vessel, it is possible to provide uniform illumination from one side and observe the culture from the other side. Fey *et al.* demonstrated that photographs of spheroids in culture could be used to determine the amount of soluble protein (or DNA or number of cells) by measuring their shadow area and using a look-up table [39, 42]. Thus, if the culture chamber is uniformly illuminated from one side and a camera is placed on the other side (**Figure 7**), it is possible to measure the sizes of the clusters without removing them from the incubator.

Even though most modern incubators have a double door, with the inner door made of glass, it is difficult to see the cell clusters clearly often because of poor illumination. The use of an integrated back-light and a camera to inspect the cultures brings yet another advantage: it is not necessary to open the incubator to see the cultures. If these shadow area measurements are repeated over time it becomes possible to follow the growth curve of the clusters. The only manipulation required is to change the media (typically this would be every 2–3 days). If the media is changed for example on a 2, 2 and 3 day (weekly) cycle, then the incubator will need to be opened only 10 times during a 21 day culture. Since a practiced person can change the media within 1 minute each time, this means that the cells need to be out of the incubator for less than 10 minutes in the 21 day period.

Thus, the construction using illumination and a camera for each cell culture vessel minimises the number of times that the incubator needs to be opened. This in turn further reduces the risk of infection, in addition to the effect gained by running the incubator 'dry'.

An extra source of illumination has been included on the same side as the camera so that it is possible to see the clusters by direct inspection and not just their silhouettes.

All of the images are displayed on (and can be captured from) a tablet that also serves to regulate the temperature, CO_2 and rpm of the culture vessels (**Figure 8**).

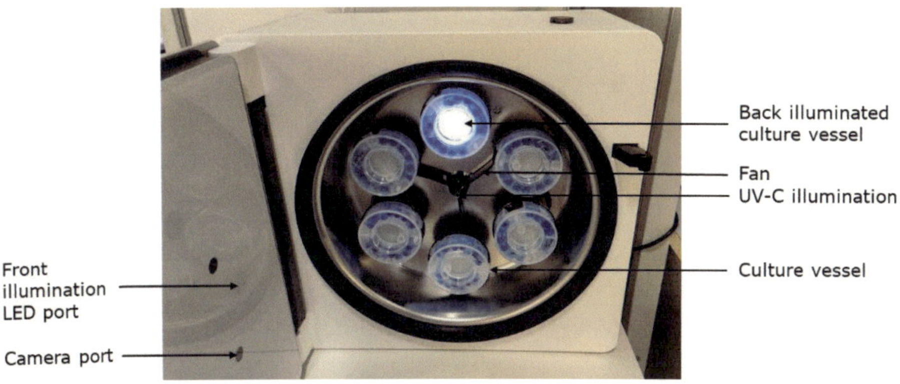

Figure 7.
A clinostat incubator, containing 6 culture vessels (one back illuminated).

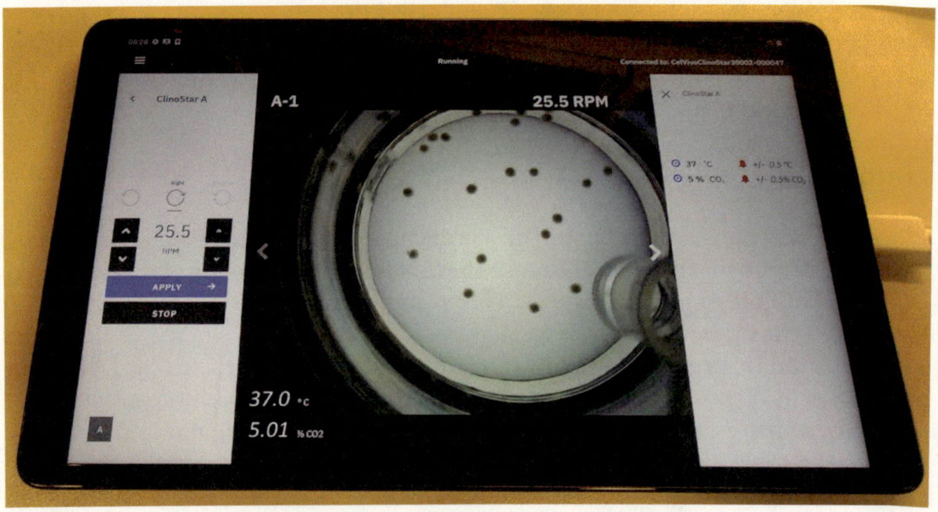

Figure 8.
The tablet display showing regulation of the rpm and set value (left panel), culture vessel (main panel), clinostat incubator number (A-1, main panel top left), actual rpm (top right), actual temperature and CO_2 (bottom left). The front access port plug can be seen at the bottom right of the culture vessel.

7. Decontamination

One final step has been taken to reduce the risk of microorganism contamination even further. A UV-C light has been built into the incubator. The UV-C LED source itself is behind the bowl of the incubator but the UV-C light is led out through a fused silica light guide which passes along the shaft of the fan. UV-C capture from the LED was calculated to be 88%. By terminating the light guide in an arrow shape (with angles of 52 and 56 °), the emitted UV-C sweeps the incubator as the fan rotates. Normally, UV-C light reflectance from stainless steel is usually about 5% but this has been increased to about 75% by using a special ePTFE coating. Thus, the UV-C irradiation is reflected in all directions and will reach all surfaces. All clinostat motors are activate during decontamination so that all sides of the culture vessel holder will also be irradiated. The inner surface of the glass door is assumed to be totally absorbing for the UV-C. According to the specifications of the LED lamp, the UV-C light emitted will provide a dose of at least 12 mJ/cm^2 everywhere in the incubator after 2 hours. This results in a log4 reduction (99.99% reduction) in viable bacteria. A log6 reduction is normally defined as sterile for medical facilities (and therefore this is classified only as a decontamination).

8. Yield and variability

One easy way to initiate spheroid cultures is to use embryoid body plates (**Figure 9**).

Here, cells are centrifuged into the bottom of inverted square-based pyramid micro-indentations in microtitre plate wells. Not surprisingly, the spheroids are somewhat squarish immediately after their release from the embryoid body plate and there is quite a lot of loose cells (seen most clearly in the 'Day 0 and 2' image in **Figure 9**).

These loose cells do not sediment down as quickly as the spheroids and thus are lost during successive media changes. The remaining spheroids become steadily

DOI: http://dx.doi.org/10.5772/intechopen.96091

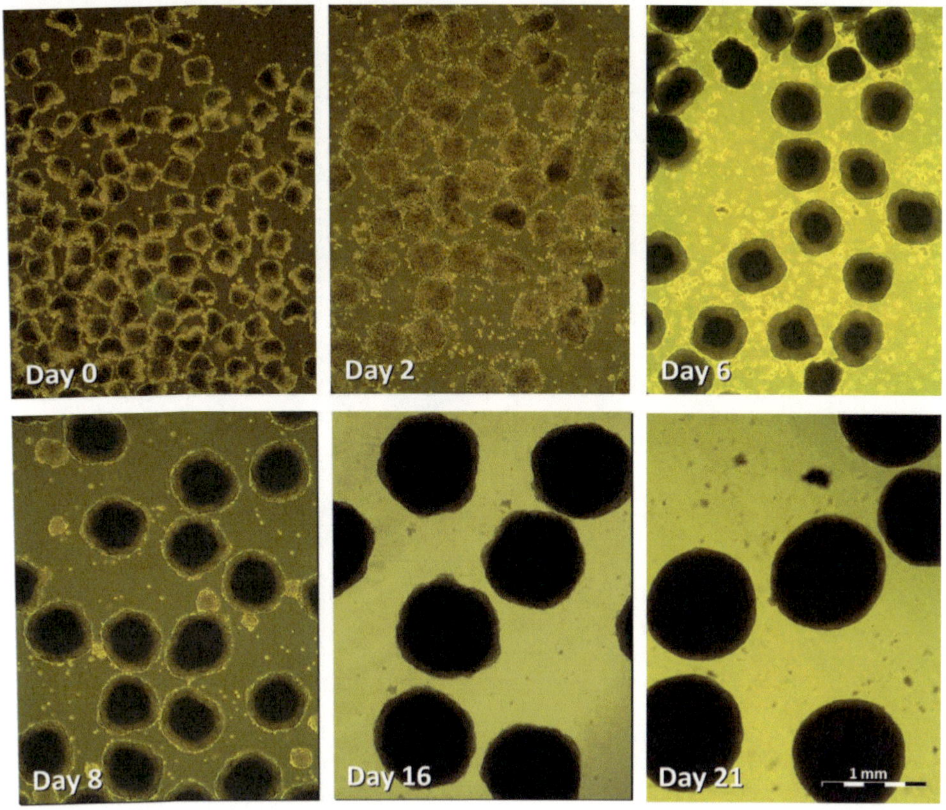

Figure 9.
C3A spheroids at various times. C3A cells (800 cells per well) are left overnight in an embryoid body plate to form a cluster and are released on day 0 and then cultured in DMEM containing 5% foetal bovine serum in a non-humidified clinostat incubator at 37 °C and 5% CO_2/95% air for the number of days shown. The same magnification has been used for all images and the scale bar in the bottom corner illustrates 1 mm.

rounder and more robust as they grow. Starting from a single embryoid body plate well, these procedures have been shown to produce large numbers of spheroids (about 1200) similar to those shown in **Figure 9** after 21 days (these would normally be cultured in four culture vessels). At this stage, each spheroid contains about 82,300 cells and contains 12.31 μg protein (C3A spheroids). The standard deviation of their diameters is less than 21% (after 21 days in culture) and this approach thus provides large numbers of very reproducible spheroids for further experimentation [39, 43].

Once C3A spheroids have recovered, they reach a metabolic equilibrium, characterised by a constant production of ATP, cholesterol and urea for at least 24 days [32]. During this period, treatment of these spheroids with for example any one of six commonly used drugs (acetaminophen (APAP), amiodarone, diclofenac, metformin, phenformin and valproic acid) causes them to respond (as shown by the increase in ATP production) and then recover to the pre-treatment conditions [43]. This can be repeated multiple times and has been proposed to be useful for assessing repeated-dose drug toxicity [39].

The liver is the primary source of many of the proteins found in the blood. To illustrate just how stable C3A spheroids are, they have been kept alive for 302 days. Even after this length of time C3A spheroids are quite capable of synthesising and post translationally modifying these blood proteins (**Figure 10**).

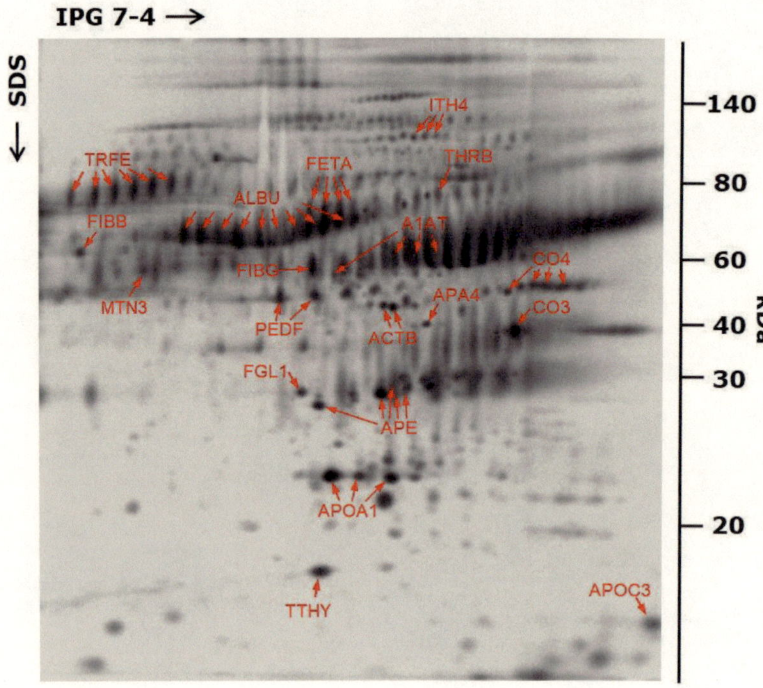

Figure 10.
Proteins secreted from 302 day old C3A spheroids. Some of the proteins are named for reference: ACTB, actin beta; ALBU, albumen; APA4, apolipoprotein a I; APA4, apolipoprotein a IV; APOC3, apolipoprotein C III; APOE, apolipoprotein E, CO3 complement C3 alpha; CO4 complement C4; FETA Foetal albumen; FGL1, fibrinogen-like protein 1; FIBB, fibrinogen beta; FIBG, fibrinogen gamma; ITH4, inter alpha trypsin inhibitor heavy chain 4; MTN3, Matrilin3; PEDF, pigment epithelium derived factor; THRB, prothrombin; TRFE, Serotransferrin; TTHY, transthyretin. 302 day old C3A spheroids were biosynthetically labelled for 20 hrs with [^{35}S]-methionine in order to be able to distinguish newly synthesised proteins from proteins present in the media. The whitish vertical streaks above ALBU indicate the presence of unlabelled BSA. Proteins in the growth media were collected by precipitation, washed, freeze dried, redissolved in lysis buffer and analysed by 2DGE according to [2]. Images were collected using AGFA phosphorimager plates and reader.

9. Applications

Already 8 years ago, clinostat spheroids constructed from C3A cells were shown to be more effective of predicting drug toxicity than primary human hepatocytes *in vitro* [43] and much of the data obtained since has been summarised from a biotransformation and toxicity perspective [44]. 3D spheroid cultures of primary human hepatocytes in chemically defined conditions have been used to evaluate the hepatotoxicity of 123 drugs in clinical drug induced liver injury (DILI) [45]. This has been followed by a demonstration that the system is a good candidate for determining repeated-dose toxicity (i.e. to detect accumulative toxicity) [39, 40].

C3A spheroids have also been used to reveal novel signalling pathways involved in drug treatment (acetaminophen) [46].

Currently one of the major weakness of testing for genotoxicity is the inability of indicator cells to express metabolic enzymes needed for the activation and detoxification of genotoxic compounds *in vitro*. C3A spheroids, cultivated in a clinostat system have been shown to express higher levels of these key metabolic enzymes from phase I and II, as well as DNA damage responsive genes. This suggests that this system can contribute significantly to a more reliable assessment of the genotoxic activities of both pure chemicals, and complex environmental samples. The system has been shown to be sensitive enough to detect genotoxicity even at the very low concentrations relevant to typical environmental exposure situations [47].

Herbal medicines are often assumed to be safe because they are 'natural products', despite the lack of data. To reduce the cost and accelerate their testing, a C3A 3D spheroid model has been developed and benchmarked against Sprague Dawley rats to test one of the most widely used extracts, (*Xysmalobium undulatum*, commonly known as Uzara). The results showed comparable toxicological data [48].

Heteromeric proteins from spheroids even been used as an internal quality control for proteomic data [49].

Epigenetic marking and histone clipping have been shown to be recovered in spheroids [38] and this has been shown to occur during intestinal differentiation *in vivo* [50]. Metabolic reprogramming,which may be a key change during cancer development is also demonstrated in 3D spheroids [9]. The cell line LS180 is a very appropriate cell line for studying colorectal cancer, having been very gently developed but its application suffers from the fact that the cells do not readily form spheroids or organoids. This has recently been overcome by encapsulating the LS180 cells in sodium alginate. These spheroids were shown to respond to standard chemotherapeutic drug, paclitaxel at expected concentrations and even show the development of resistance often seen *in vivo* during paclitaxel treatment. The LS180 alginate spheroids are now being used to screen for novel chemotherapeutic compounds for colorectal cancer [51]. Similar studies have shown that pitavastatin can inhibit stem cell proliferation in colon carcinoma [52].

Spheroids and organoids are being used to investigate the self-organisation of multicellular tissues [53]. Human induced pluripotent stem cells (hiPS cells) have been used to generate neural spheroids that contain oligodendrocytes, neurons and astrocytes [28] and to mimic the blood brain barrier [54]. Primary and stem cells have been used to recapitulate the intricate pattern and functionality of pancreatic islets, working towards regenerative medicine for diabetes [55]. Progress is also being made towards producing transplantable photoreceptor precursors using pluripotent stem cell-derived retinal organoids to treat retinal degeneration diseases [56].

Bacterial-host interactions during Salmonella infections are being studied using iPSCs organoids and stem cell enteroids to mimic the intestinal villus and crypt [57].

Multicellular, physiologically active organotypic cultures are being use to study a wide variety of human viral pathogens with a view to pre-clinical evaluation of vaccines, antivirals and therapeutics [58].

Clinostat cultures are also being used in bone research. Low dietary intake of both vitamin D and K is negatively associated with fracture risk, often seen in persons suffering from osteoporosis. Treatment of primary human osteoblasts (hOBs) 3D multicellular spheroids with a combination of vitamin D and K, enhanced gene expression of periostin and collagen (COL-1), as well as inducing extended osteoid formation. The two vitamins apparently affected bone mechanical properties differently: vitamin D enhancing stiffness and K2 conveying flexibility to bone. It is anticipated that the combination of these effects may translate to increased fracture resistance *in vivo* [59].

10. Conclusions

Clinostat bioreactors systems clearly provide readily controllable 3D cell culture conditions, needing small amounts of cells, media or other compounds and provide sufficient cellular material for a wide variety of assays. The culture vessels and clinostat incubator described here, would be beneficial for many *in vitro* cellular models.

The advantages of culture stability for months, its reproducibility and the possibility to treat and then see the response and recovery (if necessary, for multiple times on the same culture) offer a great potential for future research. The novel equipment described here, will facilitate this research.

Furthermore, the fact that the clinostat system does not require changes in media, the use of scaffolds or special growth factors will not only facilitate the transition from other systems to this clinostat approach but will also allow the cells to respond in their own natural pre-programmed manner.

Thanks to 3D cell culture, the border between basic research and clinical applications is dissolving – and this new era of self-assembling tissue mimetic structures requires a new range of purpose-built equipment.

Conflict of interest

The authors are all employees of CelVivo ApS.

Notes

The culture vessel and clinostat incubator illustrated in this chapter are sold under the ClinoReactor® and ClinoStar® trade names by CelVivo ApS.

Video materials

Video materials referenced in the text are available at: https://bit.ly/2PkiE9m.

Author details

Krzysztof Wrzesinski, Søren Alnøe, Hans H. Jochumsen, Karoline Mikkelsen, Torsten D. Bryld, Julie S. Vistisen, Peter Willems Alnøe and Stephen J. Fey*
CelVivo ApS, Odense, Denmark

*Address all correspondence to: sjf@celvivo.com

References

[1] Wrzesinski K, Rogowska-Wrzesinska A, Kanlaya R, Borkowski K, Schwammle V, Dai J, Joensen KE, Wojdyla K, Carvalho VB, Fey SJ (2014) The Cultural Divide: Exponential Growth in Classical 2D and Metabolic Equilibrium in 3D Environments. PLoS One 9 (9):e106973. doi:10.1371/journal.pone.0106973

[2] Fey SJ, Larsen PM (2001) 2D or not 2D. Two-dimensional gel electrophoresis. Curr Opin Chem Biol 5 (1):26-33. doi:10.1016/s1367-5931(00)00167-8

[3] Carreau A, El Hafny-Rahbi B, Matejuk A, Grillon C, Kieda C (2011) Why is the partial oxygen pressure of human tissues a crucial parameter? Small molecules and hypoxia. J Cell Mol Med 15 (6):1239-1253. doi:10.1111/j.1582-4934.2011.01258.x

[4] Carmeliet P, Jain RK (2000) Angiogenesis in cancer and other diseases. Nature 407 (6801):249-257. doi:10.1038/35025220

[5] Dotson RJ, Smith CR, Bueche K, Angles G, Pias SC (2017) Influence of Cholesterol on the Oxygen Permeability of Membranes: Insight from Atomistic Simulations. Biophysical journal 112 (11):2336-2347. doi:10.1016/j.bpj.2017.04.046

[6] Mueller-Klieser WF, Sutherland RM (1982) Influence of convection in the growth medium on oxygen tensions in multicellular tumor spheroids. Cancer research 42 (1):237-242

[7] Mueller-Klieser W, Freyer JP, Sutherland RM (1986) Influence of glucose and oxygen supply conditions on the oxygenation of multicellular spheroids. British journal of cancer 53 (3):345-353. doi:10.1038/bjc.1986.58

[8] Cassim S, Raymond VA, Dehbidi-Assadzadeh L, Lapierre P, Bilodeau M (2018) Metabolic reprogramming enables hepatocarcinoma cells to efficiently adapt and survive to a nutrient-restricted microenvironment. Cell cycle 17 (7):903-916. doi:10.1080/15384101.2018.1460023

[9] Wrzesinski K, Fey SJ (2018) Metabolic Reprogramming and the Recovery of Physiological Functionality in 3D Cultures in Micro-Bioreactors. Bioengineering (Basel) 5 (1). doi:10.3390/bioengineering5010022

[10] Tonon F, Giobbe GG, Zambon A, Luni C, Gagliano O, Floreani A, Grassi G, Elvassore N (2019) In vitro metabolic zonation through oxygen gradient on a chip. Sci Rep 9 (1):13557. doi:10.1038/s41598-019-49412-6

[11] Hulikova A, Swietach P (2014) Rapid CO2 permeation across biological membranes: implications for CO2 venting from tissue. Faseb J 28 (7):2762-2774. doi:10.1096/fj.13-241752

[12] Warburg O (1956) On the origin of cancer cells. Science 123 (3191):309-314. doi:10.1126/science.123.3191.309

[13] Casciari JJ, Sotirchos SV, Sutherland RM (1988) Glucose diffusivity in multicellular tumor spheroids. Cancer research 48 (14):3905-3909

[14] Li W, Li P, Li N, Du Y, Lu S, Elad D, Long M (2020) Matrix stiffness and shear stresses modulate hepatocyte functions in a fibrotic liver sinusoidal model. Am J Physiol Gastrointest Liver Physiol. doi:10.1152/ajpgi.00379.2019

[15] Limraksasin P, Kosaka Y, Zhang M, Horie N, Kondo T, Okawa H, Yamada M, Egusa H (2020) Shaking culture enhances chondrogenic differentiation of mouse induced pluripotent stem cell constructs. Sci Rep 10 (1):14996. doi:10.1038/s41598-020-72038-y

[16] Tsai AC, Liu Y, Yuan X, Chella R, Ma T (2017) Aggregation kinetics of human mesenchymal stem cells under wave motion. Biotechnology journal 12 (5). doi:10.1002/biot.201600448

[17] Kalmbach A, Bordas R, Oncul AA, Thevenin D, Genzel Y, Reichl U (2011) Experimental characterization of flow conditions in 2- and 20-L bioreactors with wave-induced motion. Biotechnology progress 27 (2):402-409. doi:10.1002/btpr.516

[18] Salinas EY, Aryaei A, Paschos N, Berson E, Kwon H, Hu JC, Athanasiou KA (2020) Shear stress induced by fluid flow produces improvements in tissue-engineered cartilage. Biofabrication 12 (4):045010. doi:10.1088/1758-5090/aba412

[19] Thuenauer R, Rodriguez-Boulan E, Romer W (2014) Microfluidic approaches for epithelial cell layer culture and characterisation. Analyst 139 (13):3206-3218. doi:10.1039/c4an00056k

[20] Arora S, Lam AJY, Cheung C, Yim EKF, Toh YC (2019) Determination of critical shear stress for maturation of human pluripotent stem cell-derived endothelial cells towards an arterial subtype. Biotechnol Bioeng 116 (5):1164-1175. doi:10.1002/bit.26910

[21] Naing MW, Williams DJ (2011) Three-dimensional culture and bioreactors for cellular therapies. Cytotherapy 13 (4):391-399. doi:10.3109/14653249.2011.556352

[22] van Putten S, Shafieyan Y, Hinz B (2016) Mechanical control of cardiac myofibroblasts. J Mol Cell Cardiol 93:133-142. doi:10.1016/j.yjmcc.2015.11.025

[23] Melke J, Zhao F, van Rietbergen B, Ito K, Hofmann S (2018) Localisation of mineralised tissue in a complex spinner flask environment correlates with predicted wall shear stress level localisation. European cells & materials 36:57-68. doi:10.22203/eCM.v036a05

[24] Croughan MS, Wang DI (1991) Hydrodynamic effects on animal cells in microcarrier bioreactors. Biotechnology 17:213-249. doi:10.1016/b978-0-409-90123-8.50015-x

[25] Ferruzza S, Rossi C, Scarino ML, Sambuy Y (2012) A protocol for differentiation of human intestinal Caco-2 cells in asymmetric serum-containing medium. Toxicol In Vitro 26 (8):1252-1255. doi:10.1016/j.tiv.2012.01.008

[26] Wrzesinski K, Fey SJ (2013) After trypsinisation, 3D spheroids of C3A hepatocytes need 18 days to re-establish similar levels of key physiological functions to those seen in the liver. Toxicology Research 2 (2):123-135. doi:10.1039/c2tx20060k

[27] Costantini D, Overi D, Casadei L, Cardinale V, Nevi L, Carpino G, Di Matteo S, Safarikia S, Valerio M, Melandro F, Bizzarri M, Manetti C, Berloco PB, Gaudio E, Alvaro D (2019) Simulated microgravity promotes the formation of tridimensional cultures and stimulates pluripotency and a glycolytic metabolism in human hepatic and biliary tree stem/progenitor cells. Sci Rep 9 (1):5559. doi:10.1038/s41598-019-41908-5

[28] Marton RM, Miura Y, Sloan SA, Li Q, Revah O, Levy RJ, Huguenard JR, Pasca SP (2019) Differentiation and maturation of oligodendrocytes in human three-dimensional neural cultures. Nat Neurosci 22 (3):484-491. doi:10.1038/s41593-018-0316-9

[29] Wang Q, Wang K, Solorzano-Vargas RS, Lin PY, Walthers CM, Thomas AL, Martin MG, Dunn JCY (2018) Bioengineered intestinal muscularis complexes with long-term spontaneous and periodic

contractions. PLoS One 13 (5):e0195315. doi:10.1371/journal.pone.0195315

[30] Haigh CL (2017) Cellular Analysis of Adult Neural Stem Cells for Investigating Prion Biology. Methods Mol Biol 1658:133-145. doi:10.1007/978-1-4939-7244-9_11

[31] Park TI, Schweder P, Lee K, DieriksBV,JungY,SmythL,RustenhovenJ, Mee E, Heppner P, Turner C, Curtis MA, Faull RLM, Montgomery JM, Dragunow M (2020) Isolation and culture of functional adult human neurons from neurosurgical brain specimens. Brain Commun 2 (2):fcaa171. doi:10.1093/braincomms/fcaa171

[32] Wrzesinski K, Magnone MC, Visby Hansen L, Kruse ME, Bergauer T, Bobadilla M, Gubler M, Mizrahi J, Zhang K, Andreasen CM, Joensen KE, Andersen SM, Olesen JB, O.B. SdM, Fey SJ (2013) HepG2/C3A 3D spheroids exhibit stable physiological functionality for at least 24 days after recovering from trypsinisation. Toxicology Research 2 (3):163-172. doi:10.1039/c3tx20086h

[33] Bressan E, Ferroni L, Gardin C, Pinton P, Stellini E, Botticelli D, Sivolella S, Zavan B (2012) Donor age-related biological properties of human dental pulp stem cells change in nanostructured scaffolds. PLoS One 7 (11):e49146. doi:10.1371/journal.pone.0049146

[34] Nathani P, Gopal P, Rich N, Yopp A, Yokoo T, John B, Marrero J, Parikh N, Singal AG (2020) Hepatocellular carcinoma tumour volume doubling time: a systemic review and meta-analysis. Gut. doi:10.1136/gutjnl-2020-321040

[35] Seim I, Ma S, Gladyshev VN (2016) Gene expression signatures of human cell and tissue longevity. NPJ Aging Mech Dis 2:16014. doi:10.1038/npjamd.2016.14

[36] Alrefai WA, Gill RK (2007) Bile acid transporters: structure, function, regulation and pathophysiological implications. Pharm Res 24 (10):1803-1823. doi:10.1007/s11095-007-9289-1

[37] Walsh DR, Nolin TD, Friedman PA (2015) Drug Transporters and Na+/H+ Exchange Regulatory Factor PSD-95/Drosophila Discs Large/ZO-1 Proteins. Pharmacol Rev 67 (3):656-680. doi:10.1124/pr.115.010728

[38] Tvardovskiy A, Wrzesinski K, Sidoli S, Fey SJ, Rogowska-Wrzesinska A, Jensen ON (2015) Top-down and middle-down protein analysis reveals that intact and clipped human histones differ in post-translational modification patterns. Molecular & cellular proteomics : MCP. doi:10.1074/mcp.M115.048975

[39] Fey SJ, Korzeniowska B, Wrzesinski K (2020) Response to and recovery from treatment in human liver-mimetic clinostat spheroids: a model for assessing repeated-dose drug toxicity. Toxicol Res (Camb) 9 (4):379-389. doi:10.1093/toxres/tfaa033

[40] Fey SJ, Wrzesinski K (2013) Determination of Acute Lethal and Chronic Lethal Dose Thresholds of Valproic Acid Using 3D Spheroids Constructed from the Immortal Human Hepatocyte Cell Line HepG2/C3A. Valproic Acid. Nova Science Publishers, Inc, New York

[41] Pinnau I, Toy LG (1996) Gas and vapor transport properties of amorphous perfluorinated copolymer membranes based on 2,2-bistrifluoromethyl-4,5-difluoro-1,3-dioxole/tetrafluoroethylene. Journal of Membrane Science 109:125-133. doi:10.1016/0376-7388(95)00193-X

[42] Fey SJ, Wrzesinski K (2013) Microgravity spheroids as a reliable, long-term tool for predictive toxicology.

Toxicol Lett 221S:S153. doi:/10.1016/j.toxlet.2013.05.318

[43] Fey SJ, Wrzesinski K (2012) Determination of drug toxicity using 3D spheroids constructed from an immortal human hepatocyte cell line. Toxicol Sci 127 (2):403-411. doi:10.1093/toxsci/kfs122

[44] Calitz C, Hamman JH, Fey SJ, Wrzesinski K, Gouws C (2018) Recent advances in three-dimensional cell culturing to assess liver function and dysfunction: from a drug biotransformation and toxicity perspective. Toxicology mechanisms and methods 28 (5):369-385. doi:10.1080/15376516.2017.1422580

[45] Vorrink SU, Zhou Y, Ingelman-Sundberg M, Lauschke VM (2018) Prediction of Drug-Induced Hepatotoxicity Using Long-Term Stable Primary Hepatic 3D Spheroid Cultures in Chemically Defined Conditions. Toxicol Sci 163 (2):655-665. doi:10.1093/toxsci/kfy058

[46] Wojdyla K, Wrzesinski K, WilliamsonJ,FeySJ,Rogowska-Wrzesinska A (2016) Acetaminophen-induced S-nitrosylation and S-sulfenylation changes in 3D cultured hepatocarcinoma cell spheroids. Toxicology Research 5:905-920. doi:10.1039/c5tx00469a

[47] Stampar M, Sedighi Frandsen H, Rogowska-Wrzesinska A, Wrzesinski K, Filipic M, Zegura B (2020) Hepatocellular carcinoma (HepG2/C3A) cell-based 3D model for genotoxicity testing of chemicals. Sci Total Environ:143255. doi:10.1016/j.scitotenv.2020.143255

[48] Calitz C, Hamman JH, Fey SJ, Viljoen AM, Gouws C, Wrzesinski K (2019) A sub-chronic Xysmalobium undulatum hepatotoxicity investigation in HepG2/C3A spheroid cultures compared to an in vivo model. J Ethnopharmacol 239:111897. doi:10.1016/j.jep.2019.111897

[49] Rogowska-Wrzesinska A, Wrzesinski K, Fey SJ (2014) Heteromer score-using internal standards to assess the quality of proteomic data. Proteomics 14 (9):1042-1047. doi:10.1002/pmic.201300457

[50] Ferrari KJ, Amato S, Noberini R, Toscani C, Fernandez-Perez D, Rossi A, Conforti P, Zanotti M, Bonaldi T, Tamburri S, Pasini D (2021) Intestinal differentiation involves cleavage of histone H3 N-terminal tails by multiple proteases. Nucleic acids research. doi:10.1093/nar/gkaa1228

[51] Smit T, Calitz C, Willers C, Svitina H, Hamman J, Fey SJ, Gouws C, Wrzesinski K (2020) Characterization of an Alginate Encapsulated LS180 Spheroid Model for Anti-colorectal Cancer Compound Screening. ACS medicinal chemistry letters 11 (5):1014-1021. doi:10.1021/acsmedchemlett.0c00076

[52] Zhang ZY, Zheng SH, Yang WG, Yang C, Yuan WT (2017) Targeting colon cancer stem cells with novel blood cholesterol drug pitavastatin. Eur Rev Med Pharmacol Sci 21 (6):1226-1233

[53] Toda S, Blauch LR, Tang SKY, Morsut L, Lim WA (2018) Programming self-organizing multicellular structures with synthetic cell-cell signaling. Science 361 (6398):156-162. doi:10.1126/science.aat0271

[54] Bergmann S, Lawler SE, Qu Y, Fadzen CM, Wolfe JM, Regan MS, Pentelute BL, Agar NYR, Cho CF (2018) Blood-brain-barrier organoids for investigating the permeability of CNS therapeutics. Nature protocols 13 (12):2827-2843. doi:10.1038/s41596-018-0066-x

[55] Dayem AA, Lee SB, Kim K, Lim KM, Jeon TI, Cho SG (2019) Recent advances in organoid culture for insulin production and diabetes therapy: methods and challenges. BMB Rep 52 (5):295-303

[56] Llonch S, Carido M, Ader M (2018) Organoid technology for retinal repair. Dev Biol 433 (2):132-143. doi:10.1016/j.ydbio.2017.09.028

[57] Yin Y, Zhou D (2018) Organoid and Enteroid Modeling of Salmonella Infection. Front Cell Infect Microbiol 8:102. doi:10.3389/fcimb.2018.00102

[58] Ramani S, Crawford SE, Blutt SE, Estes MK (2018) Human organoid cultures: transformative new tools for human virus studies. Curr Opin Virol 29:79-86. doi:10.1016/j.coviro.2018.04.001

[59] Schroder M, Riksen EA, He J, Skallerud BH, Moller ME, Lian AM, Syversen U, Reseland JE (2020) Vitamin K2 Modulates Vitamin D-Induced Mechanical Properties of Human 3D Bone Spheroids In Vitro. JBMR Plus 4 (9):e10394. doi:10.1002/jbm4.10394

Chapter 8

Current Scenario of Regenerative Medicine: Role of Cell, Scaffold and Growth Factor

Nilkamal Pramanik and Tanmoy Rath

Abstract

Impairment of the clinical tissue-implantation is due to the lack of a suitable organ donor and immunogenic rejection, which leads to the cause for the enormous loss of human life. The introduction of artificial regeneration of tissues by Langer and Vacanti in 1993, has revolutionized in the field of surgical organ transplantation, to alleviate the problem of tissue injury-related death. There is no doubt that the term "regenerative medicine" to open a new space of tissue reconstruction, but the complications that arise due to the proper machinery of the cell, supporting biomaterials and growth factors has yet to be resolved to expand its application in a versatile manner. The chapter would provide a significant overview of the artificial tissue regeneration while a triangular relationship between cells, matrixes, and growth factors should be established mentioning the necessity of biomedical tools as an alternative to organ transplantation.

Keywords: biomaterials, biocompatibility, extracellular matrix, therapeutic molecules, regenerative medicine

1. Introduction

Advances in biomaterials are implicated in the huge results as the artificial support matrices penetrate the barrier of all physicochemical properties in clinical tissue implantation, an artifact of regenerative tissue engineering applications. Unlike traditional tissue grafting, the artificial implanting process involves the replacement of any damaged tissues irrespective of age, diseases, and kinds of trauma. Based on the potential requirements, efforts in different fields that include material science, cell biology, medicine, theory and computational studies represent a versatile contribution in regenerative medicine to save thousands of lives. The preliminary idea of tissue engineering is to reconstruct the traditional surgical or mechanical device-related techniques; those though significantly prevented the untimely demises of lives. The time on demand of available organ donors and appropriate complimentary biological environments are implemented in the term 'Tissue Engineering' (TE) in 1933 by Langer and Vacanti [1]. TE is the versatile gift of scientists who have greatly remodeled and mimicked the *in vivo* biological niche through a combination of engineered biomaterials, cells of interest and biochemical factors, which are important factors for tissue development. The manufacture of the implantation of the desired shape is the key factor in TE, which could support seeding of isolated cells, cell–cell interaction, and its proliferation and migration. The cell adhesion and secretion of extracellular matrixes (ECM) are switched through growth factor-mediated signaling pathways [2]. The growth factors are the class of cytokines, at the basis of cell attachment, proliferation and migration in tissue regeneration, remodeling and other various cellular functions [3, 4]. Epithelial growth factors (EGFs), platelet-derived growth factors (PDGFs), insulin-like growth factors (IGFs), and hematopoietic cell growth factors (HCGFs) are promising types of cytokines that have played a significant role in tissue engineering.

The new generation of biomaterials has revolutionized the fields of regenerative medicine while, the development of 3D architecture could enable us to mimic the ideal *in vivo* tissue organoid. Other important parameters of the supporting scaffolds include the porosity, biodegradability, biocompatibility and good carrier of the therapeutic molecules, immobilized onto the matrixes. Due to intrinsic biological characteristics, both synthetic and natural materials have been investigated to formulate the three-dimensional support structure, but the requirements related to microbial resistance, genotoxicity, and mechanical strength remain to be questioned. Collagen, gelatin, hyaluronic acid, alginate, guar gum, chitosan, polyhydroxyalkanoates are the well-known naturally originated, biocompatible and biodegradable polymers, which have emerged as a bio-mimicking matrixes in the development of artificial 3D construct, but their mechanical as well as hydrophilicity limited its unique usages. The drawback is significantly erased by the appearance of biosynthetic technology. In particular, the discovery of carbon compounds such as carbon nanotubes, graphene oxide nanoparticles, etc., has revolutionized the fields of tissue engineering. The additional biocompatibility, antimicrobial activity and mechanical stability of such compounds are considered to fabricate the bioimitating 3D construct. Furthermore, synthetic materials such as poly (lactide-coglycolide) and poly (ethylene glycol) play an important role in the construction of the ideal scaffold [5, 6].

The challenge in tissue regeneration is the seeding of cells. The risk factors such as *in vivo* immune-rejection, viral or microbial contaminations, processing of clean healthy cells are the main obstacles in choosing of the desired cells. Keeping in mind, the allogeneic cells, i.e., cells from a healthy person is considered for the several tissue regeneration systems. A variety of stem cells has been an essential and elementary option for the *in vitro* cell growth in the regeneration of cartilage tissues [7]. Nevertheless, an ideal scaffold with interconnected porous networks, proper mechanically and biologically appropriate engineering should lead to ECM secretion with prominent adhesion, and cell transduction and proliferation are best suited for tissue engineering applications.

This chapter will explore the sources of the 3D polymer construct and its validity in the biological niche, i.e. biocompatibility and cell motility through different growth factors.

2. Why is the 3D construct in tissue regeneration (TE)?

In tissue engineering, the assessment of cell compatibility is evaluated in a *"in vitro"* model of either 2D or 3D based on the results of optimal support arrays in which cells must continually increase their colonies as the native tissue environment as shown in **Figure 1**. The trafficking of therapeutic delivery in several cases is to get rid of all kinds of forthcoming issues. Therefore, it must circumvent these obstacles by taking into account various facts such as the extracellular matrix density, the nature of the cell-tissue interaction, and the penetration of nano carriers through

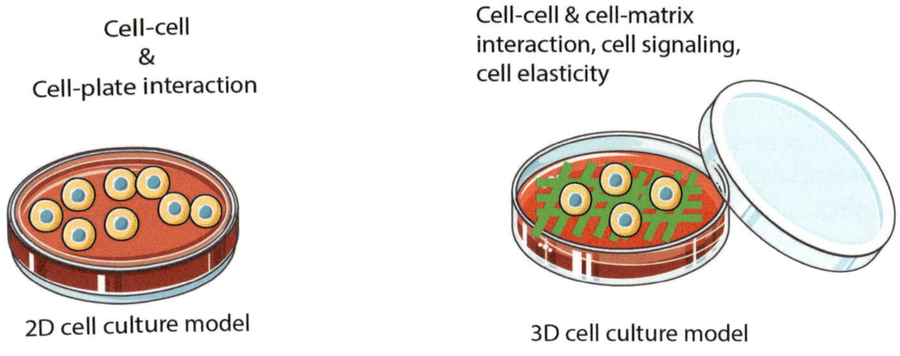

Figure 1.
Schematic comparison of 2D and 3D cell culture model.

tissue layers, etc. In 2D cell culture, the cells are grown, adhered to flat polystyrene surfaces in a thin monolayer's manner. The proliferation, migration, epigenetic and genetic expressions are varied as compared to *in vivo* tissue regeneration. Cell attachments and motility also constraint within monolayer frames and are exposed to unlimited nutrient sources. The two-dimensional culture is related to an easy and cost-effective process. However, it deprives the study of cell–cell interaction, cell-matrix interaction, cell signaling, and the nature of cell elasticity, which promotes the usefulness of the biological niche, i.e. the 3D construct.

Unlike 2D model, 3D constructs regulate the cell growth and proliferation in heterogeneity similar to *in vivo* tissue as the exposure of growth factors, oxygen, nutrients distributed unevenly in the scaffold or any other 3D construction. The cell morphology as well as the cell polarity is maintained because it greatly controls the cell-signaling, cell topology and various metabolic activities [8, 9]. However, culturing in 3D models is a lengthy and expensive process and is formulated in several ways: 3D spheroid where cells spend their survival time in layers, mimicking the correct cell–cell and cell-matrix interaction as in the environment of native tissue. The identification of biomarkers and the expression of genes that are involved in topological processes as well as the polarity changes of cancer cells are examined in the spheroid models [10]. Furthermore, it is expected that the adherence and proliferation of primary cells follow all the characteristics of *in vivo* tissue processes [11]. The 3D scaffolding systems, made of biodegradable and biocompatible materials, have demonstrated superior cell migration, proliferation through a network of porous 3D microenvironments [12]. In view of the significant advantages, the utility of bio-imitating 3D constructs is however encompassed in the niche of tissue regeneration though; 2D cell culture is still used as a reliable method before initiating the animal studies.

3. Choice of material in artificial supporting matrixes

The involvement of suitable materials, whether synthetic or naturally extracted in the fabrication of the artificial tissue environment, remains a challenge. The prerequisite in the development of 3D constructs includes biocompatibility, biodegradability, mechanical strength, interconnected and antimicrobial porous mechanical strength, antimicrobial and interconnected porous networks in which cellular activities could be performed analogously to their native tissue domicile. Taking into account the fact that biomaterials that actually contain the structural component or similar biochemical and physicochemical identity of native tissue have been granted for the processing of the platform in support of artificial cells. Meanwhile, the involvement of any unique material may or may not be able to create the imitation of equivalent tissues requires a broad understanding of the cell-matrix interaction. Therefore, the role of the combination of materials is considered as the essential means to overcome all the barriers that include bioactivity, biodegradability, microbial contamination and maximum mechanical flexibility which contribute as a key to tissue engineering.

3.1 Impact of naturally sourced biomaterials on cell-cell cross-talk

Mimicking of biological tissue environment using collagen is an attractive theme, which is due to the inherent features such as fibrous structure, biocompatibility and low antigenicity. However, the improvement of mechanical stability and biodegradability requires additional treatment that includes cross-linking or chemical modification in the presence of second party molecules. The approaches of modification of different natural biopolymer and its tuning into desired artificial tissue architecture that support the adhesion, proliferation, and migration of cells in biological niche are discussed here.

3.1.1 Collagen as base material and its derivatives

Collagen is a key component in extracellular matrixes and composed of RGD (arginine–glycine–aspartic acid) domains that plays a potential role in cell adhesion, growth and motility through its interaction with cells. But, the drawback due to poor mechanical stability and biodegradation is overcome by the modification with various natural polymers or synthetic polymers. In one approach, collagen molecules were chemically conjugated with oxidized guar gum to immobilize platelet-derived growth factor [13]. The guar gum which is a water soluble and ionic polysaccharide was oxidized to poly(dialdehyade) guar gum in presence of sodium periodate. The resultant oxidized guar gum not only promoted the cross-linking of collagen molecules but also helped to immobilize the platelet-derived growth factor, enabling the formation of biologically active hybrid 3D scaffolds with excellent swelling, thermal and biodegradable properties. FTIR, SEM analysis was performed to confirm the synthesis of the hybrid structure. SEM morphology revealed the interconnected 3D porous honeycomb structure with an average pour size of 15 ± 7 μm. The hybrid scaffold was shown to promote the release of growth factors with the increase of NIH 3 T3 cell density and proliferation and was seen as a promising candidate for tissue engineering applications.

Recently, Diogo et al. developed a method of fabrication of '*in situ*' mineralized collagen based 3D printed hydrogel. As an alternative to various traditional approaches, Co-precipitation method is used to mineralize the collagen fiber in presence of calcium chloride ($CaCl_2$) and ammonium hydrogen phosphate [$(NH_4)_2HPO_4$]. To prepare the cell laden 3D printed hydrogel, variuos raio's of mineralized collagen and alginate (a biocompatible and degradable natural polymer) mixture was treated with incubated L929, mouse fibroblast cell line and printed using a bioprinter V1 (REGEMAT 3D, Granada, Spain), resulted the cell laden 3D printed bi-oink. The cell-laden scaffold was shown to support the adhesion, growth and survival of mouse fibroblast cell line [14]. The similar kind of the cell-laden-collagen core and alginate-polyethylene oxide shell based 3D porous structure was developed using microfluidic channel and at low temperature working condition for cryopreservation (**Figure 2A**) which is subjected to maintain the shortage of cells, tissue and organs. The *in vitro* assays of two days cryo-preserved

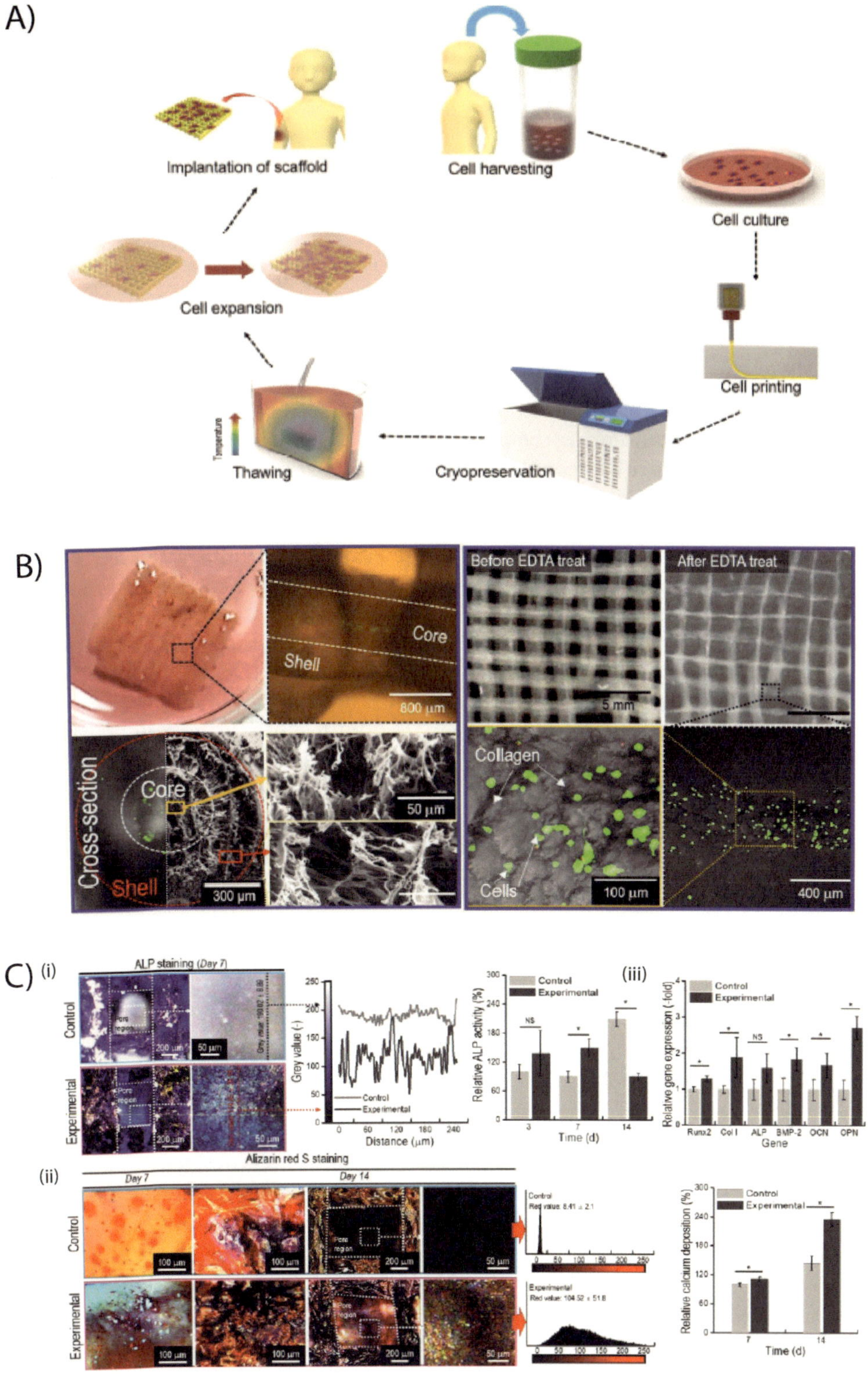

Figure 2.
(A) Application of cryopreservation/cell-printing process to tissue engineering processes. [Ref: [15], reproduced with permission from publishing authority]. (B): (a) Optical and SEM images of final scaffold with core/shell mesh structure. (b) Optical images of final scaffold before/after EDTA treatment and fluorescence images of live cells and collagen fiber in core strut after EDTA treatment. [Ref: [15], reproduced with permission from publishing authority]. (C): Osteogenic differentiation of human adipose-derived stromal cell (hASC)-laden

*structures with (experimental) or without (control) chicken bone marrow cell-conditioned medium. (i) Optical microscopy images of alkaline phosphatase (ALP) staining (at 7 days) and relative ALP activity (at 3, 7, and 14 days) of hASCs in the control and experimental structures. The experimental structure reached maximum ALP activities at 7 days (significantly higher than those of control) and then decreased at 14 days, whereas the ALP activities of the control group continued to increase at 14 days (n = 6, *p < 0.05). Decreased gray values of the magnified ALP staining, indicating that the proliferating cells in the pore were effectively mineralized. The image was captured in the pore of the experimental structure. (ii) Optical microscopy images of Alizarin Red S staining (at 14 days) and relative calcium deposition of the scaffolds (at 7 and 14 days). Calcium deposition levels of the experimental scaffolds were significantly higher than those of the control scaffolds (n = 6, *p < 0.05). Increased red staining was observed in the pore region in the experimental scaffold. (iii) Expression levels of runt-related transcription factor 2 (*Runx2*), collagen type I alpha chain 1 (*Col I*), *Alp*, bone morphogenic protein 2 (*Bmp-2*), osteocalcin (*Ocn*), and osteopontin (*Opn*) at 14 days of culture. Significantly increased expression levels of *Runx2, Bmp-2, Ocn*, and Opn *were detected in the experimental structure (n = 6, *p < 0.05). All values are expressed as mean ± SD. [Ref. [20], reproduced with the permission from publishing authority]. [Ref: [16], reproduced with permission from publishing authority].*

osteoblast cells or human adipose stem cells demonstrated good cell viability and steady growth similar to conventional 3D scaffold based cell treatment as shown in **Figure 2B**, which would bring the potential application in tissue engineering [15]. In a report, the mixture of neonatal chicken bone marrow cells (cBMCs) derived bioactive component and collagen was used to prepare the cell supporting bioink, which was further printed with human adipose tissue-derived stromal cell (hASC) lines to formulate the hASC-laden 3D scaffold [16]. The *'in vitro'* study using 3D architecture was shown to promote the growth, proliferation and osteogenesis of hASC cells. The system was further implanted in a rat mastoid obliteration model to monitor the potential effect of cBMCs derived bioactive component on the osteogenic differentiation in new bone regeneration. After 12 weeks of post transplantation, experimental groups showed excellent bone formation as compared as shown in **Figure 2C**. The modification of collagen fiber with synthetic polymer such as polycaprolactone or polylactic acid also resulted the mechanically and biologically active 3D porous cell supporting materials and which was confirmed by SEM, FTIR and proton NMR studies. In skin tissue engineering, the 3D scaffold was shown to increase the adipose tissue derived mesenchymal stem cell (AT-MSC) adhesion and growth with the formation of a tissue environment compared to only PCL or PLA-based scaffolds [17].

3.1.2 Hyaluronic acid as base material and its derivatives

As like collagen, hyaluronic acid (HA) is also a part of extracellular matrix and shown to have a potential role in modulating inflammation, cell attachment, and migration as well as tissue morphogenesis, owing to the biodegradable, biocompatible, non-immunogenicity and anti-inflamatory properties. An attempt by Gao et al. was initiated to develop the self-crosslinked hyaluronic acid-grafted collagen-I hydrogel using EDAC/NHS reaction method. Further, chondrocytes was encapsulated into the hydrogel to verify the cell-matrix interaction and which had a significant effect on the secretion of cartilage-specific matrices to promote the migration, proliferation and gene expression of chondrocytes cells. The *in-vivo* cytocompatibility and biodegradation studies on Sprague–Dawley (SD) rats (~200 g) showed the gradual decrease of the assembled nanofibre bundle and weight of the hydrogel after prolonged subcutaneous implantation [18]. Therefore, the manufactured self-crosslinking hydrogel could find significant application in tissue engineering applications.

In an approach, the injectable HA-SH/peptide hybrid hydrogels was developed based on the covalent/noncovalent supramolecular interaction between thiolated hyaluronic acid (HA-SH) and BPAA-AFF-OH short peptide to regulate the chondrogenic expression both *in vitro* and *in vivo* environments in the cartilage tissue engineering [19]. The prepared hydrogel confirmed by proton NMR, FTIR and SEM analysis was then employed to explore the cytocompatibility of chondrocyte cells. The chondrocyte cells laden hybrid scaffolds demonstrated the significant adhesion, proliferation of chondrocyte with the expression of chondrogenic specific genes such as Col II, Sox9 and AGG. The *in vivo* study based on the subcutaneous implantation of chondrocyte cells encapsulated hydrogel in New Zealand rabbit's models also revealed the abundant aggregation and proliferation of cells with the secretion of matrix after 4 weeks of post implantation period, resulting in the inhibition of hypertrophy trend of chondrocytes and tunable hyaline cartilage formation.

In order to improve the mechanical properties, methacrylated HA was modified with elastin-like polypeptide (ELP, consists of 70 repeats of the pentapeptide VPGVG) through free radical photopolymerization technique. The hydrogel made from the combination of MeHA/ELP revealed the tunable physicochemical and mechanical properties which is comparable to native tissue structure. Further, incorporation of zinc nanoparticles into the hydrogel had resulted an excellent antimicrobial platform for cell adhesion, growth, and proliferation phenomena (See **Figure 3A**). The '*in vivo*' cytocompatility experiment via subcutaneous implantation of MeHA/ELP hydrogel demonstrated that the weight of the hydrogel was significantly decreased with the generation and growth of autologous tissue without any inflammatory action [20]. This was due to the biodegradation of the transplanted hydrogel that led to the new space for the spreading and infiltration of the proliferated cells. The immunofluroescent staining study also exhibited the minor invasion and infiltration of lymphocyte and macrophages cells, assigning the potential application of the engineered hydrogel in various artificial tissue regeneration processes.

Like various tissue regeneration processes, utilizing of HAbased cell supporting materials explicated the significant output in artificial salivary gland repairing and remodeling. In an experiment, Lee et al. demonstrated the synthesis of hyaluronic acid–catechol (HACA) conjugates based platform named as NiCHE (nature-inspired catechol conjugated hyaluronic acid environment) to mimic the mesenchyme of embryonic submandibular glands (eSMGs) as shown schematically in **Figure 3B(i)** [21]. The NICHE was developed by the coating of HACA conjugates on the various polymeric scaffolds such as polycarbonate membrane, stiff agarose hydrogel, and polycaprolactone that led to cell adhesion and growth, vascular endothelial and proliferation of progeniotor of eSMGs cells isolated from ICR mice fetus [See **Figure 3B(ii&iii)**].

3.1.3 Gelatin as base material and its derivatives

Owing to the excellent biocompatibility, biodegradability and water solubility, gelatin has emerged tremendous interest for the formation of 3D hydrogel in tissue engineering application. Song et al. developed an injectable 3D printed gelatin hydrogel composed of continuous phase gelatin and gelatin microgels. The two-step cross-linked injectable gelatin was shown to exhibit the biocompatible lattice, cup-shaped, tube-shaped and rheological modified structure analogous to human anatomical features. The biocompatibility of the microgel led to the spread and expression of metabolic activities in mouse fibroblast cells, which can be attributed to the good cell-matrix interaction such as *in vivo* remodeling stages [22].

Due to the limited clinical success in repairing defective cartilage, unlike conventional surgery, the biopolymer-based tissue engineering approach such as the production of gelatin-linked electrospun, gelatin-polycaprolactone (gelatin-PCL) nanofiber-filled decellularized extracellular matrix has been investigated to monitor biological functions. The decellularized composite has shown to exhibit the

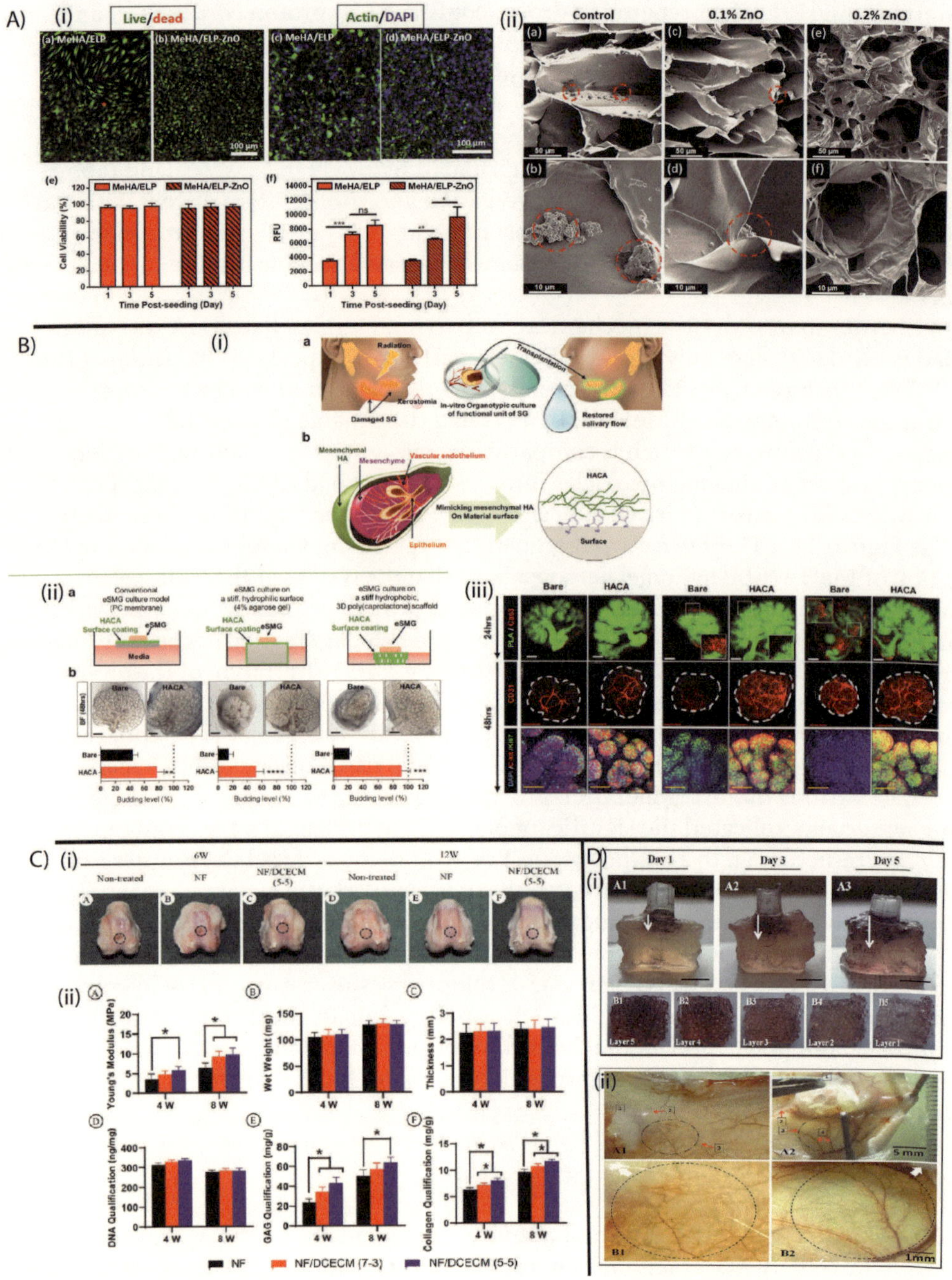

Figure 3.

(A) (i) In vitro cytocompatibility of MeHA/ELP and MeHA/ELP-ZnO hydrogels. Representative live/dead images from hMSCs seeded on (a) MeHA/ELP and (b) MeHA/ELP-ZnO hydrogels after 5 days of seeding. Representative phalloidin (green)/DAPI (blue) stained images from hMSCs seeded on (c) MeHA/ELP and (d) MeHA/ELP-ZnO hydrogels at day 5 post culture. Quantification of (e) viability and (f) metabolic activity of hMSCs seeded on hydrogels after 1, 3, and 5 days of culture. Hydrogels were formed by using 2% MeHA and 10% ELP with 0 and 0.2% (w/v) ZnO nanoparticles at 120 s UV exposure time ($p < 0.05$, ** $p < 0.01$, *** $p < 0.001$). [Ref: [20], reproduced with permission from publishing authority]. (ii) In vitro antimicrobial properties of MeHA/ELP-ZnO hydrogels with different ZnO concentrations. Representative SEM images of methicillin-resistant* Staphylococcus aureus *(MRSA) colonization on hydrogels containing (a, b) 0% ZnO, (c, d) 0.1% ZnO, and (e, f) 0.2% ZnO. Clusters of bacteria are shown in dashed circles. [Ref: [20], reproduced with permission from publishing authority]. (B): (i/a) Schematic Diagram of Salivary Gland Damage and Tissue Engineering-Based Therapeutic Approach; (i/b) Schematic Diagram of Mimicking Mesenchymal HA of Developing eSMG on Material Surfaces by Using Adhesive HACA. [Ref: [21], reproduced with permission from publishing authority]. (ii) NiCHE coating platform enhances growth of eSMGs on various substrates.*

*(b) Bright field images and budding levels of eSMGs cultured either on bare or HACA-coated materials after 48 h-culture. Average bud count of eSMGs freshly isolated from TP15 mouse fetus is considered as 100%. Scale bar = 200 μm. (iii) Apoptotic activity, VE structure, and mitotic activity of progenitor cells of eSMGs cultured either on bare or HACA-coated materials after 24 and 48 h-culture, respectively. White scale bar = 200 μm, red scale bar = 500 μm, yellow scale bar = 100 μm. [Ref: [21], reproduced with permission from publishing authority]. (C) (i) Gross view and histological evaluation of repaired region at 6 and 12 weeks postsurgery. Macroscopic images of cartilage defects regions at 6 weeks (A–C) and 12 weeks (D–F) postsurgery. (ii) Biomechanical and biochemical analyzes of the engineered cartilage tissue in vivo. Young's modulus (A), wet weight (B), thickness (C), DNA qualification (D), GAG qualification (E), and collagen qualification (F) of the in-vivo-engineered cartilage tissue. Values are expressed as mean ± SD, n = 3, *p < 0.05. [Ref: [23], adapted with permission from publishing authority]. (D) (i): (A1-A3) Spatial distribution of the purple formazan crystal inside the 5 L implant at day1(A1), 3(A2) and 5(A3). The scale bars represent 5 mm. Distribution profile of purple formazancrystal indicates an in-growth of cells inside the implant. (B1–5) Presence and distribution of MTT crystals on each bead layer. (ii) Study of the osteogenic properties of the implant in vitro. The study was carried out using human mesenchymal stem cells (hMSC). (A) Time dependent variation of alkaline phosphatase expression. ALP activity was measured in the supernatant of the culture. (B) Study of the expression of osteogenic marker through RT-PCR. The study was carried out after culturing the hMSC on different substrates in presence of osteogenic media for 14 days. (C) Fluorescent micrographs of the replated partially differentiated hMSC stained with FITCPhalloidin(green) and DAPI (blue). The cells were initially cultured on implant and control substrates. They were then trypsinized and replated on tissue culture plate. Imaging was done after 3 days of replating. [Ref: [26], reproduced with permission from publishing authority].*

excellent mechanical property and promoted the cartilage regeneration with the secretion of collagen and glycosaminoglycan as shown in **Figure 3C** [23].

The development of gelatin methacrylate (GelMA) and poly (ethylene glycol) diacrylate (PEGDA) printed three layered scaffold, modified by lysine functionalized rosette nanotubes (RNTK) significantly improved the adhesion, growth and differentiation of adipose-derived mesenchymal stem cells (ADSCs). The RNTK not only acted as a potential biomimetic layer, its presence dramatically increased the secretion of collagen II, glycosaminoglycan, and total collagen as compared to native GelMA-PEGDA scaffolds, and have an potential impact on cartilage regeneration [24].

To improve wound repair caused by burns or accidental injuries, a versatile approach has been shown to fabricate the skin tissue analogue of a mechanically stable acellular elastomeric scaffold in the presence of biodegradable polyurethane and gelatin composite. The Gel-20%PU showed the best cell infiltration and biodegradation in a mouse *in vivo* experiment. Also, it reveals negligible immunogenicity and could be accepted as a substitute for new generation tissues [25].

3.1.4 Sodium alginate as base material and its derivatives

The implementation of the osteogenic microenvironment loaded with therapeutic agents has emerged as the key pathway for bone tissue engineering in recent decades. Like various biopolymers, the utility of alginate, which is a polyionic-polysachharide comprising units of mannuronic acid and guluronic acid, has strengthened the field of next-generation polymer remodeling. The fabrication of calcium alginate bead based 3D implant made by the stacking of hexagonal closed pack (HCP) layers (**Figure 3D(i)**) in presence of glutaraldehyde crosslinker facilitated the spatiotemporal drug release in the artificial matrixes through the changes of the spatial coordinates of the drugs loaded layers. The supporting scaffold promoted the growth, progression and cytoskeletal reorganization of the osteoblast cells and triggered the expression of the alkaline phosphatase, runx2 and collagen type1 in human mesenchymal stem cells, attributed to the osteoconductive and osteogenic nature of the implant [26]. The *in vivo* assessment of the VEGF loaded implant was conducted in mice model and it revealed the regeneration of tissue with prominent existence of neovascularization as shown in **Figure 3D(iii)**, due to cohesive interaction between supportive implant and native tissue environment. A recent report [27] demonstrated the formation of mechanically stable alginate-gelatin

(ALG-GEL) hydrogels, resembling the comprehensive nonlinear and complex mechanical features of brain soft tissues. The rheology analysis also indicated that the stiffness of the hydrogel is solely dependent on the blending concentration and incubations times of the composites, assigning for the potential application in the fabrication of brain tissue supporting matrixes. Another report, where, (2, 2, 6, 6-Tetramethylpiperidin-1-yl)oxyl or (2,2,6,6-tetramethylpiperidin-1-yl) oxidanyl [TEMPO] oxidized cellulose nanofibre incorporated alginate scaffolds was investigated to enhance the biodegradability, sustainability and mechanically strengthened reactive surface area. The rheology study resulted in the recovery of 60% viscosity than that of native alginate scaffolds. The simulated body fluid (SBF) mediated mineralization evolved the nucleation of the hydroxyappetite into the hydrogel [28]. The combinatory efforts including direct writing 3D printing and freeze-drying techniques were carried out to develop the dual porous mechanically and dimensionally stable cellulose based 3D scaffolds. The dehydrothermal treatment displayed the increased surface hardness, indentation modulus and compression strength, should opened the new glimpse toward the decoration of bio-mimetic bone tissue engineering [29]. Furthermore, several studies have been conducted using cellulose or different derivatives to present an active tissue engineering tool and revealed the positive result in terms of cytocompatibility, biodegradability and flexibility of the scaffolds [30]. Similarly, Suneetha et al. [31] described the synthesis of mussel inspired polydopamine (PDA) filled sodium alginate (SA) – polyacrylamide (PDA – SA – PAM)-based hydrogel for skin tissue regeneration. The *in situ* synthesis process was conducted via two consecutive reaction steps. Initially, the dopamine molecules in the dopamine and sodium alginates blend was polymerized through alkali-induced polymerization and secondly, free radical polymerization technique was used to polymerize the acrylamide part in the processing of mechanically and biologically supporting adhesive hydrogel. The cytocompatibility assessment of the human skin fibroblasts (SFs) and keratinocytes (KTs) seeded PDA – SA – PAM-based hydrogel exhibited the higher cell adhesion, proliferation and spreading into the 3D microenvironment as compared PDA-free or 2D polystyrene plate and which is confirmed by fluorescence based live-dead assays or SEM morphology analysis as shown in **Figure 4A(i&ii)**. In addition, the effect of PDA molecules on the platelet adhesion was evaluated by the processing of porcine whole blood and it showed the higher adhesion of the platelet on the hydrogel as shown in SEM images, attributing to the potential effect of PDA in the regulation of fibrous network and adhesion of bioactive molecules.

3.1.5 Chitosan as base material and its derivatives

Chitosan, a polysaccharide with various functional groups has increased tremendous interest in biomedical applications such as tissue engineering. But, major problems due to poor solubility and biodegradability limit its monopoly use in the processing of cell supporting materials. This is avoided by the stacking or modifying with various synthetic or natural biomaterials. In a report, Li et al. developed the oxidized alginate hydrogel crosslinked with N, O-carboxymethyl chitosan with moderate swelling, degradation and porosity. The chitosan modified alginate scaffold revealed improved biocompatibility, as the number of free aldehyde groups in the oxidized alginate is reduced after crosslinking [32].

In another report [33], the methacrylated chitosan molecules were conjugated with lysozyme (an endo-carbohydrase) via riboflavin initiated photo-cross-linking to a constructed biodegradable and biocompatible hydrogel. The *in vitro* biodegradation study of the hydrogel revealed the increase of the pore size and larger fraction of outliers in cryo-SEM micrographs. Further, the mouse bone marrow

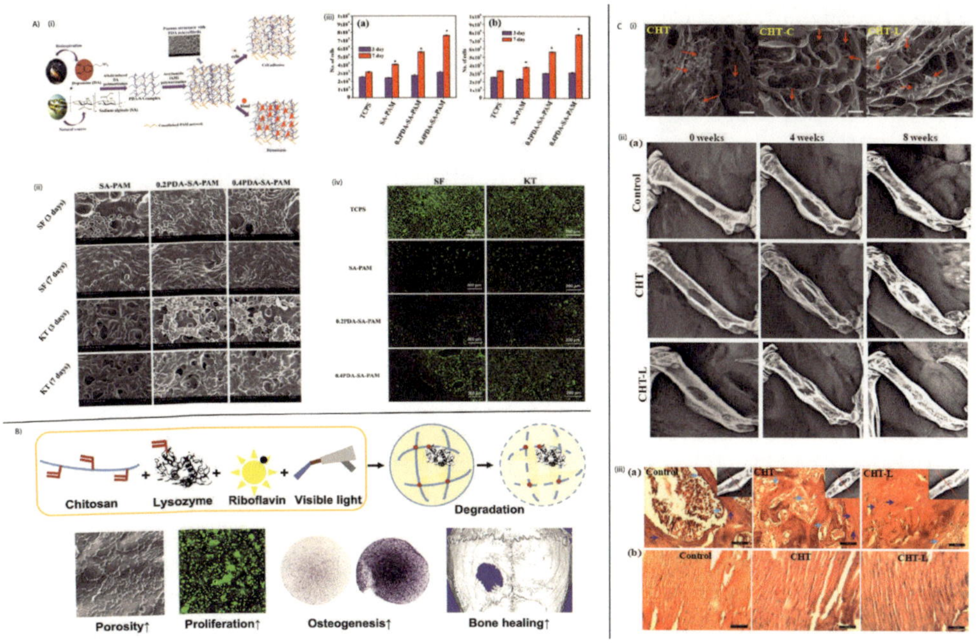

Figure 4.
*(A) (i) Schematic Representation of the Formation of Adhesive Hydrogels for Tissue Engineering Applications. (ii) SEM images of cell attachment of SF and KT cells on hydrogels in different culture conditions (3 and 7 days). (iii) MTT assay cell proliferation of hydrogels for (a) SF and (b) KT. (iv) live/dead assay fluorescence images of SF and KT cells on hydrogels under 10× magnification (scale bar 200 μm) (*p < 0.05). [Ref: [31], reproduced with permission from publishing authority]. (B) Schematic presentation of Chitosan-Lysozyme Conjugates for Enzyme-Triggered Hydrogel Degradation in bone Tissue Engineering Applications. [Ref: [33], reproduced with permission from publishing authority]. (C) (i) SEM images of the cell seeded scaffold of pure CHT and its nanohybrid. Red arrow indicates the position of the cells. Scale bar = 60 μm; (ii) (a) X-ray photographs of rat femur bone defects of control (devoid of any material), CHT (filled with pure CHT scaffold), and CHT-L (filled with nanohybrid scaffold, CHT-L) after one day, four weeks and eight weeks of implantation. Blue and cyan arrows indicate osteocyte and osteoblast cell, respectively; (iii/a) H & E stained histopathological section of the rat femur bone defects after eight weeks of implantation, inset figure of each image indicates that the section were taken from that part (indicated by dotted red lines). Scale bars represent 100 μm; (iii/b) Histopathological section of connective tissue attached with the bone, stained using H & E. Scale bar is 100 μm. [Ref: [35], reproduced with permission from publishing authority].*

stromal cell line (BMSC) loaded hydrogel exhibited the adhesion, proliferation and spreading of BMSCs with the expression of the osteogenic-specific markers throughout various layers of hydrogel as compared to chitosan based hydrogel. This may be attributed to the lysozyme mediated breaking of chitosan chains, thereby helping the penetration of cells through the disintegrated hydrogel networks. Also, as shown in **Figure 4B**, the *in vivo* bone regeneration experiment demonstrated the significant recovery of the defected bone with new bone tissues after six weeks of hydrogel post-implantation in a nude mice model with the recruitment of cells to the damaged zone. Similarly, the mechanically stable and tunable porous graphene oxide incorporated alginate-chitosan-collagen (GO/SA-CS-Col) based composite scaffolds was fabricated via Ca^{2+} mediated crosslinking and freeze-drying techniques. The composition and surface morphology were confirmed by FTIR, Raman spectra, SEM and XRD analysis. *In vitro* study of the osteoblast cell encapsulated scaffold revealed the adhesion, proliferation of the cells and osteogenic differentiation [34]. In an approach, the sulfonated graphene oxide functionalized chitosan based hybrid scaffold was prepared and FTIR, SEM, TEM and XRD analysis confirmed the synthesis of the interconnected porous chitosan/GO nanohybrid scaffolds [35]. The *in vitro* drug release assay at phosphate buffer solution at 37°C exhibited the sustained release of the drug molecules, may be due to the noncovalent interaction between drug and composites that triggering the slow diffusion of the drug molecules. The hybrid scaffold also revealed the high cell growth and spreading into the deep part of porous scaffold as compared to GO-free chitosan scaffold which was observed by fluorescence and SEM analysis as shown in **Figure 4C(i)**. Further, the *in vivo* experiment using cell laden scaffold in rat model was investigated and the 75 days of post-implantation result demonstrated the faster healing of the defected area with significant proliferation of the osteoblast cells as compared to pure chitosan scaffold (see in **Figure 4C(ii)**). Intertestingly, Zao et al., developed a glucono δ-lactone (GDL) incorporated and carboxymethyl chitosan (CMCh) stabilized calcium phosphate (ACP) (designated as CMCh-ACP hydrogel) bioactive hydrogel using freeze-drying process for mesenchymal stem cells [MSCs] based bone regeneration [36]. FTIR analysis exhibited the characteristics peaks at 1064and 547 cm^{-1} due to the presence of phosphate (PO_4^{3-}) group of spherical particles with average size of 80 nm. Next, the cytocompatability of the MCSs laden (iMAD cell line) CMCh-ACP hydrogel revealed the time dependent increase of cell density with negligible apoptotic cell morphology as in Hoechst 33258 stained, indicating the biocompatibility of the hydrogel for long-term cell friendly growth microenvironment. Like, *in vitro* assays, the *in vivo* bone regeneration experiment in presence of BMP9-(potent bone-forming factor) induced iMAD cells/CMCh-ACP hydrogel demonstrated the efficient new bone formation with the extensive vascularisation on the surface of the masses, attributing to the upregulation osteogenic-specific biomarkers and regulars, thereby enabling the BMP9 induced osteogenesis. In our several works, we demonstrated the modification of chitosan with different biomaterials such as montmorillonite clay (OMMT), hydroxyapatite, poly (ethylene glycol), polymethylmethacrylate-co-2-hydroxyethyl-methacrylate and polyvinyl alcohol. The formulated porous scaffolds were made with improved mechanical, antibacterial and biocompatible for application in bone tissue engineering [37–40].

3.1.6 Polyhydroxyalkanoates (PHA) as base material and its derivatives

Unlike different biomaterials, *polyhydroxyalkanoates (PHA)* are the class of biodegradable biopolymer extracted by the harvesting of microbial cells. Despite the cost-effective synthesis and ease of processing, the hydrophobicity, brittleness and lack of antibacterial limits it random uses in biomedical applications such drug delivery, surgical suture and supporting matrices for tissue regenerations. Efforts are being made to improve its biocompatibility, mechanical strength and antimicrobial properties by blending or modifying the surface with bioactive and high-strength nanomaterials. One approach was used to develop the biocompatible collagen-immobilized porous 3D scaffold based on poly(3-hydroxybutyrate-co-3-hydroxyvalerate) [collagen/PHBV], which allows better growth and proliferation of the rat osteogenic cell line (UMR-106 cell line) than native PHBV scaffold [41]. A similar trend was also observed when hydroxyappetite was further incorporated into the collagen grafted PHBV composite. The modified scaffolds revealed better adhesion and growth of osteoblast cells [42]. In another study, a hyaluronic acid immobilized chitosan-grafted porous PHA membrane was fabricated and it exhibited better protein adsorption and improved adhesion and proliferation of L929 fibroblasts. The supportive matrix also showed excellent antibacterial activity against several bacterial strains [43]. The mechanically and biocompatibility challenged porous PHH-mixed PHB [PHBHHs] scaffolds showed significant growth and proliferation of chondrocytes isolated from rabbit articular cartilage (RAC) as compared to only PBHs or PHB scaffolds. With the increase of the PHBHH content in the mixture, both the mechanical and the cell compatibility increased dramatically, they have a potential impetus in tissue engineering applications [44]. Recently, a group of researchers has potentially formulated the carbonaceous or conductive nonmaterial such as polyaniline, graphane oxide modified PHA based 3D porous scaffolds for tissue engineering applications. The antimicrobial and cell-stimulated active 3D constructs not only improved cell attachment, proliferation, but migratory behaviors were observed through interconnected porous networks. The magnetically active MRI scaffolds have tissue engineering applications controlled by significant bioimaging [45–47].

3.1.7 Silk as base material and its derivatives

Silk is a naturally occurring fibrous protein with biodegradability, biocompatibility, and mechanical durability that has utility in tissue engineering applications. In one study, silk fibroin-grafted polycaprolactone nanofibers were able to deliver dual growth factors such as bone morphogenetic protein-2 (BMP-2), transforming growth factor-beta (TGF-β), in the regeneration of bone tissue [48]. Li et al. also presented a similar type of biocompatibility while a PCL/silk 3D bioprinting scaffold was imposed to regenerate the meniscus tissue [49]. The computer-assisted 3D printed silk matrices have attracted significant attention and found to be improved the cell–cell and cell-matrix interaction and enable their activity in patient specific tissue architecture [50]. Similarly, the gelatin-silk composite was subjected to the fabrication of 3D bioprinting for cartilage tissue engineering in rabbit model [51].

The novel development of 4D printing hydrogel has gained significant attention in next generation biofabrication. The fabrication of 4D printing from 3D printing hydrogel was regulated by the modulation their interior or exterior properties with the proper controlled of expansion rate of the hydrogel in distilled water and salt water. The biocompatibility of assessment of the 4 D printing hydrogel was conducted in culture medium by shape change method as mentioned earlier. The results revealed the adhesion and growth of the PKH127 (green)-labeled human chondrocyte (hTBSCs) along with the deposition of cartilage extracellular matrix in the side of the construct. To verify the clinical applicability of the construct, the rabbit TBSC and chondrocytes-laden artificial 4D construct was implanted into the site of the rabbit trachea and the results of 8 weeks post-implantation revealed the regeneration of the respiratory epithelial layer and formation of neocartilage around the perichondrium. This findings proved the potential application of the cell laden 4D hydrogel in the recovery of respiratory organ, trachea regeneration [52]. A very recently, the approach of development of electrical simulation modulated polypyrrole/silk fibroin (PPy/SF) based conductive composite scaffold has been opened up the new avenue in the neuronal tissue regeneration [53]. The 3D printing electrospining method was used to fabricate for the alignment of silk fibrous, followed by the coating of polypyrrole (a mechanically stable conductive material) to get the desired silk fibroin (PPy/SF) composite scaffold as nerve guidance conduits (NGCs). Morphological tracking by SEM analysis exhibited the core-shell structure having interpenetrating PPy fibers on the smooth SF nanofibers with average diameter of 0.427 ± 0.083 μm. Resultant physicochemical properties such as mechanical stability (0.059 MPa) and conductivity (0.11446 ± 0.00145 mS/mm) of composite were comparable to ideal working in NGCs system, indicating the increase of mechanical property of the conduit by the coating of PPy. The ES controlled cell compatibility of the NGCs was evaluated with the seeding of Schwann cells (SCs) and it showed the significant growth, proliferation and migration of the cells with the expression of neurotrophic factors. Further, to investigate the effect of artificial NGCs on *in vivo* nerve tissue regeneration, the composite was implanted in defected sciatic nerve of rat and monitored for six months under ES regulation.

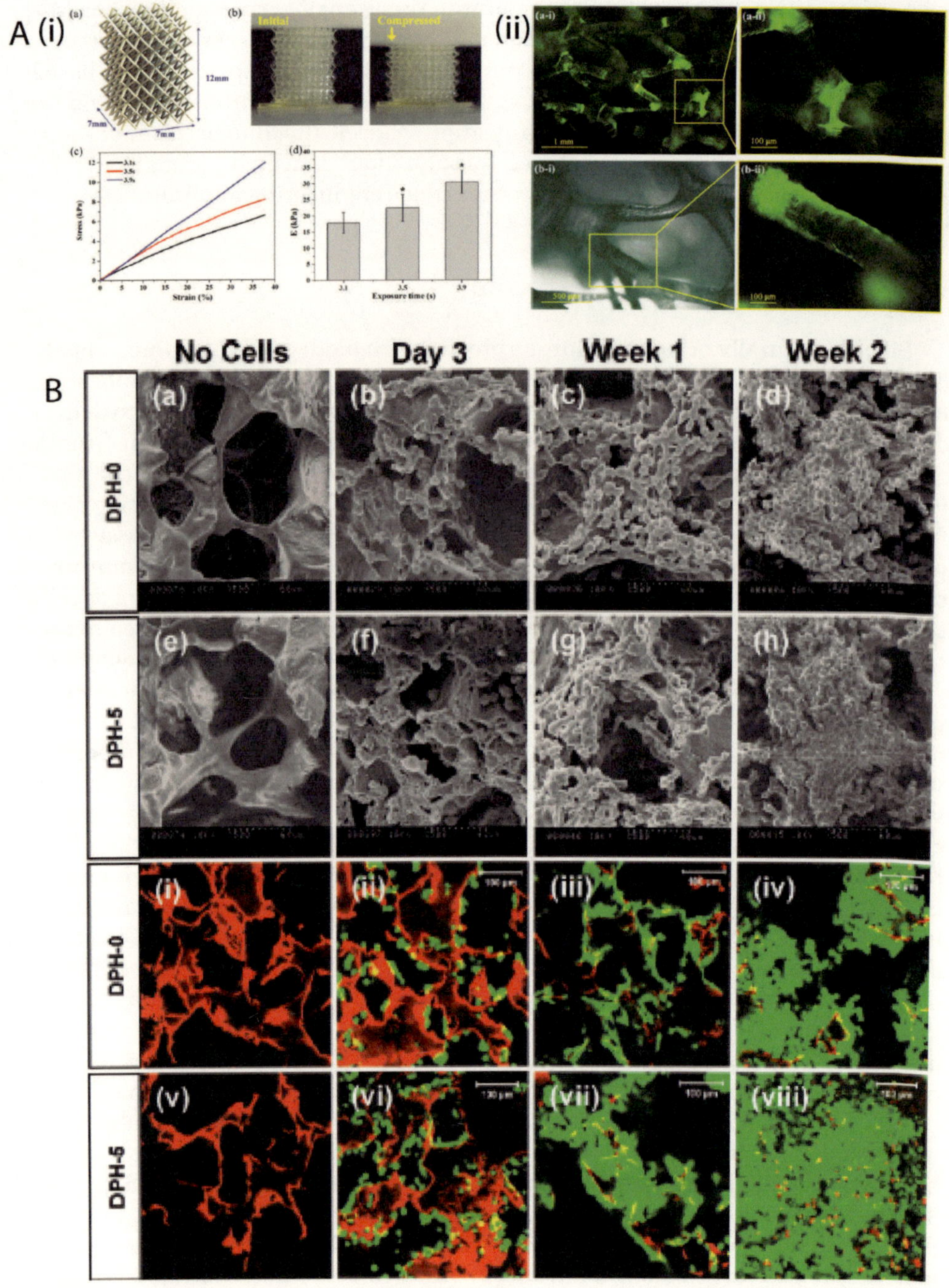

Figure 5.

(A) (i) (a) 3D model of the designed octahedral type of scaffold with marked dimensions; (b) scaffold was loaded on the compression platform; (c) strain–stress curves; (d) elastic moduli for three groups of homogeneous scaffolds; (ii) (a-i) Fluorescent microscope images taken with a 4 × objective to show the 3 T3 fibroblasts distribution in the scaffold. (a-ii) Interaction of 3 T3 fibroblasts with the joint of scaffold. (b-i) optical and fluorescent microscope images taken with a 10× objective. (b-ii) Fibrous-like cell layer formed on the frame surface of scaffold. [Ref: [54], reproduced with permission from publishing authority]. (B) Interaction of A10 VSMCs with D-PHI porous scaffolds. SEM (a-h) and live-dead (i-viii) images of D-PHI-0 (a-d and i-iv) and D-PHI-5 (e-h and v-viii) porous scaffolds in the absence of cells and following a 3 day, 1 week, and 2 week culture period with A10 VSMCs at 0 μm depth (scaffold surface). Cell-free scaffolds (i and v) fluoresce red under the microscope. All SEM images were taken at 500 × original magnification. [Ref: [55], reproduced with permission from publishing authority].

Histochemical and microscopic analysis revealed the densely regenerated myelinated fibers and mylinated axon dispersed in the fibrous networks that promoted the regeneration of the pheripheral injured nerve. Since, the cellular activities in nervous system are regulated by the expression of various neurotrophic factors (BDNF and NT-4/5) and signaling pathways. The ES modulation may activate the MAPK in the cell microenvironment and promoted the growth of the axon, correlated with nerve regeneration. Therefore, although several reports have been undergone using silk for the construction of different tissue architectures but intensive research must be conducted to find potential validity in clinical trials.

3.1.8 Different synthetic materials and their combination

The synthetic materials based 3D hydrogel have also shown to mimic the native tissue stiffness while the optimum conditions for the 3D constructions are digitally controlled. The digital light processing (DLP) based printed poly(ethylene glycol) diacrylate (PEGDA) hydrogels exhibited nearly 60% of enhanced elastic modulus, suited for the support of 3 T3 cells adhesion and proliferation as shown in **Figure 5A** [54]. In one study, degradable, polar hydrophobic and ionic porous polyurethane scaffolds were synthesized using a lysine-based crosslinker. The scaffolds demonstrated (see **Figure 5B**) the comprehensive mechanical, swelling and biocompatible properties that support the adhesion and growth of muscle cells in vascular tissue engineering [55]. Apsite et al., reported the design and fabrication of polycaprolactone and poly(N-isopropylacrylamide) based multilayerd porous electrospun mats. The self-folding 4D bio-fabrication was found to act as good cells adhesion and viability, assigning as a new perspective in new generation tissue engineering [56]. In a paper, Kutikov explained how the integration of hydrophilic polyethylene glycol into hydrophobic polyester block copolymers changes the physicochemical properties of 3D matrices. The incorporation also demonstrated the different types of cell adhesion, growth, and tissue regeneration both *in vitro* and *in vivo* experiment [57]. Therefore, the deviations in the fabrication of 3D artificial support matrices using natural biopolymer or synthetic materials individually must be compensated by the chemistry of piling or surface modification to increase any physical properties that would satisfactory fill the gaps to improve the clinical applications.

4. Effect of growth factors on cell-matrix interaction

Enormous studies have been thoroughly investigated on the interaction between cellular and bio-mimetic 3D matrices *in vitro* and *in vivo* tissue generation experiments that demonstrated the phenomena of adhesion, growth and differentiation of different cells. But, most of the study doesn't meet the pre-requisite for the successful clinical application due to the insufficient secretion of protein molecules that responsible for the biological and biochemical signaling between cell–cell and cell matrix cross-talk. The prominent small proteins that induce cell growth, proliferation, differentiation and regulate angiogenesis are encoded as growth factors. The emergence of versatility of different growth factors related to the reported mediated repair of damaged tissue tends to fall into various categories based on their functionality in tissue engineering. EGFs, NGFs, IGF, FGFs, PDGFs, interleukins etc. are the class of growth factors mainly disclosed for the cell–cell medicated trafficking of proliferation and actin-cytoskeleton in living tissue regeneration process.

Mechanically, the function of growth factors is to drive progenitor cells to its damaged target tissues by extracellularly mediated signaling pathways. In fact, therapeutic molecules bind to the cell surface transmembrane receptor and then to the internalized receptor-protein complex through phosphorylation-mediated signal transduction that triggers down-regulation of cells, followed by reduction of overwhelming responses and stimulation at the cellular level to carry out biological functions. Furthermore, the non-diffusible method leads to the binding of growth factor to the cell surface without any major internalization or downregulation in the results of long-term biological activities, as shown in **Figure 6A(i&ii)** [58]. Mimicking the *in vivo* tissue environment, various approaches have been implicated using growth factors loaded 3D biocomposite for sustained release without any dysfunction of the protein molecules. Bone morphogenesis protein-2 and 7 (BMP-2 & BMP-7) are the part of transforming growth factors enable the proliferation and osteogenic differentiation of bone marrow derived mesenchymal stem cells. The removal of bio-signaling molecules has demonstrated the deregulation of cell proliferation, differentiation and alteration of bone tissue formation [59, 60]. Co-administration of TGF-b3 and BMP-2 via alginate-based scaffolds revealed a tendency for increased osteogenesis in *in vivo* bone formation tests. A similar type of output has been observed while TGF-1 and IGF-1 are used simultaneously for bone tissue engineering [61, 62]. In a study, Kim et al., demonstrated that the inhibition of epithelial growth factor predominantly affects the cell–cell and contact based cell proliferation. In addition, over-expression of cadhreine, a transmembrane-type cell surface protein limited cell-to-cell contact with the arrest of cell cycle, resulted in spatial cell rearrangement tuned to tumor formation. Therefore, the epithelial growth factor plays an active function towards the formation of epithelial cells in tissue engineering [63].

It has been a challenge to meet the need to develop a bio-mimetic tool for vascular tissue engineering. In contrast to various soft tissues, vascular tissue controls the supply of oxygen, essential cellular nutrients, the transport of waste products and stem cells as well as progenitor cells. Therefore, it is urgent to reconstruct the

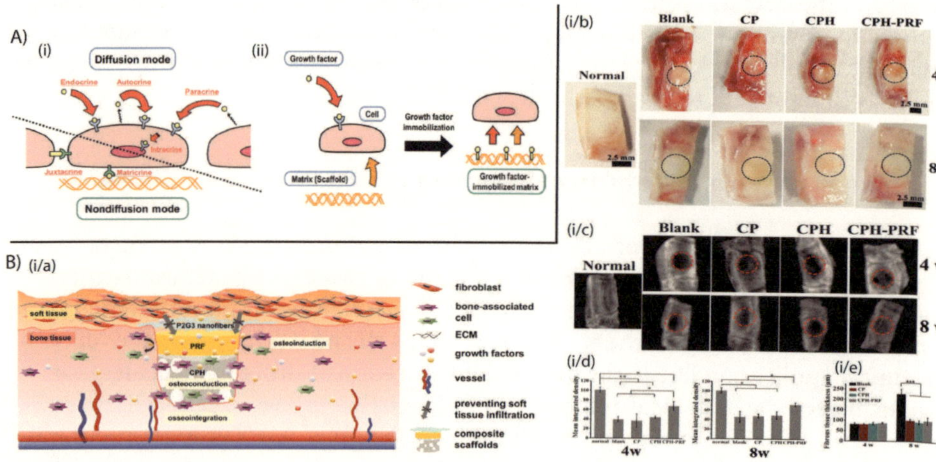

Figure 6.

*(A) (i) Modes of action of growth factors. Growth factors interact with their receptors in a diffusible manner (e.g., by endocrine, paracrine, autocrine and intracrine pathways) or in a non-diffusible manner (e.g., by juxtacrine and matricrine pathways). Some growth factors are known to act in both ways. (A) (ii) Three main factors in tissue engineering: cells, growth factors and matrices (scaffolds). The conjugation of growth factors and matrices provides a new approach for generating biofunctional substrates for regenerative medicine [Ref-58, reproduced with the permission from publishing authority]. (B) (i/a): Schematic representation of proposed mechanisms for enhanced bone regeneration in vivo. (i/b): Optical images of retrieved specimens from representative critical-sized bone defects at 4 and 8 weeks. (i/c) Micro-CT analysis. (i/d) Quantitative analysis of bone regeneration. (i/e) Fibrous tissue thickness at the defect site at 4 and 8 weeks (*P < 0.05; **P < 0.01; ***P < 0.001). [Ref. [66], adapted with permission from publishing authority].*

network of the neovascularization process with the initiation of adhesion, growth and differentiation of cells as a native tissue environment in artificial tissue engineering. Cao et al. demonstrated the therapeutic approaches of growth factors and their signal cascade that control neovascularization and the formation of neovessels using the spatiotemporally controlled 3D construct both *in vitro and in vivo* pathways. The literature also explained how vascular epithelial growth factor (VEGF) plays a critical role in vasculogenesis in stages of embryonic development from pre-existing blood vessels through consecutive signaling pathways [64, 65]. The multifunctional triple layered chitosan/poly (gamma-glutamic acid)/hydroxyapatite (CPH) hydrogels was formulated to regulate the release of platelet-rich fibrion (PRF) which was extracted from rat abdominal arota, into the site of damaged bone tissues. The PRF entrapped composite hydrogel was prepared through noncovalent electrostatic interaction and lyophilization technique to promote the osteoconductive mediated new bone tissue formation. The PRF entrapped composite hydrogel was prepared through noncovalent electrostatic interaction and lyophilization technique to promote the osteoconductive process in the formation of new bone. PRF is a combination of different growth factors such as TGF-β, PDGF, and IGF that have an abiity to induce the mineralization and the upregulation of various osteogenetic biomarkers in order to activate the osteoblast as seen in vitro and in vivo experiments. As a part of '*in vivo*' tissue regeneration study, rat calvarial defect models demonstrated the superior healing of the calvarial defect after 8 weeks post implantation period in presence of PRF/CPH composite than that of control experiment (see **Figure 6B**) [66]. In summary, the combined growth factors entrapped 3D supporting matrixes would bring a new avenue towards the cell–cell cross-talk mediated tissue generation with the advancement of bio-mimetic tools in finding the arrays of the artificial tissue engineering in the future.

5. Conclusions

Understanding the mechanism and basic criteria in the process of tissue regeneration has unveiled the secret of the communication involved in cell–cell, cell-matrix interaction that enables healing in an artificial tissue environment such as native tissue repair processes. In fact, the biocompatibility of any fabricated 3D architecture plays an important role in adhesion, proliferation, migration, and differentiation of the cells of interest to biologically mimic the signaling cascade that triggers cellular activities. Several investigations have shown that 3D constructs comprising naturally extracted and synthetic materials having a porous and mechanically stable geometry promoted integrin ligand-mediated differentiation and tailored actin-cytoskeletal cell morphology in a better way. The studies also explained how the biological and biochemical performances of cells are influenced by the different growth factors mediated signaling pathways and the active function of the ECM components. Therefore, present review provided the core thinking behind the physicochemical features of supporting matrixes that significantly control the cell–cell and cell-matrix interaction towards the implementation of clinically approved artificial 3D biocomposite for the successful clinical tissue engineering applications.

Acknowledgements

Dr. Nilkamal Pramanik and Dr. Tanmay Rath acknowledge UGC, DST, SERB- DST (NPDF), Govt. of India, for their financial supports. Dr. Nilkamal Pramanik also gratefully acknowledges Dr. Tanmay Rath, Prof. Patit Paban Kundu

(Department of Polymer Science and Technology) and Dr. Ranjan Kumar Basu (Department of Chemical Engineering), University of Calcutta for their kind guidance to carry the biomaterials based tissue engineering works.

Conflict of interest

No conflict of interest is a declaration.

Acronyms and abbreviations

TE	Tissue Engineering
ECM	Extracellular matrixes
EGFs	Epithelial growth factors
PDGFs	Platelet derived growth factors
IGFs	Insulin like growth factors
HCGFs	Hematopoietic cell growth factors
AT-MSCs	Adipose tissue-derived mesenchymal stem cells
GelMA	Gelatin methacrylate
PEGDA	Poly (ethylene glycol) diacrylate
HCP	Hexagonal closed pack
TEMPO	(2, 2, 6, 6-Tetramethylpiperidin-1-yl)oxyl or (2,2,6,6-tetramethyl-piperidin-1-yl)oxidanyl
SBF	Simulated body fluid
hBMSCs	Human bone marrow derived mesenchymal stem cells
OMMT	Montmorillonite clay
HA	Hyaluronic acid
IPN	Interpenetrating network based
BMP-2	Bone morphogenetic protein-2
PEGDA	Poly(ethylene glycol)diacrylate
VEGF	Vascular epithelial growth factor

Author details

Nilkamal Pramanik[1*] and Tanmoy Rath[2*]

1 Centre for BioSystems Science and Engineering, Indian Institute of Science, Bengaluru 560012, Karnataka, India

2 Motihari College of Engineering, Motihari, Aryabhatta Knowledge University, Bihar 845401, India

*Address all correspondence to: nilkamalorganic@gmail.com and tanmayrath@mail.com

References

[1] Langer R, Vacanti JP. Tissue Engineering. Science. 1993; 260:920-926. Doi: 10.1126/science.8493529.

[2] Vacanti JP, Langer R. Tissue engineering: the design and fabrication of living replacement devices for surgical reconstruction and transplantation. *Lancet*. 1999 l; 354; 1: SI32-4. Doi: 10.1016/s0140-6736(99)90247-7.

[3] Shi HX, Lin C, Lin BB et al. The anti-scar effects of basic fibroblast growth factor on the wound repair *in vitro* and *in vivo*. PLoS ONE. 2013; 8(4): e59966, Doi:10.1371/journal.pone.0059966.

[4] Zhang HY, Zhang X, Wang ZG et al. Exogenous basic fibroblast growth factor inhibits ER stress-induced apoptosis and improves recovery from spinal cord injury. *CNS Neuroscience and Therapeutics*. 2013; 19(1):20-29. Doi. org/10.1111/cns.12013

[5] Kim BS, Mooney DJ. Development of biocompatible synthetic extracellular matrices for tissue engineering. Trends Biotechnol.1998; 16(5):224-230. Doi: 10.1016/s0167-7799(98)01191-3.

[6] Drury JL, Mooney DJ. Hydrogels for tissue engineering: Scaffold design variables and applications. Biomaterials. 2003; 24(24):4337-4351. Doi: 10.1016/s0142-9612(03)00340-5.

[7] Grounds MD, White JD, Rosenthal N, Bogoyevitch MA. The role of stem cells in skeletal and cardiac muscle repair. J Histochem Cytochem. 2002; 50: 589-610. Doi: 10.1177/002215540205000501.

[8] Ghosh S, Spagnoli GC, Martin I, et al. Three-dimensional culture of melanoma cells profoundly affects gene expression profile: a high density oligonucleotide array study. J Cell Physiol. 2005; 204: 522-31. Doi: 10.1002/jcp.20320.

[9] Berthiaume F, Moghe PV, Toner M, Yarmush ML. Effect of extracellular matrix topology on cell structure, function, and physiological responsiveness: hepatocytes cultured in a sandwich configuration. FASEB J. 1996; 10: 1471-84. Doi: 10.1096/fasebj.10.13.8940293.

[10] Ghosh S, Spagnoli GC, Martin I, et al. Three-dimensional culture of melanoma cells profoundly affects gene expression profile: a high density oligonucleotide array study. J Cell Physiol. 2005; 204: 522-31. Doi: 10.1002/jcp.20320.

[11] Griffith LG, Swartz MA. Capturing complex 3D tissue physiology in vitro. Nat Rev Mol Cell Biol. 2006; 7: 211-24. Doi: 10.1038/nrm1858.

[12] Glicklis R, Shapiro L, Agbaria R, Merchuk JC, Cohen S. Hepatocyte behavior within three-dimensional porous alginate scaffolds. Biotechnol Bioeng. 2000; 67: 344-53. Doi: 10.1002/(sici)1097-0290(20000205)67:3<344::aid bit11>3.0.co;2-2

[13] Ragothaman M, Thanikaivelan Palanisamy T, Cheirmadurai Kalirajan C. Collagen–poly(dialdehyde) guar gum based porous 3D scaffolds immobilized with growth factor for tissue engineering applications. Carbohydrate Polymers. 2014; 114: 399-406. Doi.org/10.1016/j.carbpol.2014.08.045.

[14] Diogo GS, Marques CF, Sotelo CG, Pérez-Martín RI, Pirraco RP, Reis RL, Silva TH. Cell-Laden Biomimetically Mineralized Shark-Skin-Collagen-Based 3D Printed Hydrogels for the Engineering of Hard Tissues. ACS Biomater. Sci. Eng. 2020; 6: 3664–3672. Doi.org/10.1021/acsbiomaterials.0c00436.

[15] Lee JY, Koo YW, Kim GH. An innovative cryopreservation process using a modified core/shell cell-printing with microfluidic system for cell-laden scaffolds. ACS Applied Materials & Interfaces.2018; 10(11): 9257-9268. Doi.org/10.1021/acsami.7b18360.

[16] YANG WS, Kim WJ, Ahn JA, Lee J, Ko DW, Park S, Kim JY, Jang CH, Lim JM, Kim GH. A New Bioink Derived from Neonatal Chicken Bone Marrow Cells and its 3D-Bioprinted Niche for Osteogenic Stimulators. ACS Applied Materials & Interfaces. Doi: 10.1021/acsami.0c13905.

[17] Bakhshayesh A R D, Mostafavi E, Alizadeh E, Asadi N, Akbarzadeh A, Davaran S. Fabrication of Three-Dimensional Scaffolds Based on Nanobiomimetic Collagen Hybrid Constructs for Skin Tissue Engineering. ACS Omega. 2018; 3: 8605–8611. Doi.org/10.1021/acsomega.8b01219.

[18] Gao Y, Liu Q, Kong W, Wang J, He L, Guo L, Lin H, Fan H, Fan Y, Zhang X. Activated hyaluronic acid/collagen composite hydrogel with tunable physical properties and improved biological properties. IJBM. 2020; 164: 2186-2196. Doi:.org/10.1016/j.ijbiomac.2020.07.319.

[19] [Qing Wang,‡ Xing Li,‡ Peilei Wang, Ya Yao, Yang Xu, Yafang Chen, Yong Sun, *Qing Jiang, Yujiang Fan and Xingdong Zhang, Bionic composite hydrogel with a hybrid covalent/noncovalent network promoting phenotypic maintenance of hyaline cartilage, **J. Mater. Chem. B**, 2020, **8**, 4402-4411. Doi: 10.1039/D0TB00253D.

[20] Sani ES, Portillo-Lara R, Spencer A, Yu W, Geilich BM, Noshadi I, Webster TJ, Annabi N. Engineering Adhesive and Antimicrobial Hyaluronic Acid/Elastin-like Polypeptide Hybrid Hydrogels for Tissue Engineering Applications. ACS Biomater. Sci. Eng. 2018; 4(7): 2528-2540. Doi: 10.1021/acsbiomaterials.8b00408.

[21] Lee SW, Ji Ryu JH, Do MJ, Namkoong E, Lee H, Par K. NiCHE Platform: Nature-Inspired Catechol-Conjugated Hyaluronic Acid Environment Platform for Salivary Gland Tissue Engineering. ACS Applied Materials & Interfaces. **2020;** *12*(4): 4285-4294. Doi: 10.1021/acsami.9b20546.

[22] Song K, Compaan AM, Chai W, Huang Y. Injectable Gelatin Microgel-Based Composite Ink for 3D Bioprinting in Air. ACS Appl. Mater. Interfaces. 2020; 12: 22453–22466. Doi.org/10.1021/acsami.0c01497.

[23] Li Y, Liu Y, Xun X, Zhang W, Xu Y, Gu D. Three-Dimensional Porous Scaffolds with Biomimetic Microarchitecture and Bioactivity for Cartilage Tissue Engineering. ACS Appl. Mater. Interfaces. 2019; 11: 36359–36370. Doi.org/10.1021/acsami.9b12206.

[24] Zhou X, Tenaglio S, Esworthy T, Hann SY, Cui H, Webster TJ, Fenniri H, Zhang LG. 3D Printing Biologically-inspired DNA Based Gradient Scaffolds for Cartilage Tissue Regeneration. ACS Appl. Mater. Interfaces. Doi: 10.1021/acsami.0c07918.

[25] Sheikholeslam M, Wright MEE, Cheng N, Oh HH, Wang Y, Datu AK, Santerre JP, Amini-Nik S, Jeschke MG, Electrospun Polyurethane–Gelatin Composite: A New Tissue- Engineered Scaffold for Application in Skin Regeneration and Repair of Complex Wounds, ACS Biomater. Sci. Eng. 2020; 6: 505–516. Doi: org/10.1021/acsbiomaterials.9b00861.

[26] Agarwal T, Kabiraj P, Narayana GH, Kulanthaivel S, Kasiviswanathan U, Pal K, Giri S, Maiti TK, Banerjee I. Alginate bead based hexagonal close packed 3D implant for bone tissue

engineering. ACS Appl. Mater. Interfaces. 2016; 8 (47): 32132-32145. Doi: 10.1021/acsami.6b08512.

[27] Distlera T, Schallerb E, Steinmann P, Boccaccinia A R, Budday S. Alginate-based hydrogels show the same complex mechanical behavior as brain tissue. Journal of the Mechanical Behavior of Biomedical Materials. 2020; 111: 103979. Doi: 10.1016/j.jmbbm.2020.103979.

[28] Abou-Zeid RE, Khiari R, Beneventi D, Alain Dufresne A. Biomimetic Mineralization of 3D Printed Alginate/TEMPO-Oxidized Cellulose Nanofibril Scaffolds for Bone Tissue Engineering. Biomacromolecules. 2018; 19: 11, 4442-4452. Doi: 10.1021/acs.biomac.8b01325.

[29] Mohan T, Štiglic AD, Beaumont M, Konnerth J, Gürer F, Makuc D, Maver U, GradiŠnik L, Plavec J, Kargl R, Kleinschek KS. Generic Method for Designing Self-Standing and Dual Porous 3D Bioscaffolds from Cellulosic Nanomaterials for Tissue Engineering Applications. ACS Appl. Bio Mater. 2020; 3: 1197–1209. Doi.org/10.1021/acsabm.9b01099.

[30] Domingues RMA, Gomes ME, Reis RL. The potential of Cellulose Nanocrystals in Tissue Engineering strategies. Biomacromolecules. 2014; 15(7): 2327-2346. Doi.org/10.1021/bm500524s.

[31] Maduru Suneetha, Kummara Madhusudana Rao,* and Sung Soo Han, Mussel-Inspired Cell/Tissue-Adhesive, Hemostatic Hydrogels for Tissue Engineering Applications, ACS Omega 2019, 4, 12647–12656. Doi: 10.1021/acsomega.9b01302.

[32] Li X, Weng Y, Kong X, Zhang B, Li M, Diao K, Zhang Z, Wang X, Chen HA. Covalently Crosslinked Polysaccharide Hydrogel for Potential Applications in Drug Delivery and Tissue Engineering. J. Mater. Sci.: Mater. Med. 2012; 23: 2857-2865. Doi: 10.1007/s10856-012-4757-5.

[33] Kim S, Cui ZK, Koo B, Zheng J, Aghaloo T, Lee M. Chitosan-Lysozyme Conjugates for Enzyme-Triggered Hydrogel Degradation in Tissue Engineering Applications. ACS Appl. Mater. Interfaces. 2018; 10: 48, 41138-41145. Doi: 10.1021/acsami.8b15591.

[34] Kolanthai E, Sindu P A. Khajuria D K. Veerla S C. Kuppuswamy D. Catalani L H. Mahapatraa D R. Graphene Oxide–A Tool for Preparation of Chemically Crosslinking Free Alginate-Chitosan-Collagen Scaffold for Bone Tissue Engineering. ACS Appl. Mater. Interfaces. 2018; 10(15): 12441-12452. Doi: 10.1021/acsami.8b00699-37]10.1021/acsami.8b00699-37]

[35] Mahanta A K, Patel DK, Maiti P. Nanohybrid Scaffold of Chitosan and Functionalized Graphene Oxide for Controlled Drug Delivery and Bone Regeneration. ACS Biomater. Sci. Eng. 2019; 5: 5139–5149. Doi: 10.1021/acsbiomaterials.9b00829.

[36] Zhao C, Qazvini N T, Sadati M, Zeng et al. A pH-Triggered, Self-Assembled, and Bioprintable Hybrid Hydrogel Scaffold for Mesenchymal Stem Cell Based Bone Tissue Engineering. ACS Applied Materials & Interfaces. **2019;** *11*(9):, 8749-8762. Doi: 10.1021/acsami.8b19094.

[37] Bhowmick A, Banerjee SL, Pramanik N, Jana P, Mitra T, Gnanamani A, Das M, Kundu PP. Organically modified clay supported chitosan/hydroxyapatite-zinc oxide nanocomposites with enhanced mechanical and biological properties for the application in bone tissue engineering, International journal of biological macromolecules. 2018; 106: 11-19. Doi.org/10.1016/j.ijbiomac.2017.07.168.

[38] Bhowmick A, Pramanik N, Manna PJ, Mitra T, Selvaraj TKR, Gnanamani A, Das M, Kundu PP. Development of porous and antimicrobial CTS–PEG–HAP–ZnO nano-composites for bone tissue engineering. RSC advances. 2015; 5 (120): 99385-99393. Doi.org/10.1039/C5RA16755H.

[39] Bhowmick A, Pramanik N, Jana P, Mitra T, Gnanamani A, Das M, Kundu PP. Development of bone-like zirconium oxide nanoceramic modified chitosan based porous nanocomposites for biomedical application. International journal of biological macromolecules. 2017; 95: 348-356. Doi: 10.1016/j.ijbiomac.2016.11.052.

[40] Bhowmick A, Pramanik N, Mitra T, Gnanamani A, Das M, Patit Paban Kundu PP. Mechanical and biological investigations of chitosan–polyvinyl alcohol based ZrO2 doped porous hybrid composites for bone tissue engineering applications. New Journal of Chemistry. 2017; 41 (15): 7524-7530. Doi.org/10.1039/C7NJ01246B.

[41] Tesema Y, Raghavan D, Stubbs JJ. Bone cell viability on methacrylic acid grafted and collagen immobilized porous poly (3-hydroxybutrate-*co*-3-hydroxyvalerate). Appl. Polym. Sci. 2005; 98: 1916–1921. Doi.org/10.1002/app.22352.

[42] Baek JY, Xing ZC, Kwak G, Yoon KB, Park SY, Park LS, Kang IK. Fabrication and Characterization of Collagen-Immobilized Porous PHBV/HA Nanocomposite Scaffolds for Bone Tissue Engineering. Journal of Nanomaterials. 2012; 1–11. Article ID 171804. Doi.org/10.1155/2012/171804.

[43] Hu SG, Jou CH, Yang MC. Protein adsorption, fibroblast activity and antibacterial properties of poly (3-hydroxybutyric acid-co-3-hydroxyvaleric acid) grafted with chitosan and chitooligosaccharide after immobilized with hyaluronic acid. Biomaterials. 2003; 24: 2685-93. Doi: 10.1016/s0142-9612(03)00079-6.

[44] Zhao K, Deng Y, Chen GQ. Effects of surface morphology on the biocompatibility of polyhydroxyalkanoates. Biochem Eng J. 2003; 16: 115-123. Doi.org/10.1016/S1369-703X(03)00029-9.

[45] Pramanik N, Bhattacharya S, Rath T, De J, Adhikary A, Ranjan Kumar Basu RK, Kundu PP. Polyhydroxybutyrate-co-hydroxyvalerate copolymer modified graphite oxide based 3D scaffold for tissue engineering application. Materials Science & Engineering C. 2019; 94: 534-546. Doi: 10.1016/j.msec.2018.10.009.

[46] Pramanik N, Dutta K, Basu RK, Kundu PP. Aromatic π-Conjugated Curcumin on Surface Modified Polyaniline/Polyhydroxyalkanoate Based 3D Porous Scaffolds for Tissue Engineering Applications. *ACS Biomater. Sci. Eng.* 2016; 2(12): 2365-2377. Doi.org/10.1021/acsbiomaterials.6b00595.

[47] Pramanik N, De J. Basu RK, Rath T, Kundu PP. Fabrication of magnetite nanoparticle doped reduced graphene oxide grafted polyhydroxyalkanoate nanocomposites for tissue engineering application. RSC Adv. 2016; 6: 46116. Doi.org/10.1039/C6RA03233H.

[48] Bhattacharjee P, Naskar D, Maiti TK, Bhattacharya D, Kundu SC. Non-mulberry silk fibroin grafted poly(ϵ-caprolactone)/nanohydroxyapatite nanofibrous scaffold for dual growth factor delivery to promote bone regeneration. J. Colloid Interface Sci. 2016; 472: 16–33. Doi: 10.1016/j.jcis.2016.03.020.

[49] Li Z, Wu N, Cheng J, Sun M, Yang P, Zhao F, Zhang J, Duan X, Fu X, Zhang J, Hu X, Chen H, Ao Y. Biomechanically, structurally and functionally

meticulously tailored polycaprolactone/silk fibroin scaffold for meniscus regeneration.Theranostics.2020;10(11): 5090-5106. Doi: 10.7150/thno.44270.

[50] Mehrotra S, Moses JC, Bandyopadhyay A, Mandal BB. 3D printing/bioprinting based tailoring of *in vitro* tissue models: Recent advances and challenges. ACS Applied Bio Materials. 2019; 2(4): 1385–1405. Doi.org/10.1021/acsabm.9b00073.

[51] Shi W, Sun M, Hu X, Ren B, Cheng J, Li C, Duan X, Fu X, Zhang J, Chen H et al. Structurally and functionally optimized silk-fibroin–gelatin scaffold using 3D printing to repair cartilage injury *in vitro* and *in vivo*. Adv. Mater. 2017; 29 (29): 1701089. Doi: 10.1002/adma.201701089.

[52] Kim SH, Seo YB, Yeon YK, Lee YJ, Park HS, Sultan MT, Lee JM, Lee JS, Lee OJ, Hong H, Lee H, Ajiteru O, Suh YJ, Song S-H, Lee K-H, Park CH, 4D-bioprinted silk hydrogels for tissue engineering, Biomaterials (2020). Doi: 10.1016/j.biomaterials.2020.120281.

[53] Zhao Y, Liang Y, Ding S, Zhang K, Mao H, Yang Y. Application of conductive PPy/SF composite scaffold and electrical stimulation for neural tissue engineering. Biomaterials. 2020; 255: 120164. Doi: 10.1016/j.biomaterials.2020.120164.

[54] Xue D, Zhang J, Wang Y, Mei D. Digital Light Processing-Based 3D Printing of Cell-Seeding Hydrogel Scaffolds with Regionally Varied Stiffness. ACS Biomater. Sci. Eng. 2019; 5: 4825–4833. Doi.org/10.1021/acsbiomaterials.9b00696.

[55] Sharifpoor S, Labow RS, Santerre JP. Synthesis and Characterization of Degradable Polar Hydrophobic Ionic Polyurethane Scaffolds for Vascular Tissue Engineering Applications. Biomacromolecules. 2009; 10: 2729-2739. Doi.org/10.1021/bm9004194.

[56] Apsite I, Stoychev G, Zhang W, Jehnichen D, Xie J, Ionov L. Porous stimuli-responsive self-folding electrospun mats for 4D biofabrication. Biomacromolecules. 2017; 18: 10, 3178-3184. Doi: 10.1021/acs.biomac.7b00829.

[57] Kutikov AB, Song J. Biodegradable PEG-Based Amphiphilic Block Copolymers for Tissue Engineering Applications. ACS Biomaterials Science & Engineering. 2016; 2 (11): 1968-1975. Doi.org/10.1021/acsbiomaterials.5b00122.

[58] Tada S, Kitajima T, Ito Y. Design and Synthesis of Binding Growth Factors. Int. J. Mol. Sci. 2012; *13:* 6053-6072. Doi: 10.3390/ijms13056053.

[59] Raida M, Heymann AC, Gu¨nther C, Niederwieser D. Role of bone morphogenetic protein 2 in the crosstalk between endothelial progenitor cells and mesenchymal stem cells. Int J Mol Med. 2006; 18: 735-9. Doi: 10.3892/ijmm.18.4.735.

[60] Jin D, Pei GX, Wang K, Wei KH, Chen B, Qin Y. The regulatory effect of human bone morphogenetic protein 7 gene transfer on the proliferation and differentiation of rabbit bone marrow mesenchymal stem cells. Zhongguo Yi Xue Ke Xue Yuan Xue Bao 2003; 25: 22-5.

[61] Schmidmaier G, Wildemann B, Gabelein T, Heeger J, Kandziora F, Haas NP, et al. Synergistic effect of IGF-I and TGF-b1 on fracture healing in rats: single, versus combined application of IGF-I and TGF-b1. Acta Orthop Scand. 2003; 74: 604-10. Doi: 10.1080/00016470310018036.

[62] Simmons CA, Alsberg E, Hsiong S, Kim WJ, Mooney DJ. Dual growth factor delivery and controlled scaffold degradation enhance in vivo bone formation by transplanted bone marrow stromal cells. Bone. 2004; 35: 562-569. Doi.org/10.1016/j.bone.2004.02.027.

[63] Kima JH, Kushirob K, Grahamb NA, Asthagiric AR. Tunable interplay between epidermal growth factor and cell–cell contact governs the spatial dynamics of epithelial growth. PNAS. 2009; 106(27): 11149-11153. Doi.org/10.1073/pnas.0812651106.

[64] Cao L, Mooney DJ. Spatiotemporal control over growth factor signaling for therapeutic neovascularisation. Advanced Drug Delivery Reviews. 2007; 59: 1340-1350. Doi: 10.1016/j.addr.2007.08.012.

[65] Fischbach C, Mooney DJ. Polymers for pro- and anti-angiogenic therapy. Biomaterials. 2007; 28: 2069-2076.

[66] Zhang L, Dong Y, Xue Y, Shi J, Zhang X, Liu Y, Adam C. Midgley A C, Wang S. Multifunctional Triple-Layered Composite Scaffolds Combining Platelet-Rich Fibrin Promote Bone Regeneration. ACS Biomaterials Science & Engineering. **2019;** *5*(12): 6691-6702. Doi: 10.1021/acsbiomaterials.9b01022.

Chapter 9

Naturally Derived Carbon Dots as Bioimaging Agents

Gangaraju Gedda, Arun Bhupathi and V.L.N. Balaji Gupta Tiruveedhi

Abstract

The recent advances in nanoscience and technology have opened new avenues for carbon-based nanomaterials. Especially, Carbon dots (CDs) have gained significant attention due to their simple, economic and rapid green synthesis. These materials exhibit excellent water solubility, fluorescence emission, high fluorescence quantum yield, Ultraviolet (UV) to Infrared (IR) range absorbance and high bio-compatibility. Therefore, these materials are widely used for various biological applications including bio-imaging. With the integration and doping of surface passive agents and elements, respectively influenced the enhancement of fluorescence property of CDs. Also, the conjugation of receptor-based targeting ligands leads to targeted bioimaging. CDs in combination with other imaging contrast agents lead to the development of novel contrast agents for bimodal imaging and multimodal imaging techniques. The combination of diagnostic CDs with therapeutic agents resulted in the formation of theragnostic CDs for image guided therapies. In this chapter, a comprehensive view on the top-down and bottom–up green synthesis methods for naturally derived CDs discussed. Further, unique physical, chemical, optical and biological properties of CDs described. Finally, fluorescence based bimodal and multimodal imaging techniques also described.

Keywords: carbon dot, bioimaging, fluorescence, theragnostic, contrast agent

1. Introduction

The term 'imaging' is a perception that it is a type of photography; however, it is far from the biomedical domain. Bioimaging provides the anatomical visualization of cellular, subcellular structures, tissues, organs of multicellular organisms [1]. The biomedical imaging modalities utilize the various kind of energy sources such as light, magnetic resonance, positrons, ultrasound, electrons, and X-rays. The broad range of medical imaging modalities includes fluorescence (FL); X-ray computed tomography (CT), magnetic resonance (MR), ultrasound (US), positron emission tomography (PET) and single-photon emission computed tomography (SPECT) for diagnosis of various soft tissues and hard tissue pathologies and scientific research [2]. These techniques disclose the three-dimensional molecular information of any specimen's biological structures and physiological processes.

Optical imaging, predominantly FL imaging modality received special attention from all the imaging modalities due to their simple operation process, cost-effective armamentarium, excellent resolution, incredible sensitivity and high resolution [3–5].

Therefore, a wide range of fluorescent imaging probes has been discovered for FL imaging, such as organic dyes, semiconductor quantum dots, metal nanocluster and up-conversion nanoparticles [3, 4, 6]. Nevertheless, their limitations include high toxicity, complicated synthesis mechanisms, poor water-solubility and high cost. On the other hand, single-mode fluorescence imaging techniques were limited to depth penetration and difficulty to provide tomographic information due to light attenuation and photon scattering of biological tissue. Therefore, developing FL based multimodal imaging by integrating other imaging modalities with FL imaging modality has become an essential strategy to resolve the single mode FL imaging limitations. Interestingly, FL based multimodal imaging provides several advantages including non-invasive imaging visualization with superior depth penetration, higher sensitivity and resolution [7]. Hence, it is necessary to develop a single probe by integrating other contrast agents with fluorescent materials for FL-based multimodality imaging applications.

Nanotechnology advancements in contrast agent development are progressing rapidly either by doping/incorporating or conjugation of other contrast elements into/with fluorescent nanomaterials to obtain a multimodal imaging probe [8]. Among the various types of nanomaterials, carbon dots (CDs) gained remarkable attention due to their significant physical, chemical and biological properties [9]. The integration of several unique properties in single nanosize carbon dots (CDs), make them ideal alternative material to replace the semiconductor quantum dots, metallic nanomaterials and other forms of carbon materials in various fields. Specifically, bioimaging, drug delivery, phototherapy, anti-microbial agents, sensors, solar cells, light-emitting diodes and photocatalysis [10–13]. Specifically, CDs show significant potential in fluorescence-based multimodal imaging *in vivo* and *in vitro*. For example, FL/MR dual-modal imaging was developed by integrating iron oxide nanomaterials or doping Gd^{3+} or Mn^{2+} ions into CDs. Similarly, FL/PA, FL/CT and FL/PET etc., established by incorporating respective contrast agents. This book chapter initially discusses the top-down, bottom-up and green synthesis procedures of CDs, optical properties, and elemental doping and surface functionalization. Next, the bioimaging, importance of carbon dots application in the various medical imaging techniques, and therapeutic applications of carbon dots together as theragnostic are described. Finally, the outlook of carbon dots in bioimaging is mentioned.

2. Synthesis methods of carbon dots

In 2004, during the purification process of single-walled carbon nanotubes (SWCNTs) using gel electrophoresis, the CDs were discovered [10]. Later, various procedures established for the synthesis of CDs. Broadly, the CDs synthesis methods can be classified into as "top-down" and "bottom-up" approaches (**Figure 1**).

2.1 Top-down method

In the "top-down" approach, the breakdown of bulk carbon materials into nano size carbon occurs under relatively harsh conditions such as oxidative acid treatment, electrochemical exfoliation, laser ablation, and arc discharge [14]. The first described CDs were produced by the top-down process via laser ablation of graphite in the gaseous phase, subsequently acid oxidative treatment [15]. Later, numerous methods such as arc discharge, etching, electrochemical oxidation, ultrasonication, chemical exfoliation, and nitric acid/sulfuric acid oxidation developed to obtained CDs by reducing the size of bulk carbon materials [14, 16]. Mostly, graphite, graphene or graphene oxide (GO) sheets, carbon nanotubes (CNTs), carbon fibers

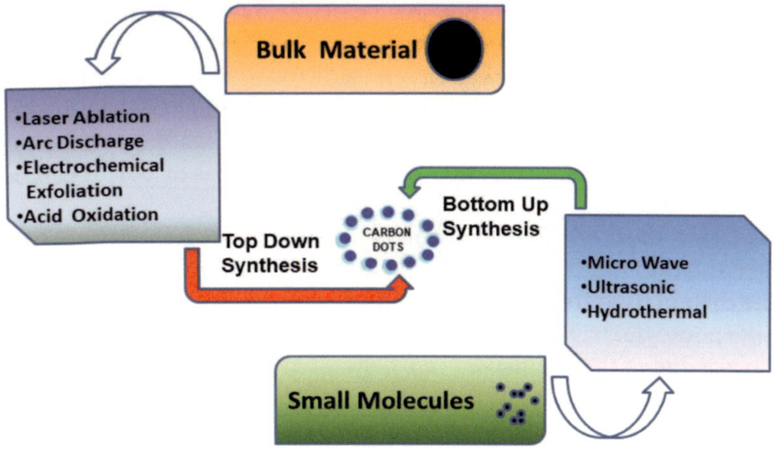

Figure 1.
Synthesis methods of carbon dots.

and carbon soot etc. used as a precursor material in these methods. Even though these methods were successfully used to prepare CDs, they are limited with harsh conditions, complicated synthesis strategies, low quantum yield, expensive, eco-unfriendly, and unsuitable for the production of CDs in industrial-scale. These methods rarely used for the preparation of CDs from natural sources.

2.1.1 Bottom-up method

In the "bottom-up" approach, the CDs are synthesized from carbon-containing small molecules in a "polymerization– carbonization" process. Several methods include combustion, hydrothermal, solvothermal, and microwave-assisted pyrolysis developed in bottom-up synthesis [16]. Typically, in these methods carbon precursor such as small organic molecules taken in a liquid or gas stage are ionized, dissociated, sublimated or evaporated and then condensed via condensation, carbonization, polymerization and passivation to form nanosize CDs. Compared with the "top-down" strategy, the "bottom-up" approach is extensively used for the green synthesis of CDs using natural renewable sources. Here, we discussed some important synthesis methods of CDs.

Acid oxidation: In this method, CDs were synthesized by exfoliation and cleaving of activated carbon, graphene oxide, carbon nanotubes, carbon fibers and soot etc. by using concentrated acids such as sulfuric acid and nitric acid [17, 18]. Typically, this method involves the decomposing of the bulk carbon into nanoparticles and simultaneously introducing hydrophilic groups on the carbon core. Generally, these raw materials are low in cost, readily available and feasible for simple operation. This method can be extended for the synthesis of hetero atom doped carbon dots. For example, the heteroatom N doped CDs prepared using activated carbon as precursor and Nitric acid as oxidizing agent [19]. However, this method limited with some disadvantages such as harsh conditions and time-consuming process to eliminate excessive acid.

Electrochemical exfoliation: This is a facile green and large-scale approach in which, CDs were prepared by avoiding excess concentrated acid, complex separation and purification process [20, 21]. In this method, high purity graphite used as anode and Pt wire used as a counter electrode. Distilled water can be used as electrolyte but the rate of reaction is very slow. In order to increase the rate of reaction, ionic liquids like 1- butyl-3 methylimidazolium tetrafluoroborate and 1-butyl

3-methylimidazolium hexafluorophosphate can be mixed with distilled water and can be used as electrolyte [22]. The electrochemical exfoliation carried by applying static potential through direct power which leads to corrosion of graphite anode and hence formation of CDs. The mechanism involves releasing carbon dots because of the electrochemical scissors OH^- and O^- ions from the water's anodic oxidation. Depending on the type of electrolyte nitrogen, phosphorus or boron can be doped in carbon dots.

Laser ablation method: The term ablation refers to the removal of surface atoms. Laser ablation method involves the absorption of highly energetic laser pulse by the carbon precursors and stripping of electrons from the atoms through a process like photoelectric effect generating a high electric field. Production of CDs takes place due to the repulsive force generated between positive ions and solid material [23, 24]. The size of the CDs can be controlled by a laser furnace. The precursors for laser ablation method are toluene, bulk graphite, graphene oxide and graphite powder etc. Laser ablation method provide high quality product with great velocity depending on the purity of the target and ambient media (gas or liquid). The size and other properties of carbon dots were controlled by irradiation time and laser fluence. The limitations of the method are requirement of high input energy and sophisticated equipment.

Ultrasonic treatment: In this green synthetic method, carbon materials can be broken down by the action of very high energy of ultrasonic waves [25, 26]. Ultrasonic waves create high pressure and low-pressure waves in liquid medium resulting in the formation, growth and violent collapse of small vacuum bubbles. The collapse of the bubbles lead to local high temperature and pressure up to 5000 K and 1000 atm respectively, producing the CDs. The precursors used for making CDs in this method are crab shell powder, glucose, active carbon, polyethylene glycol, citric acid, tri-ammonium citrate, and arginine. N, S, and P elements doped CDs can also be prepared by this method.

Microwave synthesis: This method involves the irradiation of electromagnetic radiations within a range of 1 mm to 1 m through the carbon precursor containing reaction mixture, which results from rapid and uniform heating. The microwaves absorbed by the solvent and precursor leading to the activation of molecules directly and its leads to formation of CDs [27, 28]. So, reaction volumes as such as 200 μl to >100 ml can be used without difficulty. The advantages of microwave irradiation are fast, higher efficiency and require less purification. The microwave irradiation can be controlled instantaneously so the risk of overheating is also minimized. However, the main drawback of this method is that solvents with lower boiling point cannot be used. This method widely used to convert bio-waste and natural sources such as plant materials, sea food waste and kitchen waste into CDs [29–31].

Thermal decomposition: In ordinary thermal decomposition, a carbon containing compound or substance decomposes chemically by action of heat and converted into CDs [32]. In general, CDs were synthesized from the variety of precursors like citric acid and L-cysteine etc. by simple heating under pyrolytic condition and controlled pressure using ionic liquid like 1-butyl 3-methyl imazonium bromide [33, 34]. The advantages of ionic liquid are high thermal stability, chemical stability; low melting point and low vapor pressure. At very high temperature, an irreversible thermal decomposition of organic matter takes place in inert mixture. Low cost, easy to operate, less time consuming and large-scale production are the advantages of the thermal decomposition method.

Pyrolysis: Pyrolysis is an irreversible thermal decomposition reaction in which decomposition of organic materials take place in inert atmosphere and at high pressure. Pyrolysis of the carbonaceous material is a simple, clean and inexpensive route for synthesizing CDs because no need of additives, acids or bases [35, 36].

In this method, solid residues with high carbon content were formed from organic materials by prolonged pyrolysis in an inert mixture. During pyrolysis, dehydration and fragmentation occurs. The natural precursors used for producing CDs in this method are cheap biowaste materials like rice husk, coffee grounds, watermelon peel, sago waste, peanut shells and wool etc.

Hydrothermal or solvothermal synthesis: In hydrothermal synthesis, carbon precursors undergoes "polymerization–carbonization" and leads to formation of CDs in water media taken in a sealed container under high temperature and pressure [37]. In solvothermal synthesis, organic solvents like methanol, ethanol, n-butanol and N, N- dimethylformamide etc. can be used as the solvent instead of water [38, 39]. This method was proved to be a cheap and eco-friendly route to the synthesis of carbon dots. However, solvothermal reactions can lead to an explosion in a few cases because the temperature rises rapidly in limited space. This can be avoided by taking a small quantity of solvent and reactant.

2.1.2 *Natural materials as a green precursor for preparation of CDs*

The green synthesis of CDs relies on natural precursors such as plant materials, protein products and waste materials [40]. Compared with bulk carbon materials (Graphene, Graphene Oxide and carbon tubes etc.) and toxic organic compounds including aromatic molecules, natural materials are renewable, economical, eco-friendly, safer and easier to get industrial-scale production. Mostly, "bottom-up" methods adopted for the synthesis of CDs due to the existing small organic molecules in natural sources can be carbonized into CDs at a specific temperature. A few top-down methods developed for the waste bulk carbon materials or bio-waste are broken down/cut into small-sized CDs. Among the various techniques, hydrothermal and microwave approaches are extensively used to prepare CDs from multiple natural materials. Most natural sources or biomass materials are made with small organic molecules, converted into CDs by carbonization and pyrolysis.

In recent years, various kind of plant material such as coriander leaves, ginger, garlic, grass, coffee beans, lemon, orange juice etc. due to the existence of various carbon containing organic molecules including carbohydrates, cellulose and phenolic compounds [41]. Compared with commercial precursors, the plant material derived CDs showed enhanced fluorescence emission with high quantum yield due to heteroatoms such as nitrogen, sulfur and phosphorus. Hence, the optical and structural properties of CDs are mainly relying on the selection of natural precursors. Besides this, with the growing concern about environmental pollution and sustainability, variety of waste materials including different kind of agriculture, kitchen, fruit peel and seafood waste etc. used as a starting material for the preparation of CDs [30, 42, 43]. These waste resources, also containing organic molecules, can be polymerized and followed by carbonized to form CDs.

2.2 General properties

The general properties of CDs illustrated in **Figure 2**. Structurally, CDs belongs to the quasi-spherical zero-dimension carbon nanomaterials class with a size of less than 10 nm [44, 45]. They are amorphous or nanocrystalline cores with a typical sp^2 carbon hybridization. The absorption band of CDs exhibits UV–Visible region to the NIR region and contains various functional groups. The electrifying properties of CDs are their excitation wavelength-dependent emission spectrum, high photostability and resisting to photobleaching, which permits CDs for multicolour and long-term imaging applications, respectively [45]. The cytotoxicity and pre-clinical biocompatibility of CDs on various models such as cell lines, zebrafish, mice

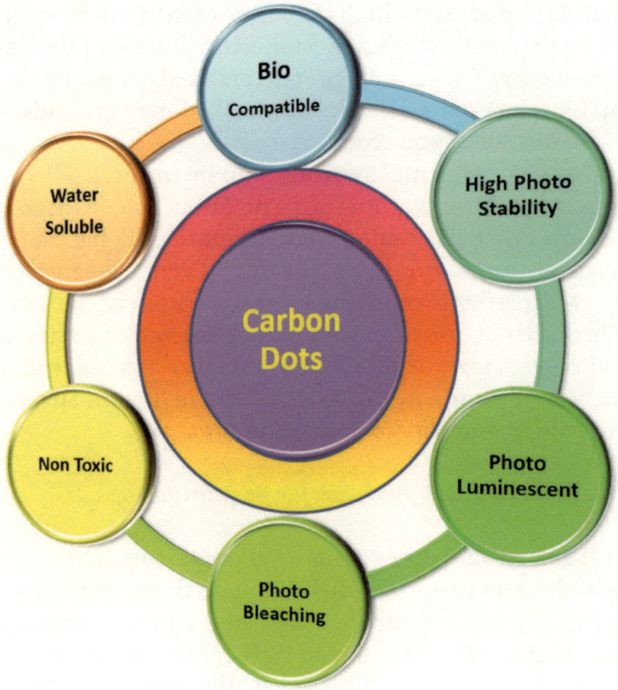

Figure 2.
Properties of carbon dots.

displayed CDs have no apparent toxic effects. Extensive studies are to be done on the toxicological and biocompatibility properties to translate from preclinical to clinical application. For targeted bio-imaging, the surface functional groups such as hydroxyl, amine and carboxylic groups allow conjugation with targeting agents.

2.2.1 Optical properties

Among all the CDs' properties, optical properties such as absorbance and fluorescence are vital for bio-imaging applications [45, 46]. Usually, CDs exhibited a strong absorption band at UV region with a falling intensity absorption tail increased to the visible light region. Usually, absorption peak around 230–340 nm was typically ascribed due to π-π^* transition of the C=C bonds of the carbon core. Similarly, the absorption band of 350–550 nm is ascribed to the surface functional groups on the carbon core. Besides this, one exciting feature of CDs is their excitation wavelength-dependent emission spectrum by varying excitation light wavelength, which is commonly observed in most CDs, which allows for multicolour imaging applications. CDs' exact PL mechanism is currently debatable due to the various methods available for the preparation of CDs and the lack of consistency in CDs' PL behavior. Nevertheless, three main mechanisms have been proposed to explain the PL of CDs: (1) The intrinsic band gap arising from the quantum confinement effect or the conjugated π domains, determined by CDs carbon core. (2) The creation of trap states (such as surface defects) in the band gap due to the surface functionalization and CDs doping. (3) The presence of individual fluorescent molecules (fluorophores) on or within the CDs. According to these theories, the wide tunable emissions of CDs have been attributed to their broad size distribution, variable surface chemistry, and the uncontrolled preparation conditions. Another fascinating PL property about CDs is that they generally exhibit high photostability, resisting photobleaching, which is very important for long-term imaging applications.

2.2.2 Elemental doping and surface functionalization

Usually, most of the bare CDs showed comparatively weak FL ability than traditional semiconductor quantum dots or organic dyes. In this line, CDs' structure altered by incorporating elements or surface functionalization strategies to improve fluorescence properties which are essential for fluorescence-based bio-imaging applications. So far, a variety of element doping is adopted to obtain CDs with charming FL properties. At present, heteroatoms such as N, S, Si, P, B, Ga, halogen (Cl, Br, I), Se, Ge, Mg, Cu, Zn, Tb, Ru and Mn incorporated into CDs during the synthesis process [47, 48]. Besides this, large functional groups such as carboxylic acid, amine, hydroxyl and amide groups presence on the surface of CDs facilitate the opportunity to conjugate with various passivate agents [38, 49]. Therefore, several groups focused on improving the fluorescence efficiency through conjugation with variety of passivating agents such as Polyethylene glycol, polyethyleneimine, poly (propionyl ethyleneimine co-ethyleneimine), 4,7,10-trioxa-1,13-tridecane-diamine, 1-hexadecylamine, poly(ethylenimide)-b-poly(ethyleneglycol)-b-poly (ethylene imide) and amino acids etc. Generally, these passivating conjugate with CDs via electrostatic interactions, covalent bonds, and hydrogen bonds. More interestingly hetero element doped or surface modified CDs also improved water solubility, photostability, biocompatibility, NIR absorbance and multicolour fluorescence emission, which are the vital parameters for bioimaging. Moreover, unique surface functional CDs have been prepared based on individual cell membrane lipids, proteins, targeting ligands and biomarkers of different cells to develop impactful imaging applications. Furthermore, variety of targeting moieties including peptides (transferrin), aptamers, antibodies and small molecules (folic acid) which have been selected to integrate on the surface of CD through N-hydroxy succinimide (NHS) or 1- ethyl-3-(3-dimethyl-aminopropyl) carbodiimide hydrochloride (EDC) chemistry [50]. These targeting moieties offer the internalization of CDs into cells or tissues via a ligand-receptor interaction. Remarkable specific cell targeting bioimaging besides adequate circulation of CDs avoid the side effects originating from the nonspecific interactions. The targeting moiety linked to CDs improves the specificity of bioimaging. Moreover, various cancer therapeutic drugs, anti-microbial agents and photosensitizers were conjugated with the CDs' surface for image guided therapeutic applications.

3. Bio-imaging

Bioimaging is an emerging field of biomedical science that comprises of the development and application of various materials for imaging technologies [51, 52]. The bioimaging techniques principles are mainly based on optics, magnetic resonance, nuclear medicine, radiation, ultrasonics, photonics and spectroscopy. The anatomical and physiological quantification of clinical parameters is measured with the image processing and analysis. With the recent development of biomedical science and emerging newer technologies, the *in vivo* or *ex vivo* biological tissue characterization of imaging properties aids in discerning its structure and function through visualization at several resolutions, extending from organ and cellular to molecular level. FL, near IR CT, PET, MRI and ultrasound images are commonly used for clinical diagnosis and research (**Figure 3**). The characteristic 'energy-matter' interaction is utilized by most bioimaging techniques to provide precise particulars of the biological processes. The imaging modality's uniqueness defines in terms of anatomical and molecular details, spatial and temporal resolution, depth of imaging and properties of contrast agents of augmented imaging. In many clinical

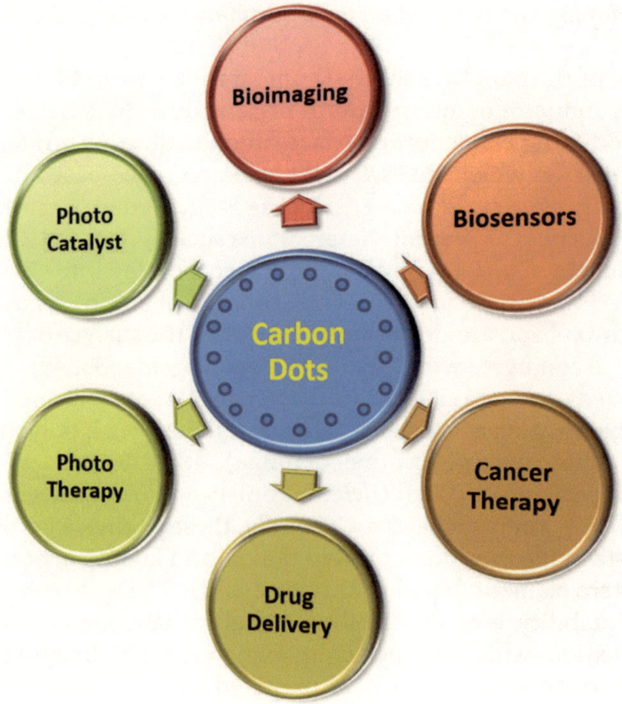

Figure 3.
Applications of carbon dots.

scenarios, the application of multimodal imaging techniques is advantageous for a simultaneous, faster and more accurate diagnosis. Exogenous contrast agents which are used in many imaging modalities enhances the signal to noise ratio. So, the development of multimodal contrast agents is essential to achieve better efficacy and accuracy in diagnosis and therapeutics.

4. Importance of carbon dot in bio-imaging

For clinical imaging application, good biocompatibility and low cytotoxicity of imaging probes are essential. The traditional quantum dots (QDs) such as CdSe, CdTe, CdS, and PbS were applied in *invitro* and *in vivo* optical bioimaging procedures [53]. But their bioimaging application is restricted due to heavy toxic metals which may cause toxicological and pathological problems for health and the environment. The silicon quantum dots (Si QDs) can be considered alternatives to heavy metal QDs in bioimaging [54]. But they undergo oxidative biodegradation in biological systems and are slightly toxic. The gold and silver nanoclusters were deemed to be alternative, non-toxic, photo luminescent nanomaterials, but suffering with poor water solubility and photostability [55]. So, there is a requirement for biocompatible imaging probes with low toxicity for bioimaging. Some CDs such as low toxicity, good biocompatibility, excellent photoluminescence and high photo stability makes them a novel nanoprobe for bioimaging.

4.1 Fluorescence imaging

FL imaging is a promising technique for observing and assessing various cells, tissues and organisms, by the high fluorescence emission with biocompatible fluorescent agents [56, 57]. Currently, fluorescent CDs are considered as a significant alternative ideal contrast agent for fluorescence imaging. Several reports revealed that cells incubated with CDs emitted fluorescence mainly due to accumulation of CDs in the cells. Generally, unmodified/bare CDs are majorly identified in the cell membrane and cytoplasmic region without reaching the nuclei. To resolve this issue, excessive effort have been devoted to surface modify the CDs with targeting agents including antibodies, peptides and other biomolecules to enhance the specific targeted bioimaging. These target ligands modified CDs showed a significant capacity to bind to the overexpressed reprehensive receptor/biomarker on cells. In addition, to resolve the issues related to deep tissue fluorescence imaging, the NIR receptive CDs were designed with longer excitation/emission wavelengths that enhanced fluorescence imaging ability [58] for *in vivo* applications. Under suitable excitation wavelength the NIR emitting CDs can be well differentiated from the auto-fluorescence background (green) with good optical contrast.

4.2 Multimodal imaging

Every imaging technique has its unique advantages in consort with integral limitations such as insufficient sensitivity or spatial resolution (**Figure 4**) [59]. Even the fluorescence imaging provides high sensitivity but lacks of sufficient resolution. To compensate this drawback, the combination of fluorescence imaging techniques with other modalities, such as FL/MRI has gained attention to enhance the currently used imaging techniques for diagnosis [58]. Multimodal imaging is a combination of two or more imaging techniques to overcome individual limitations. The development of multi-modality imaging with the FL imaging is

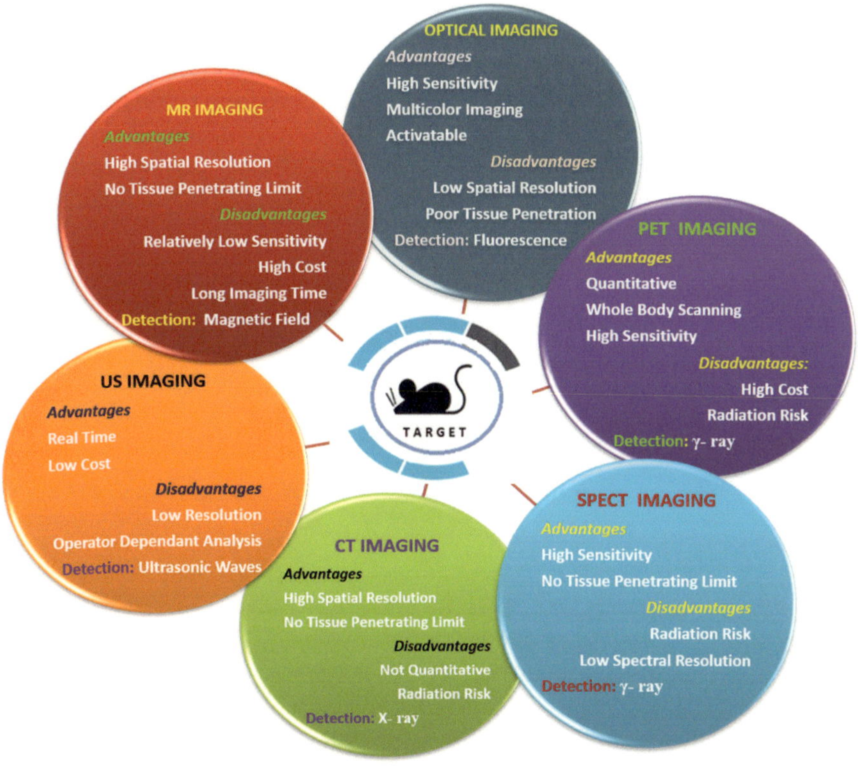
OPTICAL IMAGING
Advantages
High Sensitivity
Multicolor Imaging
Activatable
Disadvantages
Low Spatial Resolution
Poor Tissue Penetration
Detection: Fluorescence
MR IMAGING
Advantages
High Spatial Resolution
No Tissue Penetrating Limit
Disadvantages
Relatively Low Sensitivity
High Cost
Long Imaging Time
Detection: Magnetic Field
PET IMAGING
Advantages
Quantitative
Whole Body Scanning
High Sensitivity
Disadvantages:
High Cost
Radiation Risk
Detection: γ- ray
US IMAGING
Advantages
Real Time
Low Cost
Disadvantages
Low Resolution
Operator Dependant Analysis
Detection: Ultrasonic Waves
TARGET
SPECT IMAGING
Advantages
High Sensitivity
No Tissue Penetrating Limit
Disadvantages
Radiation Risk
Low Spectral Resolution
Detection: γ- ray
CT IMAGING
Advantages
High Spatial Resolution
No Tissue Penetrating Limit
Disadvantages
Not Quantitative
Radiation Risk
Detection: X- ray

Figure 4.
Advantages and disadvantages of various imaging techniques.

to achieve non-invasive imaging at greater depths of penetration, sensitivity and higher resolution required for an accurate diagnosis. Thus, optical imaging assisted multi-modalities has emerged as potent tools, which can improve the detection sensitivity, precise identification and provide more detailed anatomical or biological information of the pathology. Each imaging technique uses different contrast agents with distinctive functional, chemical compositions and sizes. In designing and developing a multi modal contrast agent, the researchers should judiciously forbid the overlay of pros and somewhat counterbalance each modality's limitations to enhance the synergistic effect. Thus, the FL imaging modality with high sensitivity is frequently combined with other imaging modalities with a high spatial resolution modality such as MR, CT, and PA etc. (**Figure 5**). Hence, multimodal contrast agents' development and application are clinically significant for enhanced imagery from desirable imaging modality. Multimodal imaging agents based on fluorescent CDs are the recent cutting-edge technologies where CDs' advantages are maximized. CDs based multimodal imaging agents are prepared by conjugating or incorporating one or more imaging agents into CDs. Here we have discussed various kinds of fluorescent CDs' based multi-modality imaging approaches such as FL/PA, FL/MR and FL/CT imaging.

4.2.1 Fluorescence/photoacoustic imaging

Photoacoustic (PA) imaging is a non-invasive, hybrid, optical and ultrasound imaging modality. The PA imaging is performed at varying depths with high depth to resolution ratio with rich optical contrast beyond the optical detection limit. The CDs have shown significant PA imaging application because of the NIR absorption, high extinction coefficient, and non-radiative heat generation. Wang, *et al.* synthesized dual-mode FL/PA imaging agent based on CDs [60]. Within the NIR spectrum, the imaging agent exhibited a maximum optical absorption at 710 nm approximately. In *in vivo* PA imaging of mice tumor model, enhancement of signal and clear demarcation of the tumor was observed due to long circulation time and increased tumor accumulation of CDs. Hence, the combination of fluorescence and photoacoustic imaging into a single probe based on CDs enabled deeper tissue penetration for tumor identification. Compared with single optical imaging, the

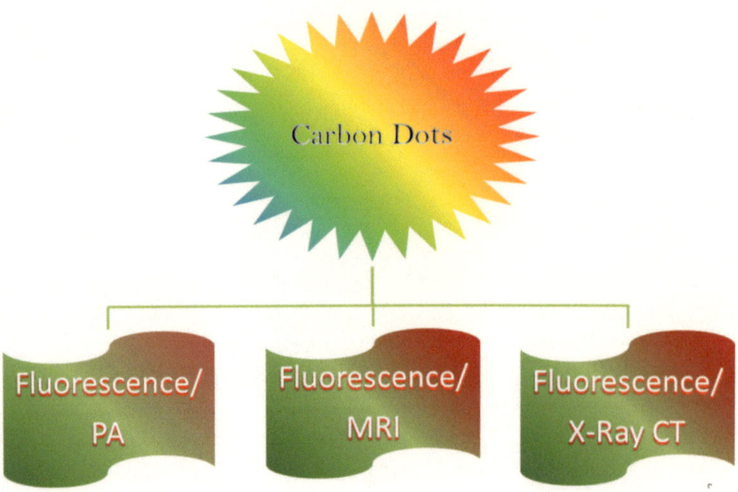

Figure 5.
Carbon dots integrated multi-modal bio imaging.

dual-mode FL/PA imaging upholds the sensitivity and provides higher-resolution anatomical images. Porphyrin implanted CDs developed by selective pyrolysis with good aqueous dispersibility displayed a strong PA signal at 686 nm in a slightly acidic or neutral environment and somewhat alkaline conditions pH 7–8 the signal was weak [61]. In breast cancer, the sentinel lymph nodes detection, the application of photo acoustic visualization of CDs was reported by Wu, *et al.* [62]. After injection the CDs exhibited rapid signal enhancement and relatively fast clearance from the lymph nodes.

4.2.2 Fluorescence/magnetic resonance imaging

Magnetic resonance imaging (MRI), is a radiation-free and non-invasive imaging technique widely used to detect various diseases including clinical cancer diagnosis and therapeutic response assessment [63]. With an external radiofrequency pulse magnetic field applied on the body, it simultaneously obtains anatomical and physiological information of regions of interests with a high spatial resolution by manipulating magnetic nucleus's resonance (^1H). Further, the integration of FL imaging with MR imaging considered as most effective non-invasive imaging tool in diagnosis and clinical research due its excellent spatial resolution, high temporal and sensitivity. Hence, the CDs assisted FL/MR dual modality potentiality can take benefits of the spatial resolution, outstanding soft-tissue contrast with MR imaging as well as superior sensitivity and the rapid data acquiring with FL imaging. This dual imaging modality is facilitated precise diagnosis with effective treatment based on corresponding imaging evidence. The CDs-relayed FL/MR dual-mode imaging modality probe can be obtained by the doping/ conjugation of magnetic elements. Specifically, extremely paramagnetic ions including Gd^{3+}, Mn^{2+}, and Fe^{3+} employed as dopant for the preparation of FL/MR bimodal contrast agent such as Gd or Mn elements into CDs. For example, Gd^{3+} doped CDs were synthesized from Gd^{3+} containing precursors and sucrose as carbon precursors via microwave assisted method polyol by Gong Ningqiang, *et al.* The attained Gd-CDs showed green fluorescence emission, low cytotoxicity and optically label cells. Meanwhile, the r_1 relaxivity of Gd-CDs was measured to be 11.356 $mM^{-1}\,s^{-1}$. This high r_1 value together with the r_2/r_1 ratio approximately 1. These results indicating that Gd-CDs is not only significant fluorescent imaging agent but also remarkable T_1 contrast agent for MR imaging [64].

Further, Jia Qingyan, *et al.* demonstrated the magneto-fluorescent Mn-doped CDs for bimodal FL/MR imaging in a single probe. The study reported the development of ultrafine Mn-doped CDs with a concurrent bimodal imaging ability through the solvothermal procedure of the precursor manganese (II) phthalocyanine [65]. The Mn-doped CDs showed strong T_1-weighted MRI signals and low cytotoxicity. The MRI signal intensities increased with the concentration, exhibiting a clear difference in brightness with a measured relaxation (r_1) value of ≈6.97 $mM^{-1}\,s^{-1}$. Furthermore, the *in vivo* T1-weighted results fortified the high retention rate of the Mn-doped CDs in tumors. The MRI signal intensity at the tumor site increased quantitatively by ≈320%, after 6 hrs injection while the MRI signal remained nearly unchanged for the analogous CDs without manganese (II) doping. CDs doped with dysprosium for a magneto-fluorescent bimodal imaging agent showed strong blue-green fluorescence at 452 nm. The excellent transverse relaxivity r_2 makes them also suitable for T_2 weighted imaging of live cells [66].

4.2.3 Fluorescence/X-ray computed tomography

X-ray computed tomography (CT) is a non-invasive medical imaging technique for disease diagnosis. The CT has intrinsic advantages such as high spatial resolution and good density; it still has inherent drawbacks of low sensitivity. On the other hand, the fluorescence imaging has high sensitivity, facile operation and low cost, but its application was hampered due to the low spatial resolution and limited penetration depth. To improve clinical diagnostic accuracy and sensitivity, the FL and CT imaging are combined for a synergistic effect. The CDs doped with Hafnium (Hf) was used for diagnostic imaging of the orthotopic liver cancer preclinical model [67]. Rapid imaging was achieved with Hafnium doped CDs due to preferential tumor accumulation within 1 min. These imaging nanoprobes with efficient renal clearance offers good biocompatibility. Iodine doped CDs conjugated with a chemotherapeutic agent like cetuximab simultaneously rendered the cancer diagnosis and targeted anti-cancer therapeutic potential in lung cancer cells [68].

5. Imaging guided therapeutic application

Nanotechnology provides the possibility of developing non-toxic CDs nanoprobes with enhanced sensitivity, accuracy and advanced functionalities for imaging-guided synergistic therapy [69, 70]. The unique advantages of CDs include high relaxivity, prolonged blood circulation time, multiple functionalities for accurate accumulation in the target site, good biocompatibility and renal clearance. The inherent radio resistance of tumors and inaccurate positioning of the radiotherapeutic equipment leads to decreased radiotherapy effectiveness. Du Fengyi, *et al.* reported the theragnostic Gd-CDs with stable photoluminescence at the visible region, relatively long circulation time, efficient passive tumor targeting ability and renal clearance for MRI-guided radiotherapy a tumor [71]. Changhong Zhao *et al.* developed red-emitting wavelength multifunctional CDs for cancer theragnostic with *in vivo* bimodal imaging of tumor tissues and anti-cancer chemo-dynamic treatment (CDT). The functionalization of red CDs was done with Ethylene di amine tetra-acetic acid, $Fe^{2+}$and Gd^{3+}exhibited strong T1 weighted MR imaging and excellent bright and stable fluorescence. The anticancer CDT effect was based on Fenton reaction, by releasing Fe^{2+} into the tumor both *invitro* and *in vivo* [72].

6. Conclusions and outlook

Naturally, renewable sources derived CDs are kind of newly born luminescent carbon-based nanomaterials in this decade. They gained great potential in bio-imaging not only because of their cost-effective and eco-friendly green synthetic approaches but also their physical, chemical and biological properties. We have elaborately discussed various synthesis methods, significant properties. Furthermore, the recent development of CD in multimodal bio-imaging. Their strong fluorescence emission, high fluorescent quantum yield, and good absorbance are widely used for fluorescence imaging. Specific CDs also allow for multicolour bioimaging due to their multicolour emission capability. Further, numerous surface functional groups provide an opportunity to conjugate with targeting moieties such folic acid for targeting imaging. Accordingly, CDs conjugation with targeted moieties can precisely transport imaging contrast agents to internal organelles or cell membranes to attain the goal of targeted bio-imaging. In the meantime, the large surface area of CDs permits them to have a more quantity of hetero atom loading ability, consequently showing remarkable multimodal imaging ability. Finally, the nano size of CDs (typically >10 nm) facilitates their navigation in tissues, endocytosis, and intracellular trafficking. Even though significant efforts have devoted to improving the multimodal imaging effect of CDs, several limitations hinder the application of CDs in bio-imaging. Primarily, the emission from most of the natural sources derived CDs showed blue or green, thus developing the methods and finding suitable natural precursor for yellow or red emissive CDs is highly desired. CDs exhibit excellent biocompatibility; however, majority studies are confined to cellular and preclinical experiments, but translation into clinical investigations is still unclear. In summary, more research still needs to be made for the effective and real-time clinical application of CDs in multimodal imaging.

Author details

Gangaraju Gedda[1]*, Arun Bhupathi[2] and V.L.N. Balaji Gupta Tiruveedhi[1]

1 Department of Basic Science, Vishnu Institute of Technology, Vishnupur, Bhimavaram, A.P, India

2 Department of Orthodontics and Dentofacial Orthopedics, Vishnu Dental College, Vishnupur, Bhimavaram, A.P, India

*Address all correspondence to: raju.analy@gmail.com

References

[1] T.-L. Liu, S. Upadhyayula, D.E. Milkie, V. Singh, K. Wang, I.A. Swinburne, K.R. Mosaliganti, Z.M. Collins, T.W. Hiscock, J. Shea, A.Q. Kohrman, T.N. Medwig, D. Dambournet, R. Forster, B. Cunniff, Y. Ruan, H. Yashiro, S. Scholpp, E.M. Meyerowitz, D. Hockemeyer, D.G. Drubin, B.L. Martin, D.Q. Matus, M. Koyama, S.G. Megason, T. Kirchhausen, E. Betzig, Observing the cell in its native state: Imaging subcellular dynamics in multicellular organisms, Science 360(6386) (2018) eaaq1392.

[2] J. Kim, Y. Piao, T. Hyeon, Multifunctional nanostructured materials for multimodal imaging, and simultaneous imaging and therapy, Chemical Society Reviews 38(2) (2009) 372-390.

[3] J. Rao, A. Dragulescu-Andrasi, H. Yao, Fluorescence imaging in vivo: recent advances, Current opinion in biotechnology 18(1) (2007) 17-25.

[4] M. Schäferling, The art of fluorescence imaging with chemical sensors, Angewandte Chemie International Edition 51(15) (2012) 3532-3554.

[5] P.P. Laissue, R.A. Alghamdi, P. Tomancak, E.G. Reynaud, H. Shroff, Assessing phototoxicity in live fluorescence imaging, Nature methods 14(7) (2017) 657-661.

[6] X. Li, L. Que, Fluorescence Enhancement Enabled by Nanomaterials and Nanostructured Substrates: A Brief Review, Reviews in Nanoscience and Nanotechnology 3(3) (2014) 161-176.

[7] J. Zhao, J. Chen, S. Ma, Q. Liu, L. Huang, X. Chen, K. Lou, W. Wang, Recent developments in multimodality fluorescence imaging probes, Acta Pharmaceutica Sinica B 8(3) (2018) 320-338.

[8] Z. Liu, F. Kiessling, J. Gätjens, Advanced Nanomaterials in Multimodal Imaging: Design, Functionalization, and Biomedical Applications, Journal of Nanomaterials 2010 (2010) 894303.

[9] J. Wang, J. Qiu, A review of carbon dots in biological applications, Journal of Materials Science 51(10) (2016) 4728-4738.

[10] P. Zuo, X. Lu, Z. Sun, Y. Guo, H. He, A review on syntheses, properties, characterization and bioanalytical applications of fluorescent carbon dots, Microchimica Acta 183(2) (2016) 519-542.

[11] J. Zuo, T. Jiang, X. Zhao, X. Xiong, S. Xiao, Z. Zhu, Preparation and application of fluorescent carbon dots, Journal of Nanomaterials 2015 (2015).

[12] X. Zhang, Q. Zeng, Y. Xiong, T. Ji, C. Wang, X. Shen, M. Lu, H. Wang, S. Wen, Y. Zhang, Energy Level Modification with Carbon Dot Interlayers Enables Efficient Perovskite Solar Cells and Quantum Dot Based Light-Emitting Diodes, Advanced Functional Materials 30(11) (2020) 1910530.

[13] X. Dong, W. Liang, M.J. Meziani, Y.-P. Sun, L. Yang, Carbon dots as potent antimicrobial agents, Theranostics 10(2) (2020) 671.

[14] J.-H. Qu, Q. Wei, D.-W. Sun, Carbon dots: Principles and their applications in food quality and safety detection, Critical reviews in food science and nutrition 58(14) (2018) 2466-2475.

[15] L.S. Chu K-W, Chang C-J, Liu L. Recent Progress of Carbon Dot Precursors and Photocatalysis Applications., Polymers (Basel) 11(4):689 (2019).

[16] R. Jelinek, Carbon-Dot Synthesis, Carbon Quantum Dots: Synthesis,

Properties and Applications, Springer International Publishing, Cham, 2017, pp. 5-27.

[17] J.C.E. da Silva, H.M. Gonçalves, Analytical and bioanalytical applications of carbon dots, TrAC Trends in Analytical Chemistry 30(8) (2011) 1327-1336.

[18] V. Mishra, A. Patil, S. Thakur, P. Kesharwani, Carbon dots: emerging theranostic nanoarchitectures, Drug discovery today 23(6) (2018) 1219-1232.

[19] Z.-A. Qiao, Y. Wang, Y. Gao, H. Li, T. Dai, Y. Liu, Q. Huo, Commercially activated carbon as the source for producing multicolor photoluminescent carbon dots by chemical oxidation, Chemical Communications 46(46) (2010) 8812-8814.

[20] J. Joseph, A.A. Anappara, White-Light-Emitting Carbon Dots Prepared by the Electrochemical Exfoliation of Graphite, ChemPhysChem 18(3) (2017) 292-298.

[21] X. Li, Z. Zhao, C. Pan, Electrochemical exfoliation of carbon dots with the narrowest full width at half maximum in their fluorescence spectra in the ultraviolet region using only water as electrolyte, Chemical Communications 52(60) (2016) 9406-9409.

[22] X. Li, Z. Zhao, C. Pan, Ionic liquid-assisted electrochemical exfoliation of carbon dots of different size for fluorescent imaging of bacteria by tuning the water fraction in electrolyte, Microchimica Acta 183(9) (2016) 2525-2532.

[23] D. Reyes, M. Camacho, M. Camacho, M. Mayorga, D. Weathers, G. Salamo, Z. Wang, A. Neogi, Laser ablated carbon nanodots for light emission, Nanoscale research letters 11(1) (2016) 1-11.

[24] D. Reyes-Contreras, M. Camacho-López, M.A. Camacho-López, S. Camacho-López, R.I. Rodríguez-Beltrán, M. Mayorga-Rojas, Influence of the per pulse laser fluence on the optical properties of carbon nanoparticles synthesized by laser ablation of solids in liquids, Optics & Laser Technology 74 (2015) 48-52.

[25] K. Dehvari, K.Y. Liu, P.-J. Tseng, G. Gedda, W.M. Girma, J.-Y. Chang, Sonochemical-assisted green synthesis of nitrogen-doped carbon dots from crab shell as targeted nanoprobes for cell imaging, Journal of the Taiwan Institute of Chemical Engineers 95 (2019) 495-503.

[26] S.K. Das, R. Gawas, S. Chakrabarty, G. Harini, R. Patidar, K. Jasuja, An unexpected transformation of organic solvents into 2D fluorescent quantum dots during ultrasonication-assisted liquid-phase exfoliation, The Journal of Physical Chemistry C 123(41) (2019) 25412-25421.

[27] X. Zhai, P. Zhang, C. Liu, T. Bai, W. Li, L. Dai, W. Liu, Highly luminescent carbon nanodots by microwave-assisted pyrolysis, Chemical Communications 48(64) (2012) 7955-7957.

[28] V. Hinterberger, W. Wang, C. Damm, S. Wawra, M. Thoma, W. Peukert, Microwave-assisted one-step synthesis of white light-emitting carbon dot suspensions, Optical Materials 80 (2018) 110-119.

[29] A. Tangy, V.B. Kumar, I.N. Pulidindi, Y. Kinel-Tahan, Y. Yehoshua, A. Gedanken, In-situ transesterification of *Chlorella vulgaris* using carbon-dot functionalized strontium oxide as a heterogeneous catalyst under microwave irradiation, Energy & Fuels 30(12) (2016) 10602-10610.

[30] H. Fan, M. Zhang, B. Bhandari, C.-h. Yang, Food waste as a carbon source in carbon quantum dots

technology and their applications in food safety detection, Trends in Food Science & Technology 95 (2020) 86-96.

[31] A. Himaja, P.S. Karthik, B. Sreedhar, S.P. Singh, Synthesis of carbon dots from kitchen waste: conversion of waste to value added product, Journal of fluorescence 24(6) (2014) 1767-1773.

[32] X.W. Tan, A.N.B. Romainor, S.F. Chin, S.M. Ng, Carbon dots production via pyrolysis of sago waste as potential probe for metal ions sensing, Journal of analytical and applied pyrolysis 105 (2014) 157-165.

[33] J.-Y. Wan, Z. Yang, Z.-G. Liu, H.-X. Wang, Ionic liquid-assisted thermal decomposition synthesis of carbon dots and graphene-like carbon sheets for optoelectronic application, RSC advances 6(66) (2016) 61292-61300.

[34] A. Zheng, T. Guo, F. Guan, X. Chen, Y. Shu, J. Wang, Ionic liquid mediated carbon dots: Preparations, properties and applications, TrAC Trends in Analytical Chemistry 119 (2019) 115638.

[35] W. Shang, T. Cai, Y. Zhang, D. Liu, S. Liu, Facile one pot pyrolysis synthesis of carbon quantum dots and graphene oxide nanomaterials: all carbon hybrids as eco-environmental lubricants for low friction and remarkable wear-resistance, Tribology International 118 (2018) 373-380.

[36] M. Rong, Y. Feng, Y. Wang, X. Chen, One-pot solid phase pyrolysis synthesis of nitrogen-doped carbon dots for Fe3+ sensing and bioimaging, Sensors and Actuators B: Chemical 245 (2017) 868-874.

[37] C. Wang, Z. Xu, H. Cheng, H. Lin, M.G. Humphrey, C. Zhang, A hydrothermal route to water-stable luminescent carbon dots as nanosensors for pH and temperature, Carbon 82 (2015) 87-95.

[38] *S. mitra*, S. Chandra, S.H. Pathan, N. Sikdar, P. Pramanik, A. Goswami, Room temperature and solvothermal green synthesis of self passivated carbon quantum dots, RSC Advances 3(10) (2013) 3189-3193.

[39] M. Li, C. Yu, C. Hu, W. Yang, C. Zhao, S. Wang, M. Zhang, J. Zhao, X. Wang, J. Qiu, Solvothermal conversion of coal into nitrogen-doped carbon dots with singlet oxygen generation and high quantum yield, Chemical Engineering Journal 320 (2017) 570-575.

[40] X. Guo, H. Zhang, H. Sun, M.O. Tade, S. Wang, Green Synthesis of Carbon Quantum Dots for Sensitized Solar Cells, ChemPhotoChem 1(4) (2017) 116-119.

[41] A.H. Zulfajri M, Sudewi S, Dayalan S, Rasool A, Habib A, Huang GG. Plant Part-Derived Carbon Dots for Biosensing, Biosensors 10(6):68. (2020).

[42] P. Kaur, S. Singh, G. Verma, Facile synthesis of mesoporous carbon material from treated kitchen waste for energy applications, Materials for Renewable and Sustainable Energy 7(2) (2018) 9.

[43] V. Sharma, P. Tiwari, S.M. Mobin, Sustainable carbon-dots: recent advances in green carbon dots for sensing and bioimaging, Journal of Materials Chemistry B 5(45) (2017) 8904-8924.

[44] X.T. Zheng, A. Ananthanarayanan, K.Q. Luo, P. Chen, Glowing Graphene Quantum Dots and Carbon Dots: Properties, Syntheses, and Biological Applications, Small 11(14) (2015) 1620-1636.

[45] M. Semeniuk, Z. Yi, V. Poursorkhabi, J. Tjong, S. Jaffer, Z.-H. Lu, M. Sain, Future Perspectives and Review on Organic Carbon Dots in Electronic Applications, ACS Nano 13(6) (2019) 6224-6255.

[46] P. Namdari, B. Negahdari, A. Eatemadi, Synthesis, properties and biomedical applications of carbon-based quantum dots: An updated review, Biomedicine & Pharmacotherapy 87 (2017) 209-222.

[47] Q. Xu, T. Kuang, Y. Liu, L. Cai, X. Peng, T. Sreenivasan Sreeprasad, P. Zhao, Z. Yu, N. Li, Heteroatom-doped carbon dots: synthesis, characterization, properties, photoluminescence mechanism and biological applications, Journal of Materials Chemistry B 4(45) (2016) 7204-7219.

[48] S. Miao, K. Liang, J. Zhu, B. Yang, D. Zhao, B. Kong, Hetero-atom-doped carbon dots: Doping strategies, properties and applications, Nano Today 33 (2020) 100879.

[49] J. Pan, Z. Zheng, J. Yang, Y. Wu, F. Lu, Y. Chen, W. Gao, A novel and sensitive fluorescence sensor for glutathione detection by controlling the surface passivation degree of carbon quantum dots, Talanta 166 (2017) 1-7.

[50] Y. Song, S. Zhu, B. Yang, Bioimaging based on fluorescent carbon dots, RSC Advances 4(52) (2014) 27184-27200.

[51] Q. Le Trequesser, H. Seznec, M.-H. Delville, Functionalized nanomaterials: their use as contrast agents in bioimaging: mono- and multimodal approaches, Nanotechnology Reviews 2(2) (2013) 125-169.

[52] R. Bilan, I. Nabiev, A. Sukhanova, Quantum Dot-Based Nanotools for Bioimaging, Diagnostics, and Drug Delivery, ChemBioChem 17(22) (2016) 2103-2114.

[53] I.L. Medintz, H.T. Uyeda, E.R. Goldman, H. Mattoussi, Quantum dot bioconjugates for imaging, labelling and sensing, Nature materials 4(6) (2005) 435-446.

[54] F. Erogbogbo, K.-T. Yong, I. Roy, G. Xu, P.N. Prasad, M.T. Swihart, Biocompatible luminescent silicon quantum dots for imaging of cancer cells, ACS nano 2(5) (2008) 873-878.

[55] Y.-C. Shiang, C.-C. Huang, W.-Y. Chen, P.-C. Chen, H.-T. Chang, Fluorescent gold and silver nanoclusters for the analysis of biopolymers and cell imaging, Journal of Materials Chemistry 22(26) (2012) 12972-12982.

[56] X. Wu, F. Tian, W. Wang, J. Chen, M. Wu, J.X. Zhao, Fabrication of highly fluorescent graphene quantum dots using L-glutamic acid for in vitro/in vivo imaging and sensing, Journal of Materials Chemistry C 1(31) (2013) 4676-4684.

[57] T.-s. Chu, R. Lü, B.-t. Liu, Reversibly monitoring oxidation and reduction events in living biological systems: recent development of redox-responsive reversible NIR biosensors and their applications in in vitro/in vivo fluorescence imaging, Biosensors and Bioelectronics 86 (2016) 643-655.

[58] J.H. Lee, Y.w. Jun, S.I. Yeon, J.S. Shin, J. Cheon, Dual-mode nanoparticle probes for high-performance magnetic resonance and fluorescence imaging of neuroblastoma, Angewandte Chemie International Edition 45(48) (2006) 8160-8162.

[59] D.-E. Lee, H. Koo, I.-C. Sun, J.H. Ryu, K. Kim, I.C. Kwon, Multifunctional nanoparticles for multimodal imaging and theragnosis, Chemical Society Reviews 41(7) (2012) 2656-2672.

[60] J. Ge, Q. Jia, W. Liu, L. Guo, Q. Liu, M. Lan, H. Zhang, X. Meng, *P. Wang*, Red-emissive carbon dots for fluorescent, photoacoustic, and thermal theranostics in living mice, Advanced Materials 27(28) (2015) 4169-4177.

[61] F. Wu, H. Su, Y. Cai, W.-K. Wong, W. Jiang, X. Zhu, Porphyrin-implanted carbon nanodots for photoacoustic

imaging and in vivo breast cancer ablation, ACS Applied Bio Materials 1(1) (2018) 110-117.

[62] L. Wu, X. Cai, K. Nelson, W. Xing, J. Xia, R. Zhang, A.J. Stacy, M. Luderer, G.M. Lanza, L.V. Wang, A green synthesis of carbon nanoparticles from honey and their use in real-time photoacoustic imaging, Nano research 6(5) (2013) 312-325.

[63] A. Shukla-Dave, H. Hricak, Role of MRI in prostate cancer detection, NMR in Biomedicine 27(1) (2014) 16-24.

[64] N. Gong, H. Wang, S. Li, Y. Deng, X.a. Chen, L. Ye, W. Gu, Microwave-assisted polyol synthesis of gadolinium-doped green luminescent carbon dots as a bimodal nanoprobe, Langmuir 30(36) (2014) 10933-10939.

[65] Q. Jia, J. Ge, W. Liu, X. Zheng, S. Chen, Y. Wen, H. Zhang, *P. Wang*, A magnetofluorescent carbon dot assembly as an acidic H2O2-driven oxygenerator to regulate tumor hypoxia for simultaneous bimodal imaging and enhanced photodynamic therapy, Advanced Materials 30(13) (2018) 1706090.

[66] T.S. Atabaev, Z. Piao, A. Molkenova, Carbon dots doped with dysprosium: a bimodal nanoprobe for MRI and fluorescence imaging, Journal of functional biomaterials 9(2) (2018) 35.

[67] Y. Su, S. Liu, Y. Guan, Z. Xie, M. Zheng, X. Jing, Renal clearable Hafnium-doped carbon dots for CT/Fluorescence imaging of orthotopic liver cancer, Biomaterials 255 (2020) 120110.

[68] H. Su, Y. Liao, F. Wu, X. Sun, H. Liu, K. Wang, X. Zhu, Cetuximab-conjugated iodine doped carbon dots as a dual fluorescent/CT probe for targeted imaging of lung cancer cells, Colloids and Surfaces B: Biointerfaces 170 (2018) 194-200.

[69] R. Mohammadinejad, A. Dadashzadeh, S. Moghassemi, M. Ashrafizadeh, A. Dehshahri, A. Pardakhty, H. Sassan, S.-M. Sohrevardi, A. Mandegary, Shedding light on gene therapy: Carbon dots for the minimally invasive image-guided delivery of plasmids and noncoding RNAs-A review, Journal of advanced research 18 (2019) 81-93.

[70] B.B. Chen, M.L. Liu, C.Z. Huang, Recent advances of carbon dots in imaging-guided theranostics, TrAC Trends in Analytical Chemistry (2020) 116116.

[71] F. Du, L. Zhang, L. Zhang, M. Zhang, A. Gong, Y. Tan, J. Miao, Y. Gong, M. Sun, H. Ju, Engineered gadolinium-doped carbon dots for magnetic resonance imaging-guided radiotherapy of tumors, Biomaterials 121 (2017) 109-120.

[72] W. Wang, Q. Zhang, M. Zhang, Y. Liu, J. Shen, N. Zhou, X. Lu, C. Zhao, Multifunctional red carbon dots: a theranostic platform for magnetic resonance imaging and fluorescence imaging-guided chemodynamic therapy, Analyst 145(10) (2020) 3592-3597.

Chapter 10

Advances in Tissue Engineering Approaches for Craniomaxillofacial Bone Reconstruction

Geetanjali B. Tomar, Jay Dave, Sayali Chandekar, Nandika Bhattacharya, Sharvari Naik, Shravani Kulkarni, Suraj Math, Kaushik Desai and Neha Sapkal

Abstract

Trauma, congenital abnormalities and pathologies such as cancer can cause significant defects in craniofacial bone. Regeneration of the bone in the craniofacial area presents a unique set of challenges due to its complexity and association with various other tissues. Bone grafts and bone cement are the traditional treatment options but pose their own issues with regards to integration and morbidity. This has driven the search for materials which mimic the natural bone and can act as scaffolds to guide bone growth. Novel technology and computer aided manufacturing have allowed us to control material parameters such as mechanical strength and pore geometry. In this chapter, we elaborate the current status of materials and techniques used in fabrication of scaffolds for craniomaxillofacial bone tissue engineering and discuss the future prospects for advancements.

Keywords: tissue engineering, regenerative medicine, bone regeneration, 3D printing, craniomaxillofacial, additive manufacturing, scaffold, polymer, synthetic polymer, biopolymer, bone defect

1. Introduction

The incredible capacity of human body to regenerate is governed by factors such as size of the defect, requirement of growth hormones and the type of the tissue [1]. Any injury to a tissue beyond the critical size needs external support for regeneration. A defect is considered as a critical size defect when it does not spontaneously heal on its own and requires intervention [2]. This approach of mitigating and reconstructing the damaged or injured tissue is referred to as regenerative medicine or tissue engineering [1].

Bone is considered to be the second most engineered tissue, which undergoes degeneration due to tumor surgeries, osteoporosis, trauma etc. [3]. Natural bone matrix is composed of organic (collagen) and inorganic (apatite) materials. By weight bone contains 30% collagen matrix, 60% mineral and 10% water. The unique modulus of bone, falls between conventional plastics and ceramics, and

IntechOpen

is primarily determined by a unique interpenetrating arrangement of collagen and apatite at the nanoscale. Naturally, the process of bone healing is determined by the size of the wound. This process in turn is directed and stimulated by well-balanced biological and microenvironmental cues. In case of large bone defects the fibrous tissue regenerates faster than the bone tissue and becomes dominant at the defect site. Excess of fibrous tissue does not compensate for the loss of mechanical strength. Therefore, repair of large bone defects necessitates implantation of a replacement material to facilitate bone healing [4].

Calvarial and long bones are unique and distinct from each other in terms of development, structure and function. From a developmental point of view, intramembranous ossification is dominant in skull bone formation whereas long bone formation majorly occurs via endochondral ossification. These distinctions require customized tailoring of specific strategies for either calvaria or long bone repair. Calvarial bones are required to withstand impact forces whereas long bones must withstand the bending and twisting movements and therefore horizontal grafting and vertical bone augmentation techniques need to be developed for reconstruction purposes respectively [5, 6].

The craniofacial region includes facial skin, muscles, bone, tendons, ligaments, nerves and blood vessels. The craniomaxillofacial bones consist of cranial and facial bones. Cranial bones enclose the brain and protect it, whereas facial bones such maxillary and mandible act as load bearing bones for dental region [7]. The bone tissue thus encompasses mandible, auditory ossicles, neuro cranium (protects the brain) and splanchnocranium (supports the face) [8]. Whereas, the cartilaginous part of the craniomaxillofacial region is primarily constituted by temporomandibular joint disc, auricle and nasal regions of the craniofacial cavity [3]. Moreover, the dental tissue in the craniofacial region includes both hard structures (enamel, cementum and dentin) and soft tissue component (pulp cavity) [7], which together make up the structure of tooth. Tooth is embedded into the maxillary and mandibular bones, which together constitutes the alveolar bone. It has been found that the cortical thickness of the alveolar bone is 2.1–2.4 mm and a density is 1.64–1.75 mg/cm^3 whereas the compressive strength of cancellous bone in the mandibular region is in the range of 0.2–10.44 MPa (average 3.9 ± 2.7 MPa, depending on the bone density, age and gender) [9].

Tooth defects or tooth loss caused by endodontic diseases, periodontal disease, tumor, trauma and variety of genetic disorders require dentin and dental pulp tissue regeneration. However, the current available treatments involve replacement of lost tooth by artificial dentition or dental implants. Thus, extensive research is required to achieve reconstruction of such craniofacial and dental tissue defects [10]. The reconstruction therapy for critical bone defects should address the post-surgical side effects of slow or deficient bone recovery, graft rejection and low osseointegration [11].

Periostium is a major source for osteoprogenitor cells whereas dura mater contains multipotent mesenchymal stem cells that facilitate skull bone healing through paracrine signaling, indicating that the indigenous surrounding tissues of the craniomaxillofacial skeleton such as dura mater, periostium, suture and bone marrow themselves play an important role in healing processes [5]. As the craniomaxillofacial region is associated with a variety of vital functions such as vision, hearing, speech, mastication, breathing and normal brain function, the injuries of this region caused due to trauma, tumor surgery or genetic defects results in critical defects which are difficult to reconstruct because of complexity of anatomical structure, variety of tissue specific requirements and restoration of esthetic facial features, seeking for facial harmony and most perfect symmetry [8, 12–14]. Furthermore, maxillectomy defects are more complex when critical structures such as the orbit, globe and cranial base are involved [12]. Moreover, applications of tissue engineering procedures in this region require additional understanding of complex developmental processes, physiology, molecular pathways and remodeling characteristics [14]. Thus, an ideal tissue engineering approach to repair craniomaxillofacial defects should result in a complete biological tissue capable of adapting to physiological cues and overcoming the limitation of prosthetics [15].

Extensive research in the field of tissue engineering over the last two decades has revolutionized our approach toward regenerative therapies. Over the years, this approach has progressed in terms of biologically relevant implant materials and technologies for fabrication of scaffolds. There have been tremendous advancements with respect to scaffold synthesis. The earlier researches had focused on replicating the 3D structure of the defect site, where as the recent researchers are capable of performing *in situ* fabrication of the implant. Moreover, further improvements in our know-how have enabled development of live grafts by utilizing stem cells for the purpose.

In the following sections the authors have attempted to summarize the need for addressing bone tissue engineering with special emphasis on craniomaxillofacial regeneration. However, the approach was not diluted and the focus was maintained on discussing the advancement in technologies over the recent years that have opened up new avenues of scaffold fabrication in the field of regenerative medicine.

Methods: After a thorough literature survey, the authors concluded to focus this chapter about the advancements in the technologies for fabrication of bone implants. The authors formulated the basic design of the chapter and targeted their search to the specific keywords, to avoid deviation from the theme. In order to provide an exhaustive but concise overview of the recent developments in methodologies for creation of craniomaxillofacial implants, the authors used various search engines including PubMed, Scopus, Google Scholar and Web of Science. The shortlisted research articles were carefully curated on the basis of their relevance. The authors selected majority of recent articles that highlight the current advances in implant fabrication techniques. To inculcate the basic concepts of materials and techniques, some of the archaic references were also incorporated in the article. The data from these reference articles was then extracted to prepare a summary of advanced techniques of scaffold fabrication, which have gained popularity due to their efficacy and cost effectiveness.

2. Craniomaxillofacial bone defects and reconstruction strategies

Earlier it was assumed that strategies developed to augment appendicular skeletal repair can be directly translated for craniofacial reconstruction. But the use of advanced techniques such as intravital imaging, fluorescence trapping and whole-body optical imaging has revealed that calvarial bone possess a larger normalized blood volume fraction and enhanced bone remodeling activity as compared to long bones [5]. However, the traditional therapeutic modalities of reconstruction such as autologous bone grafting present myriad limitations of restricted availability of donor-site, morbidity and significant complications in restoring the three-dimensional structure of craniomaxillofacial bone [14, 16].

For instance, cleft lip/palates, the most common oral and craniomaxillofacial birth defects are addressed by the standard clinical procedures of surgery involving reconstruction of the mouth roof to separate the nasal cavity from the oral cavity. Two flap palatoplasty and Furlow double-opposing Z-plasty are the two common surgical procedures that involve suturing of soft tissues to close the wound. However, complete restoration of severe cleft palate still remains a challenge due to non-availability of autologous soft tissues [17].

Furthermore, craniomaxillofacial osseous reconstructive surgeries are performed using autologous reconstruction techniques such as free flaps (fibula and ilia crest) instead of regional flaps (pectoralis major muscle with ribs, trapezius, temporalis muscle with calvaria), because of problems associated with morbidity of regional flaps, though the regional flaps provide for the best candidate in terms of tissue matching [12]. Therefore, membranes have gained extensive importance in the field of oral and maxillofacial surgery, for their use in guided bone regeneration (GBR). These membranes function as a barrier between the fast proliferating soft tissues (fibrous connective tissue or epithelium) and slow proliferating hard tissue (bone) [18]. Membrane systems that are clinically applied do not sufficiently prevent bacterial infections. To address this problem the membranes were fabricated using film casting method, which generates a mechanical barrier to prevent bacterial transmigration through the membrane [19]. Furthermore, as these membranes are either allogenic or xenogenic, a potential risk of transmission of infection along with legal, ethical or religious limitations should be taken into consideration [18].

It has been suggested that the use of scaffold with tailored geometries and surfaces may promote bone regeneration in GBR [18]. Furthermore, finite element analysis of dental implants during mastication has revealed that the surrounding alveolar bone, that supports the dental implant, experiences a compressive stress of 62 MPa while experiencing an applied bite force of 146 N. These compressive forces may go as high as 122 MPa and therefore the bone graft is expected to fully integrate and eventually replace by the host bone tissue [9].

The last decade has seen an extensive progress in craniofacial bone tissue engineering modalities that couple biomaterials with growth factors or stem cell-based therapies [14]. Basically, the bone grafting materials can be divided into autologous, allogenic, xenogenic and alloplastic [9]. However, transplantation of autograft or allograft has limited applicability due to low availability, donor site morbidity, risk of infection, persistent pain, hemorrhage and subsequent graft failure [4, 20, 21]. Also autografts, allografts and xenografts are brittle due to the post extraction processing [9]. Additionally, the traditional procedures of implantation employed metal and metal alloys for repairing of bone defects due to their excellent mechanical properties. However, it was lately realized that the elastic modulus of these metals including stainless steel and titanium-based alloys was much higher than that of human bones, leading to stress-shielding. Moreover, corrosion and release of ionic species from these metal implants has also been found to induce inflammatory responses, cell apoptosis and foreign body reaction [22]. One of the studies demonstrated that a significant amount of time spent in contouring the titanium or absorbable scaffolds (to fit the irregularity of craniomaxillofacial bones), increases the overall risk due to extended operation time. Moreover, over-bending and lack of passive fitting of titanium eventually leads to fatigue fractures [23].

Tissue engineering has been found to address some of these limitations through development of biomimicking 3D matrices [4]. The repair of complex craniofacial bone defects is challenging and the success mainly depends on the choice of reconstructive method [24]. In order to design, develop, recreate and reconstruct a tissue defect, bioimplants (cell-based or cell-free) have emerged as a promising tool. Strategies of bioimplantations require exhaustive knowledge of diverse field such as chemistry, material science, biology, medicine, and engineering. Additionally, the actual designing requires a scaffold material, cells and cell growth factors in place. We have summarized both the knowledge based and material-based requirements in **Figure 1**.

However, placement of implants in the oral cavity encounters a major challenge of insufficient bone volume, as the dental implants cannot be placed in atrophic jaw bone. Therefore, the success of bone reconstruction/regeneration procedures extensively depends on the fact that whether the implant site can firmly support the bone graft material [25]. Moreover, the dentoalveolar defects require a rapidly resorbing matrix to avoid wound dehiscence, exposure and subsequent microbial contamination [26].

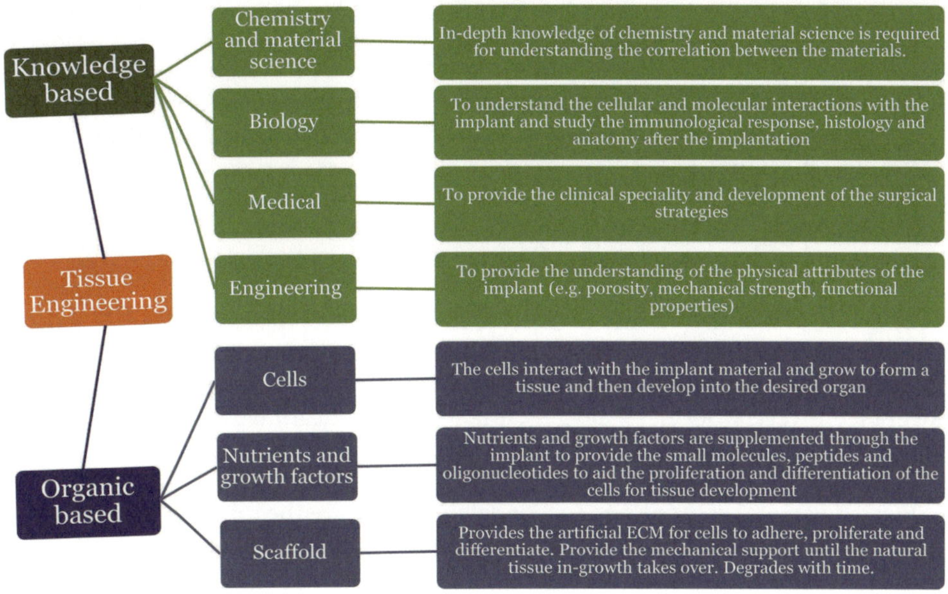

Figure 1.
Pre-requisites for tissue engineering.

Based on several such investigations and observations the specific expectations from a craniofacial scaffold can be enlisted as follows:

a. The scaffolds must have mechanical properties close to that of human bones [22].

b. The scaffold should be three-dimensional, porous with highly interconnected pore structure (to guide bone in-growth, nutrient transport, metabolic waste removal, deliver bioactive agents) to act as bioreactor for growth of cells [13, 22, 27].

c. The use of natural polymers should be preferred for the fabrication of implant to achieve better interaction with cells and eliminate the risk of immunological reaction [4].

d. The implant should appropriately fit into the complex 3D anatomical defects [13].

e. The implant should have spongy like inner part to facilitate scaffold adaptability, integration into the surrounding tissue and vascular invasion [28]. A slow or incomplete vascularization at the site of implantation could result in inadequate supply of oxygen and nutrients and problems in waste product removal, leading to hypoxia and cell death in the surrounding region [29].

f. The scaffold material should be such that it could sustain the masticatory forces of maxillofacial region and protect the implant structure from constant brain pressure until the regenerate acquires the responsibilities [13, 28].

g. The implant material should be biodegradable and bioresorbable (if the bioimplant is meant to temporarily replace an organ) [30].

h. It should be free from contamination and should be easily moldable into various shapes and sizes [30].

i. The implant should be able to develop functional groups on its surface upon appropriate treatments so that it encourages cellular attachment, differentiation and proliferation [30].

j. These implants could be an equivalent alternative to autologous bone when combined with growth factors (BMP2, TGFβ) and/or cells [4].

The choice of biomaterial and method of fabrication are the two critical factors that shape the use of scaffold. Biomaterials are the materials that interface with biological systems and can be classified on the basis of chemical and physical composition, biodegradability, type of origin and generations of modifications. Based on chemical composition biomaterials are classified into ceramics, polymers and composites [1].

i. Inorganic metal compounds and/or calcium salts are the major components of ceramics and are primarily used in orthodontal applications [1].

ii. Polymers on the other hand mimic the connective tissues and are majorly used for soft tissue engineering [1].

iii. The composites that have major applications in orthopedic and dental tissue engineering can be ceramic-based or hydrogel based; are a blend of ceramics-polymers, polymer-polymer; and can incorporate biomolecules, carbon nanotubes and metals [1, 3].

The methods of fabrication are directly dependent on the bulk and surface characteristics of the biomaterials and the projected function of the scaffold. The techniques should be capable of processing different microstructures with strict monitoring of pore size, porosity and pore interconnectivity [31]. The fabrication approach should include design techniques that can rigorously control both the exterior shape of the scaffold and interior porous architecture, to provide the right balance between load bearing strength and delivery of biomolecules [13].

3. Biomaterials for bone tissue engineering

As mentioned in the previous section the biomaterials used for bone tissue engineering are classified as ceramic, polymers and composites. According to the International Union of Pure and Applied Chemistry, the materials are further are classified into three categories: microporous (< 2 nm), mesoporous (2–50 nm) and macroporous (> 50 nm), on the basis of porosity. The porous materials suitable for fabrication of bone implants should have pore sizes ranging from micropore to mesopore scale [32]. Their porous structure provides them a higher surface area to volume ratio, thus enhancing their drug loading capacity [33].

3.1 Bioceramics

Bioceramics such as hydroxyapatite (HA), α and β tri-calcium phosphate, demineralized bone matrices, calcium carbonates, calcium sulfates and bioactive glasses have recently gained importance as novel treatment for craniomaxillofacial bone reconstruction and cleft lip/palate repair [13].

1. Hydroxyapatite (HA, $Ca_{10}(OH)_2(PO_4)_6$), due to its chemical and crystallographic similarities to inorganic components of the bone matrix is popularly used as bioactive coating on dental and orthopedic implants, where it enables adhesion and proliferation of osteoblast on the prosthetic surface and eventually results in biological fixation of implant with the bone tissues [34]. Octacalcium phosphate has also recently emerged as a biological precursor of hydroxyapatite in bone and teeth [16].

2. Calcium phosphate cement is a promising material for dental and craniofacial applications due to its injectability, moldability, bioactivity and bone replacement capability. Incorporation of RGD in calcium phosphate cement has been suggested to enhance formation of microcapillary-like structures by endothelial cells [29]. A synthetic bone substitute material fabricated by mixing alginate-fibrin microfibers and calcium phosphate cement is an aqueous phase that can be injected into osseous defects and allowed to set in-situ during dental, craniofacial and orthopedic procedures [35].

3. Tricalcium phosphate (TCP) is a commonly used bone implant material. Its low bending strength makes it suitable for engineering of maxillofacial bone instead of load-bearing bones. Particle size, depowering efficiency, binder droplet size and scaffold geometry govern the resolution, porosity and strength of 3D printed TCP scaffolds. Its partial dissolution and release of calcium and phosphate ions results in formation of biological apatite precipitate on the surface of bioceramic scaffolds [36]. One such composite scaffold of microstructure β-TCP granules embedded in glycerol matrix has been reported to induce bone formation when implanted at heterotopic sites in bilateral alveolar goat cleft model [13]. One of the major challenges while working with β-TCP is to maintain a low temperature of sintering to avoid transformation of β-TCP to chemically unstable α-TCP [26].

4. Biphasic calcium phosphate (BCP) ceramics exhibit controlled degradation rate, high porosity and low mechanical properties, thus limiting their application for non-load-bearing bones [36]. BCP implant, fabricated using custom-designed 3D microprinting, was demonstrated to induce new bone formation when implanted in critical-sized alveolar bone defects of rats [16].

5. Calcium silicate ceramics possess excellent mechanical properties and compressive strength. But their high dissolution and degradation rate results in increased pH of the surrounding environment thereby hampering cell growth and osseointegration [36]. Wollastonite ($CaSiO_3$) is an attractive bioceramic for repair of craniomaxillofacial defects because of its biological performance and improved mechanical properties by foreign ion doping [37].

6. HAB, a triphasic bioceramic developed by incorporation of hydroxyapatite, β-tricalcium phosphate, calcium silicates and traces of magnesium has been suggested to be a suitable material for craniofacial bone tissue engineering due to its osteoconductive, osteoinductive and proangiogenic properties [38].

7. Phosphate glasses (PG) contain phosphate rather than silicate and have a highly asymmetric structure. Orthophosphate (PO_4) tetrahydrone forms the basic unit of these glasses. Calcium PGs have gained importance because they can be tailored to have a composition similar to the mineral phase of the bone [39]. These bioglasses have a higher rate of dissolution in aqueous medium (due to

ease of P-O-P bond hydration), that is strongly dependent on their composition. Their dissolution rate can be tailored by adding appropriate metal oxides (TiO_2, CuO, NiO, MnO, Fe_2O_3) and these bioglasses can be utilized as controlled release vehicles [33]. Calcium PGs scaffolds have been demonstrated to regenerate bone and cementum when implanted in 1-wall intrabony alveolar defects of beagle dogs [39].

8. Mesoporous materials such as bioactive glasses (BG) are popularly used as implant materials for alveolar bone regeneration. For synthesis of mesoporous BGs, surfactant is introduced as the structure directing agent, during the sol-gel process of the glass. The surfactant is removed at the end of the process by calcination or extraction and the micelles previously occupied by the surfactant are replaced by mesopores. For the purpose of tissue engineering mesoporous bioglass can be coated on the surface of polymeric scaffold; incorporated in a polymeric matrix in the form of particles; fabricated as scaffold and coated with a polymer [33]. Mesoporous BG nanolayers (thickness 100 nm), created by spin coating on the surface of β-TCP scaffolds have been found to significantly improve osteogenesis [40].

3.2 Polymers

Polymer materials are composed of chemical compounds typically formed from monomers of carbon, hydrogen, oxygen and nitrogen. These monomer structures repeat and bind with themselves to create long molecular chains. Polymers have gained importance for fabrication of scaffolds as they are inexpensive, biocompatible, biodegradable and can be easily manipulated for their chemical, mechanical and biological properties. The commonly used polymers in craniofacial tissue engineering include natural polymers and synthetic polymers [3]. Natural polymers can be categorized into two main subgroups e.g. polysaccharides (alginate, cellulose, starch, chitosan) and polypeptides and proteins (collagen, silk fibroin, albumin) [31], whereas synthetic polymers majorly include polycaprolactone (PCL), poly lactic acid (PLA), poly(l-lactic) acid (PLLA), poly D, L-lactide-co-glycolic acid (PLGA), polyvinylidene fluoride (PVDF) and magneto-responsive polymeric systems [3, 41, 42].

Synthetic materials such as PVDF (poly (vinylidene fluoride)), P(VDF-TrFE) co-polymer of vinylidene fluoride (VDF) and trifluoroethylene (TrFE), PHBV (poly-3-hydroxybutyrate-3-hydroxy valerate), poly-l-lactic acid (PLLA) and natural polymers such as cellulose, collagen, silk and chitin, exhibit piezoelectric properties and hold a great promise in the field of bone tissue engineering [33].

3.2.1 Natural polymers

1. Collagen is extracted from animal (bovine and porcine skin or bone) and marine sources. However, animal derived collagen poses risk to public health and safety [22]. Collagen is the main organic component of dentin matrix and presents a good alternative for dental implantations [41].

Adhesion of calcium salts to a suspension of collagen and glycosaminoglycan in phosphorous acid results in precipitation of brushite form of calcium phosphate into the collagen network, which upon subsequent lyophilization form porous foam. A portion of calcium and phosphate ions from these mineralized scaffolds are released and accelerate osteogenesis. As craniofacial bones rely on intramembranous ossification, these mineralized collagen scaffolds are shown to promote osteogenesis in rabbit calvaria and sub-critical sized porcine mandible [43].

2. Silk fibroin is a natural, low-cost, biodegradable and biocompatible polymer obtained from cocoons of *Bombyx mori*, *Antheraea pernyi* (tussah), *Antheraea mylitta* (tasar) and *Philosamia ricini* (eri). Being a natural polymer, it offers good permeation for oxygen and water but has a low compressive strength [44].

Silk can be manipulated into various forms for fabrication of scaffolds for craniomaxillofacial tissue engineering applications. Addition of methacrylate groups to amine-containing side groups of silk gives rise to silk methacrylate (SilMA) scaffolds, whereas combing methacrylate groups with amine-containing side groups of gelatin results in gelatin methacrylate (GelMA), that becomes photo-cross linkable in the presence of photoinitiator [9].

3. Chitosan is a deacetylated form of chitin and is the second largest natural polysaccharide after cellulose. It is extracted from crustacean shells and marine sponges. It exhibits fungicidal and anti-microbial activities [24, 41]. Its biodegradability, biocompatibility and excellent cell adhesive properties make it a popular choice for implant material [41]. But its weak mechanical strength and high rate of biodegradability requires crosslinking with other natural or synthetic polymers (e.g. blends) for orthopedic or periodontal applications [24]. For example, chitosan is crosslinked with polyethylene glycol diacrylate (PEGDA) to produce photocrosslinkable blends [9].

3.2.2 Synthetic polymers

1. PCL is a biodegradable thermoplastic (with a low melting point of 59–64°C) that is widely used for drug delivery in dental implants owing to its low cost and physico-chemical properties, enabling its application in nanometric scale processing and prototyping [41, 45]. PCL also finds its application in prevention of bacterial accumulation on dental implants [41]. Incorporation of fibroin and nano-HA in PCL have been found to enhance compressive modulus, cellular adhesion and calcium deposition after 14 weeks of implantation in large scale calvarial defect model [46].

2. PLA is a degradable polymer that can be adapted to different morphologies. However, its degradation results in production of acidic by-products and therefore requires blending with other materials such as tricalcium phosphate [41].

3. PLLA is fast degrading polymer that possesses good physical and mechanical properties and supports cell adhesion and proliferation [41].

4. PLGA is a biodegradable and biocompatible polymer that exhibit close resemblance with natural proteins and is metabolically hydrolyzed to monomers of lactic acid and glycolic acid [41]. A functionally gradient three layered PLGA construct with low macroporosity and high mechanical properties was demonstrated to successfully bring about periodontal regeneration [47].

5. PVDF is also a biocompatible, flexible material with high mechanical strength and good anti-bacterial properties [41].

6. Magneto-responsive polymeric systems are comprised of polymer networks that are physically or chemically functionalized with magnetic nanoparticles (of magnetic elements such as iron, cobalt, nickel or their oxides). When these particles are covalently immobilized or physically entrapped (by blending, in situ precipitation or dip coating), they respond to magnetic field. This property enables spatio-temporal control over the physical, structural and mechanical properties of the polymeric scaffold. Leaching out of magnetic nanoparticles (< 50 nm) from these materials and their ability to cross the biological membrane, thus inducing inflammation, generating ROS, impeding DNA function and driving cell apoptosis limits them incorporation in the polymeric networks [42].

3.3 Composites

The composites are a blend of ceramics-polymers, polymer-polymer; and can incorporate biomolecules, carbon nanotubes and metals [1, 3].

Various ceramics, polymers as well as composites are subjected to functionalization of their surfaces to improve their compatibility with the biological microenvironment. In order to modify the surface hydrophobicity of polymers, to make them more hydrophilic and biocompatible, various surface modification techniques are employed [30, 48].

Graft polymerization technique: Polymer grafting and graft polymerization are achieved by chemical, photochemical, plasma induced and enzymatic grafting methods [30].

Nanoindentation method: This method is used to increase roughness by micropatterning to promote cell adhesion, but it is difficult to implement on large scale [30].

Surface modification by self-assembled monolayer formation: Metal surface modified by ligands through metal ligand bond formation [30].

Corona discharge: Electrically induced stream of ionized air is bombarded on the polymeric surface resulting in generation of oxygen containing functional groups. As this method does not operate in vacuum, it is prone to contamination by local moisture and humidity [30].

Flame treatment: Bombardment of polymer surface with ionized air resulting in surface functionalization of top several layers of polymer with hydroxyl, aldehyde and carboxylic functional groups. Although the method increases printability, wettability and adhesiveness of the polymer surface, it reduces the optical clarity [30].

UV irradiation: UV irradiation of polymer results in generation of reactive sites and can initiate graft polymerization of bioactive molecules such as N-vinyl pyrrolidinone [30].

Wet Chemical treatment: treatment of polyethylene and polypropylene surfaces with concentrated acid such as chromic acid in presence potassium permanganate and concentrated sulfuric acid results in development of reactive oxygen of functional group. This method generates hazardous chemical waste and surface etching and is therefore difficult to scale up [30].

Plasma treatment: Plasma is a high energy state of matter in which gas is partially ionized into charged particles, electrons and neutral molecule. Such ions when bombarded on a polymer surface results in functionalization of molecules in contact [30].

Graphene coating: Graphene is a 1-atom thick film with a honeycomb structure and is composed of carbon atoms created by sp2 hybridization [10]. The materials of graphene family have been widely applied in diverse medical applications owing to their nanoscale size photoluminescence properties, large specific surface area and anti-bacterial activity [49]. High elasticity and flexibility of graphene and its derivatives (graphene oxide (GO) and reduced graphene oxide (rGO)) presents them as a promising mechanical filler for biomaterials [34]. It is widely used as surface modification coating or dopant in scaffolds, to enhance biocompatibility and promote osteogenic differentiation of stem cells [44].

4. Fabrication techniques

Tissue engineering is a multidisciplinary field that imbibes the principles, knowledge and methods of chemistry, physics, engineering and biology. It involves three fundamental elements: cells, scaffold and cell signaling [7].

The fabrication of scaffolds requires pre-treatment of the graft material with various solvents, which facilitates the dissolution of the biomaterial. It is a general observation that processing and storage of scaffolds in the presence of solvent, hampers the control of spatial distribution of the bioactive agent in the porous structure of the scaffold. The final processing involves removal of these toxic organic solvents or any other residual porogen species by leaching or solvent extraction methods. This results in loss of the medically important bioactive agents. However, the methods employed for processing of scaffolds should also be evaluated from an environmental point of view. Therefore, E-factors (the actual amount of waste product produced in the process per gram of product) and low carbon footprint methods are the two parameters that deserve attention. Thus, processing technologies such as melt molding (compression, injection and extrusion molding); 3D printing; fused deposition modeling; sintering of solid particles (heat, compressed CO_2 and selective laser sintering); gas foaming and compressed or supercritical CO_2 foaming, operating in the absence of solvent during assembly of 3D scaffolds, present ideal strategies for development of medicated scaffolds [11].

The use of natural fiber composites over synthetic fibers also needs substantial attention from green synthesis point of view. Glass or carbon fiber-reinforced composites, belonging to the category of synthetic composites have been well researched for last 20 years. However, due to environmental and economic considerations the focus of research has diverted to natural fiber-reinforced composites. The advent of 3D and 4D printing provides huge opportunity for development of natural biocomposites, for the first time on the same time scale as their synthetic counterparts [50].

In the sections below, we will be discussing various techniques employed for fabrication of biomaterial implants for craniomaxillofacial bone reconstruction/ regeneration.

4.1 Electrospinning

Electrospinning was first applied in 1934 by Anton Formhals and represents a combination of electrospray and spinning of fibers [51]. A typical electrospinning apparatus includes a capillary tube with a spinneret, a high voltage power supply and a collector (**Figure 2**). During electrospinning, polymer droplets are generated by extruding polymer solution from the electrically conductive spinneret. A high voltage is applied between the spinneret and the grounded collector. The polymer solution ejects from the spinneret when the potential between the solution breaks through the surface tension of the droplets, resulting in fibrous polymer scaffold (diameter ranging from 100 nm to several micrometers)

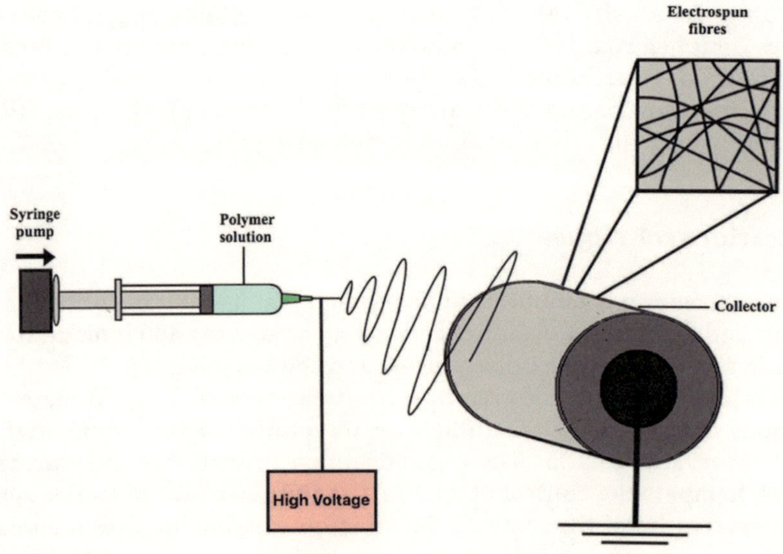

Figure 2.
A typical electrospinning apparatus for fabrication of scaffolds.

[52]. Introduction of a liquid bath collector in an electrospinning setup results in production of fluffy morphologies such as yarn or spongiform fabric. For example, the collector may contain ethanol and water-ethanol (non-solvents), for spinning of polysaccharides such as cellulose/heparin (blend) and cellulose/multiwall carbon nanotubes (core/sheath) [20]. In addition, antibiotics can also be incorporated into the electrospun scaffold to prevent bacterial colonization after implantation [53].

The electrospun scaffold is physically like a tissue paper with easy handling and therefore is well adapted for critical bone defects in craniomaxillofacial region [54]. On the basis of initial state of polymer electrospinning can be categorized as solution electrospinning, emulsion electrospinning and melt electrospinning writing [18, 55].

a. In solution electrospinning, polymer is dissolved in organic solvent (e.g. chloroform or dimethyl formamide), which evaporates when the polymer jet is ejected toward the collector [18]. A lower flow rate is preferred for proper evaporation of the solvent [51]. But the solvent residues left on the fibers limits its applications [18]. An increase in fiber diameter and pore diameter (the void portion) is observed by increasing the polymer flow rate that also alters the morphological structures [51].

b. In emulsion electrospinning core-shell nanofibers are constructed without a specific needle setup, by emulsifying the drug aqueous protein solution in the polymer solution. In this technique an emulsion is created within a single solution, where the emulsified droplets get organized in two separate phases, consequently as a result of evaporation of the solvent form the electrospun fibers [55].

c. Melt electrospinning writing utilizes melting of medical grade polymers such as PCL, thus eliminating the risk of residual toxic solvent [18]. This technique has been used for fabrication of well-defined surface layers with different geometries, that are individualized for attachment of osteoblast on one side and keratinocytes and fibroblast on the other side [19].

Ceramic, metallic, glass-based fibers can be produced by electrospinning, by injecting the polymers to a simple syringe with metallic tip of different diameters [47]. PCL and nano-HA composite scaffolds fabricated using similar technique holds potential for repairing of critical bone in craniomaxillofacial region [54]. These scaffolds not only have superior mechanical properties but also possess ability to carry growth factors and drugs [56]. It was demonstrated that trigeminal ganglion when added to ε-PCL membranes synthesized by electrospinning and functionalized with nerve growth factor nanoreservoirs, were able to regenerate peripheral axons in the pulp cavity, two weeks after implantation [57].

Melt spinning and wet spinning: Melt spinning involves melting of the polymer followed by its extrusion through small holes resulting in formation of solidified fibers after cooling. The resulting fibers are collected by a take-up wheel to form continuous fiber strands. Wet spinning involves dissolution of polymer in appropriate solvent followed by extrusion of polymer solution through a spinneret into a coagulation bath containing a non-solvent [22].

4.2 Electron beam melting (EBM)

EBM was developed and patented by Swedish Arcam Company. The equipment is mainly composed of an electron beam gun compartment and a specimen-fabrication compartment, both kept in high vacuum. The technology employs high energy electron beam to melt the metal powder. The electron beam preheats the powder bed to reach a slight-sintering state by scanning the powder layer quickly before EBM. This step is followed by selective scanning of powder layer by electron beam based on the 3D hierarchical data, causing the preheated powder to melt and solidify together. The high beam-material coupling efficiency makes it a method of choice for processing of metals with extremely high melting points. One of the case studies demonstrated fabrication of 3D titanium scaffold with EBM for reconstruction of whole mandible defect [52].

4.3 Gas foaming

The principle of gas foaming is to generate pores in a polymeric matrix through a nucleation-growth mechanism of gas bubbles that results in formation of microporous material after venting out of the bubbles. This process is compatible with both hydrophobic and hydrophilic polymeric matrices and is usually performed under mild temperatures [11]. This solvent free technique consists of 3 steps

Step 1: dispersion of porogen (chemical blowing agent e.g. Sodium Bicarbonate and Ammonium Bicarbonate or physical blowing agent e.g. inert gas - Nitrogen, Argon or Carbon dioxide) [11].

Step 2: generation of gas bubbles due to porogen removal resulting in nucleation growth mechanism and pore formation [11].

Step 3: rapid lowering of temperature to allow vitrification of the material by freezing and avoid destabilization of resulting foam [11]. The foaming process carried out using molds can be used to cast the foam to a shape that can fit into an anatomical defect.

Supercritical CO_2 ($scCO_2$) foaming and compressed CO_2 foaming are two of the green technology processes that utilize the valorization [11] and plasticizing effect of CO_2 under super critical conditions (temperature and pressure above the critical point of CO_2, 31.1°C and 72.8 bar) for reducing the apparent glass transition (T_g) and the melting temperature of the polymers. When the pressure is reduced, CO_2 dissolved in the polymer matrix gets super saturated resulting in formation of pores from growing nucleation sites. This method employs mild conditions and avoids the use of organic solvents, thus retaining the activity of thermally sensitive compounds such as growth factors [46].

4.4 Freeze-drying technique

In this method a water-soluble polymer is frozen such that interpenetrating ice crystals are created which are later removed by sublimation, resulting in formation of porous scaffold [22].

4.5 Particle leaching and phase inversion

In this process PLGA was dissolved in DMSO, and then the PLGA solution was thoroughly mixed with CaP particles in a ratio of 1:3 (w/w). This sticky mixture of CaP/PLGA was then poured into an aluminum foil mold filled with sugar crystals at a weight of 3 times the DMSO volume. The mixture diffuses throughout the mass of porogen crystals. After 2–3 minutes the mold was transferred to a refrigerator at −18°C for 1 h to set the mixture. The PLGA was precipitated and the sugar crystals were leached out of the precipitated CaP/PLGA mixture in ddH_2O at room temperature (20°C) for 3 days, during which time the ddH_2O was changed approximately 4 times each day. Every time a scaffold block was produced [58]. Thus, PLGA and two calcium phosphate phases (first is a particulate within the structure and second is a thin ubiquitous coating) get fabricated into a composite scaffold with a pore size and interconnecting macroporosity similar to that of human trabecular bone. The osteoconductive surface of calcium phosphate abrogates the putative foreign body giant cell response to the underlying polymer, whereas the internal calcium phosphate phase provides dimensional stability. The highly interconnected microporosity and the ability to wick up blood make the scaffold a clot-retention device and an osteoconductive support for growth of host bone. Such scaffold has been implemented in human patients for maintenance of alveolar bone height following tooth extraction. These scaffolds also augment alveolar bone height through standard sinus lift approaches. It was also observed that these scaffolds regenerated sufficient bone tissue in the wound site and provided good foundation for dental implant placement [16].

4.6 Phase separation

It is a solvent based technique that employs change in temperature to induce phase separation of homogenous polymer-solvent solution through solid-liquid demixing or liquid-liquid phase separation [22, 47]. On this basis it is mainly divided into two types liquid-solid and liquid-liquid phase separation. The method is conducted by reducing the temperature of solution and extraction of solvent phase, till it reaches a porous polymer scaffold [47]. The phase separation majorly involves formation of a polymer-rich phase and polymer-poor phase upon rapid cooling of polymer-solvent solution by freeze-drying or freeze-extraction [4, 22]. As a result, the polymer-poor phase is eventually removed [22]. The solvent system utilized is usually a mixture of 1,4-dioxane and water and the temperature and time for the process is around 60°C for two hours. It has been observed that strong polymer-solvent interaction leads to solid-liquid phase separation, whereas weak polymer-solvent interactions results in liquid-liquid phase separation. The role of non-solvent such as water is to lower the degree of polymer-solvent interaction so as to induce liquid-liquid phase separation [4].

4.7 Computer-aided techniques

The Computer-aided designing (CAD) is gaining popularity with respect to construction of model on the basis of constructive solid geometry or boundary representation principle. Models obtained by boundary representation require more storage space compared to constructive solid geometry. Therefore, as the model becomes larger or more detailed in internal structure the size of the file containing boundary-representation-derived-model drastically increases causing difficulty in operation. CAD methods are realized by utilizing various tools such as UG, CATIA and Pro/E. Some dedicated design software's such as Magics (3D printing preprocessing software developed by Belgium Materialize Company), have been recently developed in which the designer can directly instruct various integrated unit cells. MATERAILAS and computer-aided system for tissue scaffolds (CASTS) are some of the software and parametric library respectively that are used to design algorithms for minute detailing of the desired scaffold [52]. Implementation of CAD/CAM softwares along with radiology procedures for easy acquisition and transfer of DICOM3 (Digital Imaging and Communications in Medicine) data allows the surgeon to perform three-dimensional measurements and reconstruct the deformed or missing anatomy by segmentation [59].

Computer assisted textile-based technologies constitute an attractive route to strategize scaffolding (including stitching, braided, woven, non-woven and knitted) of more complex fibrous 3D scaffolds suitable for engineering of soft tissue such as ligament in the craniofacial regions [28].

With advancements in our knowledge about materials along with a boon in computer-aided technologies, several methods have evolved recently that increases the precision and accessibility of craniomaxillofacial bone reconstruction (**Figure 3**).

Recently rapid prototyping has emerged as an effective tool for 3D printing of porous scaffolds with interconnected porous network [42], complex geometries, well defined and reproducible architectures [22]. The basic concept of rapid prototyping involves presentation of cycles of cross-sectional sheets from where the data is exerted into the solid free form fabrication machine to produce the physical model. As the layers are built from bottom to top, each newly manufactured layer sticks to the previous. Several techniques originate from this principle of rapid prototyping. We have discussed some of the major types of this technique in the following sections [42].

4.7.1 3D printing

3D printing has emerged as a promising tool of additive manufacturing (AM) that enables us to optimize the processes of preoperative planning, develop intraoperative guidance tools, reduce operative time and improve bifunctional and esthetic outcome [12, 60]. Liu et.al fabricated Al_2O_3 scaffolds with a through-hole structure using 3D printing and sol-gel technology. Alumina (Al_2O_3) is a bioinert ceramic and exhibit negligible tissue reaction and therefore several researchers incorporate other components into Al_2O_3 to enhance the mechanical strength of the scaffold. Fabrication of Al_2O_3 / borosilicate glass scaffolds using urea- formaldehyde resin as in-powder adhesive by 3D printing has been demonstrated to maximize the tensile

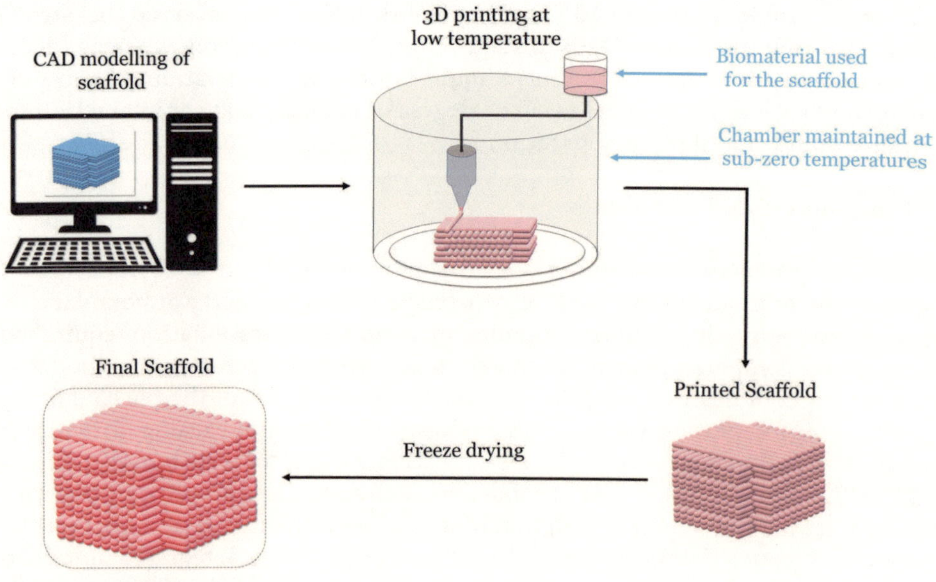

Figure 3.
Computer-assisted scaffold modeling for fabrication of implants.

strength [40]. In the last decade, investigators have reported 3D-printed prostheses of nose, ears, eyes, face, and hand [12]. With the help of direct writing technology tricalcium phosphate scaffolds have been fabricated and used to repair rabbit trephine defects [61].

Significant improvements in clinical imaging and user-friendly 3D software with progression of open source platforms, associated with recent hardware developments have enabled 3D printer to build layers as small as 16 μm thickness for stereolithography (Polyjet, Stratasys); 178 μm thickness for fused deposition modeling (Fortus 900 mc, Stratasys); 80 μm thickness for selective laser sintering (sPro 230 HS, 3D systems) and 75 μm resolution for stereolithography (3D systems) [12, 62]. These 3D printing techniques including stereolithography, multi jet modeling, selective laser sintering, binder jet technique and fused deposition modeling provide appreciation of visuospatial relationship between the anatomical structures created and craniomaxillofacial reconstructive surgery [12].

1. Inkjet printing was the first bioprinting technology of AM that was developed by Hewlett Packard company in 1970s as a 2D printing technology [42]. Later in 1992 an elevator platform that can move along Z axis was added to it to develop a 3D bioprinting system [42]. It offers the option of creating complex spatial patterns without fabricating purpose-specific lithographic masks. Structural and conformal cell printing methods have been used to create cell constructs from bottom to upward (layer-by-layer or cell-by-cell), resulting in heterogeneous cell and biomolecular 3D structure. Structural cell printing requires simultaneous or sequential printing of cells and biomolecules whereas conformal cell printing is a hybrid approach where biomolecules are printed on top of thin layers of prefabricated scaffolding. This method is beneficial for fabrication of implants that facilitates vascularization and therefore promises their role in oral and maxillofacial bone regeneration [63].

2. Piezo inkjet printing: In powder bed inkjet printing, droplets of dilute solutions or biomaterials act as binder to the bulk material positioned within the

powder bed. These droplets are dispensed and driven either by thermal or piezoelectric processes into a powder bed. The thermal inkjet printing employs temperature between 100 and 300°C to nucleate a bubble and eject the droplets, which produces shear and thermal stress on natural polymer inks, resulting in inconsistent droplet volume. Piezoelectric technology utilizes pressure or acoustic waves produced via piezoelectric actuator to generate the drops and therefore can be used with a range of polar and non-polar solvents [52].

A wide range of powder materials such as polymers, ceramics, proteins and cells can be processed using this technique. However, the ink's viscosity is limited to 5 to 20 Pa.s to avoid high ejection pressure or continuous flow of material [3].

3. Selective laser sintering (SLS) is an additive manufacturing technique which utilizes high power laser for sintering of metals or ceramic powders for scaffold synthesis [40, 42]. This technique was developed and patented by Carl Deckard and Joe Beaman in 1989 [42]. The method employs a computer-controlled CO_2 laser beam to induce a local increase of temperature (above the T_g of the selected polymer) and selectively fuse and sinter polymer composite powders in a layer-by-layer manner to build a 3D scaffold [11, 22, 40]. After the fabrication is completed excess powder is removed either by brushing or application of compressed air [42]. SLS is a single step process that offers products with high resolution due to laser precision [11]. The method is associated with certain disadvantages due to its working requirements. (a) since the scaffold is created by fusion of spherical particles, there is certain degree of roughness on its surface that requires polishing [42]; (b) use of high temperature renders it unsuitable for natural polymers [3]; (c) at industrial scale standard SLS machines require large quantities of material in adequate powder form, thus making the process very expensive [11]. This method extensively finds its application in regeneration and repair of periodontal, craniofacial bone and osteochondral defects that possess complex anatomy and can be used to work with a variety of powder materials including metals, bioceramics and synthetic polymers such as PLA, PCL, poly ethyl ether ketone and poly ether ketone ketone [3].

4. Stereolithography or vat polymerization fabricates the products through selectively curing photo reactive resin. The method involves formulation and polymerization of photopolymer liquid in a vat by ultra violet light irradiation on the surface with designed pattern. As the platform moves the parts that are built downward after each new layer are cured. The steps are repeated to form the entire object and the excessive resin is drained out. SLA utilizes two types of polymerization reaction – free radical polymerization and cationic polymerization. On the basis of irradiation type SLA is further categorized into vector scan approach (irradiation through ultra violet beam and projection on liquid surface through optics and scanning galvanometer) and mask projection approach (the radiation source creates large area pattern through digital micromirror device and harden one layer at a time) [52].

UV radiation is the most common curating agent in SLA. When a two-dimensional layer of gelatin methacrylate (GelMA) and different concentration of photoinitiator were cured with UV exposure, it was found that the concentration of photoinitiator affected the porosity of GelMA hydrogel by polymerization-induced phase separation. Similarly, fabrication of poly(propylene fumarate) (PPF) was carried out by embedding PPF/diethyl fumarate photopolymer with PLGA microspheres loaded with bone morphogenetic proteins (BMPs). PPF is known to form cross linked polymer network when combined with photoinitiator bisacrylphosphrine oxide and exposed to UV light [9]. Cha et al. utilized nano-SLA to print micropillar and microridge patterns on the scaffold and investigated the effect of these patterns on cell adhesion, proliferation and osteogentic differentiation [36]. PolyHIPEs (poly high internal phase emulsion) are the class of material where porosity is created due to phase separation between two immiscible liquids in presence an emulsifier. 2-ethylhexyl acrylates (EHA) and isobornyl acrylate (IBOA), when mixed together and combined with the photoinitiators (diphenyl(2,4,6-trimethylbenzoyl) phosphine oxide/2-hydroxy-2-methylpropiophenone) formed a porous structure in presence of water, upon curation and photopolymerization by laser. In this method the curation is carried out by laser instead of UV radiation. Similarly methacrylated poly(D,L-lactide) (PDLLA) scaffolds were prepared using Irgacure 2959 as photoinitiator [9].

Ceramics are known to be non-photocurable and therefore, they require photocurable resin to bind the particles together [9]. Ceramic materials are primarily made up of metals with inorganic calcium or phosphate salts and are generally osteoconductive and osteoinductive [3]. The scientists investigated that bioceramic slurry of HA and TCP, mixed with photocurable FA1260T resin, cured with SLA and sintered at 1400°C (to remove the solidified photocurable resin and fuse the bioceramic particles together), resulted in fabrication of biocompatible osteoinductive scaffold. In one of the studies, researchers investigated the utility of thiol-ene reactions to produce photopolymer networks, as an alternative to the use of photoinitiators. These reactions occur between alkene and thiol-monomers to form an alkyl sulfide group that is regarded to photo-trigger the chemical reaction, thus eliminating the need of photoinitiator. A 1:1 ratio of thiol (pentaerythritol tetrakis(3-mercaptopropionate) (PETMP)) and alkene (poly (ethylene glycol)divinyl ether (PEG-DVE)), has been shown to crosslink without the presence of photoinitiator and was also biocompatible [9].

5. Laser-assisted 3D printing also known as laser-assisted bioprinting (LAB) basically has three main components (a) a pulsed laser source, (b) a transparent glass slide or ribbon, as a target, serving as a support for the printing material and (c) a receiving substrate to collect the materials. While printing, a focused laser pulse stimulates a small area of the target which is mainly made up of an energy absorbing layer on the surface and bioink solution underlay. Evaporation of a portion of the energy absorbing layer results in formation of a droplet that is collected by the receiving substrate and crosslinked [3]. Pure calcium silicate and dilute magnesium doped scaffolds of different layer thickness and macropore sizes, prepared by varying the layer deposition mode from single-layer printing to double layer printing, have been demonstrated to improve bone tissue ingrowth in craniomaxillofacial bone defect treatment [37]. Varying the layer configuration from single to double layer printed versions has been shown to significantly enhance side-wall pore size and strut thickness [37].

As, LABs are not equipped with nozzle and obviate direct contact between dispenser and bioink, they minimize the problem of material or cell clogging [3, 42].

6. Fused deposition modeling (FDM) was developed and patented by Scott Crump and is one of the most popular rapid prototyping technique [42]. It is the most widely used extrusion based additive manufacturing technique that fabricates scaffolds without the use of toxic organic solvents [22]. Extrusion based printing uses pneumatic, piston or screw driven system to create

pressure and push out the suspension, solution or emulsion [1]. FDM is a heat utilizing technique, where the thermoplastic filament is guided into a liquefier for melting through rollers and extruded from the computer-controlled nozzle in a layer-by-layer manner to create a scaffold [22, 25]. Thus, the fabrication process involves movement of computer-controlled nozzle in X-Y plane in order to create the desired pattern after which the nozzle move upward along the Z axis to a predefined distance, to print the next layer [42]. The thermoplastic polymers used for fabrication of scaffolds are called as bioinks [1]. To ensure good interlayer adhesion, the previously formed layer is kept at temperatures just below the solidification peak of thermoplastic material [34]. The process temperature depends on the melting temperature of the building material, which is generally very high for biological molecules [25].

The efficacy of FDM largely depends on the parameters such as nozzle temperature, nozzle diameter, extrusion speed, layer thickness and raster angle [22]. Its solvent free technology cost effectiveness and high speed renders some advantages to this technique [42]. Since this process is carried out at high temperature incorporation of biological molecules becomes impossible [34]. Furthermore, this technique faces a limitation in terms of availability of a medical grade biocompatible thermoplastic material with viscosity that is adequately low for extrusion but at the same time high enough for scaffolding [42]. PCL/HA bone scaffolds fabricated using CT-guided FDM have been found to exhibit cortical bone like features, displayed close mechanics to that of natural bone and integrated tightly with the surrounded tissue [52]. Scientists have developed computer-aided low-temperature deposition manufacturing system that has been successfully demonstrated to fabricate 3D scaffolds identical to the patient-specific alveolar bone defects. But as the resulting bone substitutes are in the form of blocks or granules, they face limitations in clinical applications requiring restoration of complex structure in craniomaxillofacial region [16].

7. Fused filament fabrication (FFF): Similar to other 3D printing techniques, the FFF also involves layer-by-layer deposition of thermoplastic material through a heated nozzle onto the platform or previously printed layers. FFF has certain advantages that include (a) minimizing the cost of production runs (b) reducing the production waste (c) shortening the design manufacture cycle (d) ability to build intricate geometries and (e) ability to tailor microstructure and properties in each layer. The mechanical performance of FFF is controlled by slicing and printing parameters. The slicing parameters include raster angle (in-plane angle), the inter-filament distance, layer height, filament orientation, nozzle diameter, filling pattern (e.g. honeycomb, hexagonal, triangular) and the build orientation (out-of-plane). The printing parameters include nozzle geometry, nozzle temperature, printing speed, printing trajectory, bed temperature and calibration. Though development of fiber-reinforced composites developed using FFF have enhanced mechanical properties, the major limitation of these printed composites are inherent extrusion-induced defects, such as porosity (due to poor interfacial bonding between the fibers and the polymer and between the printed beads or the printed layers) [50].

No matter which specific technique is used to produce the 3D biomodel, the following are proven advantages of using 3D printing for reconstructive surgery [12]:

a. 3D printing involves direct visualization of anatomic structures and their spatial relationships, thus improving the understanding of complex underlying conditions which significantly enhance the quality of diagnosis and treatment planning [12].

b. 3D modeling helps the plastic surgeon to provide better preoperative counseling to their patients [12].

c. 3D biomodel allows the assessment of bony defects for grafting and the adaptation/prebending of reconstruction plates. This results in improvement in preoperative surgical planning by designing incisions and surgical resection margins [12].

d. 3D modeling facilitates development of intraoperative guidance tools to improve communication among surgeons. This shortens the operative time; reduces time under general anesthesia; shortens the duration of wound exposure; and reduces intraoperative blood loss, errors, and risks [12].

e. 3D printing helps in the production of patient-specific implants/prosthetics in everyday surgical practice such as temporomandibular joint prostheses, distraction devices, and fixation devices. This improves the esthetic outcomes as a result of individual fitting and complements individual anatomical needs. Furthermore, in contrast to the standard implants, these customized implants avoid the need for intraoperative modification and adjustments resulting in improved clinical outcomes and a decreased risk of complications, such as infections. These custom made implants yield superior functional and esthetic outcomes [12].

f. The 3D printing is more predictable and provides accurate surgical outcomes [12].

g. Typical 3D printing materials can be sterilized using chemicals, such as Food and Drug Administration–approved glutaraldehyde protocols, steam and gas for intraoperative handling [12].

h. 3D printing enables accessibility of physical models that can be realistically held and rotated and can be used as an educational tool for medical students and residents. These models can be interactively manipulated regardless of complexity and are accessible without the need for computers or advanced training [12].

i. As 3D printing allows use of a variety of materials, its utility is not only limited for bone reconstruction but can also be extended for replacing soft tissues [12].

It has been a general observation that 3D printed biocomposites have low fiber content (< 30 wf%) and a very low aspect ratio (L/d), that reduces their overall viscosity and improves printability. In addition, discontinuous or short fiber-reinforcement exhibit high porosity of biocomposite because of low pressure applied during printing. Therefore, the future trends in 3D printing are expected to deliver higher mechanical properties with improved material selection. The use of continuous natural fiber for biocomposites could bring about drastic improvements in mechanical performance due to high fiber content and better control of anisotropy by fiber orientation [50].

With advent of 3D printing technology, it is now possible to fabricate cell-based 3D scaffolds. The use of stem cells for clinical applications must fulfill Good Manufacturing Practice (GMP) requirements to ensure safety and quality of the treatment [63]. Bone marrow stromal and adipose derived stem cells find preferred applicability for orthopedic and maxillofacial tissue regeneration [61]. Hamlet and colleagues investigated a cell-based approach for alveolar bone regeneration using hydrogel as bioink for cell delivery. Bioprinting of periodontal ligament cells has also been performed to create a 3D hydrogel microarray. The process of bioprinting the cells using a pressure-assisted valve-based bioprinting system is carried out within a sterile hood and controlled by a computer [3].

4.7.2 4D bioprinting

The director of the Self-Assembly lab at the Massachusetts Institute of Technology (MIT), Skylar Tibbits, demonstrated the concept of 4D printing for the first time in 2014 [64]. 4D printing is an invasive and robust [42] technique that involves the development of raw printing materials and design of the mechanism and multilayer architecture of printed structures that directly incorporate a pre-programmed transformation [50]. With the rapid progress of nanotechnology 4D bioprinting has been developed to incorporate time as the fourth dimension in combination to the 3D bioprinting strategies, to bring about changes in confirmation, shape and functionalities (shape, property, self-assembly or self-repair) of the printed objects [22, 50]. So, basically 4D printing can be defined as the ability of 3D printed material to actuate when an external stimulus is applied [50]. The types of stimuli can be physical (e.g. temperature, pressure, electricity, light and magnetic field), chemical (e.g. humidity and pH) [42] and biological (cell traction force-CTF). Mechanisms of CTF have been utilized for cell origami technology in which 3D constructs of cell are developed by folding two-dimensional elements into predefined shapes. Currently the stimuli-responsive biomaterials have largely replaced CTF-based and manual folding approaches for 4D printing [64].

A case study: Maxillo-orbital surgery for placement of titanium implants to anatomically reduce bone fracture presents several challenges. In many cases deep insertion of titanium mesh implant to the orbital floor may result in damage to optic nerve and vision loss. However, if the mesh is not inserted deep enough, the reconstruction of orbital floor will not deplete and the eye will lack support. Therefore, titanium mesh implants must be inserted into the orbital wall and should tightly fit the surface of orbital floor. Under certain circumstances the titanium mesh may deviate from its position, thus increasing or decreasing the volume of orbital cavity, and as a result symptom such as diplopia, exophthalmos and enophthalmos are not relieved [23]. 4D printing has revolutionized our approach to address such complicated issues by empowering the surgeons to place and modify of scaffold in real-time during the surgical procedure. This technique enables actuation of a 3D material by application of external stimulus and can be performed after the scaffold has been placed at the site of injury/defect.

A 3D printed product should exhibit smart behavior such as "Shape memory" or "Self-actuation", to be considered for 4D printing [42]. A variety of materials have been developed for this purpose such as shape memory polymer (SMP), electro-active polymer (EAP) and hygromorph composites (moisture induced morphine – that utilizes moisture induced anisotropic swelling of natural fibers to drive actuation in development of hygromorph composites) [50].

Shape memory is defined as ability of materials to "remember" and recover their original shape. This suggests that the original shape of a material can be deformed to fix into a secondary form, by application of an external physical force. The material retains this new shape until a specific stimulus (e.g. temperature, ultraviolet light, humidity, electric and magnetic field) is applied that triggers the transformation of matter and the original shape is regained. Humidity is utilized as one such stimulus for shape changing materials, and this increases the utility of hydrogels for 4D printing. Since, hydrogels have relatively low stiffness, natural fibers are preferred for fabrication of scaffolds. Hygromorphs biocomposites are the natural fiber biocomposites, making their mark as the new class of smart materials and can be used in 4D printing [50].

Currently two design strategies are employed for generating actuation with 4D printed hygromorph biocomposites: mono-material printing and multi-material printing deposition. The mono-material printing approach presumes that a given material possesses different mechanical properties and different coefficients of expansions in different directions (anisotropy), induced by the orientation of the fibers within the filament and the printing process itself [50].

Scientists have synthesized renewable bioscaffolds by utilizing PCL and cross-linkers with castor oil which displayed both shape memory and shape recovery at physiological temperatures. Additionally, scaffolds made from epoxidized acrylate material based on renewable soyabean oil, using 3D laser printing, have been shown to express temperature-responsive shape memory. The major disadvantage of solid-state SMP in terms of 4D bioprinting is that the cells can only be seeded on the surface but cannot be uniformly dispersed within it. Moreover, the incitation mechanisms utilized to trigger deformation procedures also pose substantial restrictions. For example, dramatic changes in physical and chemical parameters such as UV and pH may have possible negative effects on cell viability but variation in temperature (between 4 and 40°C) and Ca^{2+} concentration does not have any detrimental effect on living cells [64].

The main factors influencing the process of 4D printing are: (a) type of additive manufacturing process utilized; (b) the nature of the responsive material; (c) type of stimulus; (d) mechanism of interaction between the material and stimulus; and (e) mathematical modeling of the material transformation [42]. The stimuli-responsive biomaterials have made it possible to realize spatio-temporal distributions and release of bioactive cues and cells for heterogenous tissue regeneration. The Project Cyborg software designed by MIT is a platform that offers abilities to simulate self-assembly and optimization of design constructs of programmable materials [64].

4.7.3 Reverse modeling

Reverse modeling design is an image-based technique that reconstructs bone tissue microstructure based on its CT or MRI image. This technique employs binary value method to analyze slice information, where element "1" represents the solid and "0" represents the void. The 2D model thus created is transformed into STL (standard tessellation language) files and transmitted to AM equipment to construct 2D layer. Layer-by-layer method is then used to obtain the 3D structure. This method combines advanced medical imaging system, powerful image analysis software and rapid AM technique to mimic microarchitecture of bone tissue [52].

Cutting et al. in 1986 elaborated the use of 3D computed tomography (CT) images in planning virtual surgeries, and these principles have now been extrapolated to develop customized 3D scaffolds for craniofacial reconstruction [14].

4.7.4 Mathematical modeling

This method mainly utilizes shape functions to construct porous scaffold with implicit function surfaces or irregular polygonal models. Triply periodic minimal surface (TPMS) method uses trigonometric functions to derive complex porous structure with minimal surface, in which the curvature at any point is zero. It is similar to the natural surface geometries of beetle shells, butterfly wings and crustacean bones, where periodicity exists in three independent directions and no sealed cavities are present in the geometry. TPMS based method has been used for designing tissue scaffolds and a simple primitive (P-type) unit. Other types of TPMS units such as diamond (D-type) and gyroid (G-type) have also been proposed for bone scaffold designing. Capfer et al. studied two types of TPMS-based structures including network solids and sheet solids. (a) In network solids the minimal surface makes the solid void interface, whereas in (b) sheet solids minimal surfaces to sheets with predefined thickness are inflated to construct porous solids. The latter was found to possess considerably higher mechanical stiffness and Poisson's ratio [52].

5. Conclusion

Tissue engineering is a multidisciplinary field that focuses on the development of materials and strategies for tissue reconstruction/regeneration. Recent developments in technology has improved the ways in which engineering of tissues are performed. The main requirement for tissue engineering is the selection of material and technique used for fabrication of scaffold with the given material. However, the advancements in fabrication technology have dramatically improved the amalgamation of biomaterial and cell-based scaffolds. Such drastic improvement in our understanding and implementation of material science along with cell biology has empowered surgeons to approach the challenging regions such as craniofacial sites for reconstructive surgeries.

Innovative and multidisciplinary approaches including advanced materials, nanobiotechnology, cell biology, computer assisted techniques, robotics and tools of artificial intelligence offer huge potential for augmentation of craniomaxillofacial tissue engineering [65]. Such rapid progress in technologies bestows great promise for large scale manufacturing and implementation of these scaffolds for reconstructive surgeries. This would also make the process economic and affordable for clinical applications.

Acknowledgements

The corresponding author expresses gratitude to all the contributing authors and anonymous reviewers for their valuable contribution and suggestions of the received manuscripts. The authors also thank Savitribai Phule Pune University, Pune, India for providing the necessary infrastructure during the compilation of this chapter. We also thank our colleagues, whose work has been cited in this article, for their inspiration. Jay Dave and Sayali Chandekar thank Lady Tata Memorial Trust and Savitribai Phule Pune University, India for doctoral fellowship respectively.

Conflict of interest

The authors declare no conflict of interest with relation to this study.

Author details

Geetanjali B. Tomar*, Jay Dave†, Sayali Chandekar†, Nandika Bhattacharya, Sharvari Naik, Shravani Kulkarni, Suraj Math, Kaushik Desai and Neha Sapkal
Institute of Bioinformatics and Biotechnology, Savitribai Phule Pune University, Pune, Maharashtra, India

*Address all correspondence to: geetanjalitomar13@gmail.com; joshigeet@gmail.com

† Both authors have contributed equally.

References

[1] Jammalamadaka U, Tappa K. Recent advances in biomaterials for 3D printing and tissue engineering. J Funct Biomater. 2018;9(1).

[2] Frohbergh ME, Katsman A, Mondrinos MJ, Stabler CT, Hankenson KD, Oristaglio JT, et al. Osseointegrative properties of electrospun hydroxyapatite-containing nanofibrous chitosan scaffolds. Tissue Eng - Part A. 2015;21(5-6):970-81.

[3] Tao O, Kort-Mascort J, Lin Y, Pham HM, Charbonneau AM, ElKashty OA, et al. The applications of 3D printing for craniofacial tissue engineering. Micromachines. 2019;10(7).

[4] Akbarzadeh R, Yousefi A. Effects of processing parameters in thermally induced phase separation technique on porous architecture of scaffolds for bone tissue engineering. J Biomed Mater Res Part B Appl Biomater. 2014 Aug;102(6):1304-15.

[5] Wang D, Gilbert JR, Zhang X, Zhao B, Ker DFE, Cooper GM. Calvarial Versus Long Bone: Implications for Tailoring Skeletal Tissue Engineering. Tissue Eng - Part B Rev. 2020;26(1):46-63.

[6] Asaad F, Pagni G, Pilipchuk SP, Giannì AB, Giannobile W V., Rasperini G. 3D-Printed Scaffolds and Biomaterials: Review of Alveolar Bone Augmentation and Periodontal Regeneration Applications. Int J Dent. 2016;2016.

[7] Gaihre B, Uswatta S, Jayasuriya A. Reconstruction of Craniomaxillofacial Bone Defects Using Tissue-Engineering Strategies with Injectable and Non-Injectable Scaffolds. J Funct Biomater. 2017;8(4):49.

[8] Gupte MJ, Ma PX. Nanofibrous scaffolds for dental and craniofacial applications. J Dent Res. 2012;91(3):227-34.

[9] Rider P, Kačarević ŽP, Alkildani S, Retnasingh S, Schnettler R, Barbeck M. Additive manufacturing for guided bone regeneration: A perspective for alveolar ridge augmentation. Vol. 19, International Journal of Molecular Sciences. 2018. 1-35 p.

[10] Li G, Zhou T, Lin S, Shi S, Lin Y. Nanomaterials for Craniofacial and Dental Tissue Engineering. J Dent Res. 2017;96(7):725-32.

[11] Santos-Rosales V, Iglesias-Mejuto A, García-González CA. Solvent-free approaches for the processing of scaffolds in regenerative medicine. Polymers (Basel). 2020;12(3).

[12] Matias M, Zenha H, Costa H. Three-Dimensional Printing: Custom-Made Implants for Craniomaxillofacial Reconstructive Surgery. Craniomaxillofac Trauma Reconstr. 2017;10(2):089-98.

[13] Martín-Del-Campo M, Rosales-Ibañez R, Rojo L. Biomaterials for cleft lip and palate regeneration. Int J Mol Sci. 2019;20(9).

[14] Tevlin R, McArdle A, Atashroo D, Walmsley GG, Senarath-Yapa K, Zielins ER, et al. Biomaterials for craniofacial bone engineering. J Dent Res. 2014;93(12):1187-95.

[15] Hung BP, Naved BA, Nyberg EL, Dias M, Holmes CA, Elisseeff JH, et al. Three-Dimensional Printing of Bone Extracellular Matrix for Craniofacial Regeneration. ACS Biomater Sci Eng. 2016;2(10):1806-16.

[16] Kinoshita Y, Maeda H. Recent developments of functional scaffolds for craniomaxillofacial bone tissue engineering applications. Sci World J. 2013;2013.

[17] Li W, Fu Y, Jiang B, Lo AY, Ameer GA, Barnett C, et al.

Polymer-integrated amnion scaffold significantly improves cleft palate repair. Acta Biomater. 2019;92:104-14.

[18] Fuchs A, Youssef A, Seher A, Hochleitner G, Dalton PD, Hartmann S, et al. Medical-grade polycaprolactone scaffolds made by melt electrospinning writing for oral bone regeneration - A pilot study in vitro. BMC Oral Health. 2019;19(1):1-11.

[19] Fuchs A, Youssef A, Seher A, Hartmann S, Brands RC, Müller-Richter UDA, et al. A new multilayered membrane for tissue engineering of oral hard- and soft tissue by means of melt electrospinning writing and film casting – An in vitro study. J Cranio-Maxillofacial Surg. 2019;47(4):695-703.

[20] Chakrapani VY, Kumar TSS, Raj DK, Kumary T V. Electrospun 3D composite scaffolds for craniofacial critical size defects. J Mater Sci Mater Med. 2017;28(8):1-10.

[21] Zumarán C, Parra M, Olate S, Fernández E, Muñoz F, Haidar Z. The 3 R's for Platelet-Rich Fibrin: A "Super" Tri-Dimensional Biomaterial for Contemporary Naturally-Guided Oro-Maxillo-Facial Soft and Hard Tissue Repair, Reconstruction and Regeneration. Materials (Basel). 2018 Jul 26;11(8):1293.

[22] Li Y, Liao C, Tjong SC. Synthetic biodegradable aliphatic polyester nanocomposites reinforced with nanohydroxyapatite and/or graphene oxide for bone tissue engineering applications. Nanomaterials. 2019;9(4).

[23] Xue R, Lai Q, Sun S, Lai L, Tang X, Ci J, et al. Application of three-dimensional printing technology for improved orbital-maxillary-zygomatic reconstruction. J Craniofac Surg. 2019;30(2):E127-31.

[24] Rodríguez-Méndez I, Fernández-Gutiérrez M, Rodríguez-Navarrete A, Rosales-Ibáñez R, Benito-Garzón L, Vázquez-Lasa B, et al. Bioactive Sr.(II)/chitosan/poly(ε-caprolactone) scaffolds for craniofacial tissue regeneration. In vitro and in vivo behavior. Polymers (Basel). 2018;10(3):1-26.

[25] Park SA, Lee HJ, Kim KS, Lee SJ, Lee JT, Kim SY, et al. In vivo evaluation of 3D-printed polycaprolactone scaffold implantation combined with β-TCP powder for alveolar bone augmentation in a beagle defect model. Materials (Basel). 2018;11(2).

[26] Maroulakos M, Kamperos G, Tayebi L, Halazonetis D, Ren Y. Applications of 3D printing on craniofacial bone repair: A systematic review. J Dent. 2019;80(May):1-14.

[27] Roberge J, Norato J. Computational design of curvilinear bone scaffolds fabricated via direct ink writing. Comput Des. 2018 Feb;95:1-13.

[28] Ribeiro VP, Silva-Correia J, Nascimento AI, da Silva Morais A, Marques AP, Ribeiro AS, et al. Silk-based anisotropical 3D biotextiles for bone regeneration. Biomaterials. 2017;123:92-106.

[29] Chena W, Thein-Hanb W, Weirb MD, Chena Q, Hockin HKX. Prevascularization of biofunctional calcium phosphate cement for dental and craniofacial repairs. Dent Mater. 2015;30(5):535-44.

[30] Sengupta P, Prasad BLV. Surface Modification of Polymeric Scaffolds for Tissue Engineering Applications. Regen Eng Transl Med. 2018;4(2):75-91.

[31] Raeisdasteh Hokmabad V, Davaran S, Ramazani A, Salehi R. Design and fabrication of porous biodegradable scaffolds: a strategy for tissue engineering. J Biomater Sci Polym Ed. 2017;28(16):1797-825.

[32] Shadjou N, Hasanzadeh M. Silica-based mesoporous nanobiomaterials as promoter of bone regeneration process. J Biomed Mater Res - Part A. 2015;103(11):3703-16.

[33] Aslankoohi N, Mondal D, Rizkalla AS, Mequanint K. Bone repair and regenerative biomaterials: Towards recapitulating the microenvironment. Polymers (Basel). 2019;11(9).

[34] Li M, Xiong P, Yan F, Li S, Ren C, Yin Z, et al. An overview of graphene-based hydroxyapatite composites for orthopedic applications. Bioact Mater. 2018;3(1):1-18.

[35] Song Y, Zhang C, Wang P, Wang L, Bao C, Weir MD, et al. Engineering bone regeneration with novel cell-laden hydrogel microfiber-injectable calcium phosphate scaffold. Mater Sci Eng C. 2017;75:895-905.

[36] Ma H, Feng C, Chang J, Wu C. 3D-printed bioceramic scaffolds: From bone tissue engineering to tumor therapy. Acta Biomater. 2018;79:37-59.

[37] Shao H, Ke X, Liu A, Sun M, He Y, Yang X, et al. Bone regeneration in 3D printing bioactive ceramic scaffolds with improved tissue/material interface pore architecture in thin-wall bone defect. Biofabrication. 2017;9(2).

[38] Prabha RD, Kraft DCE, Harkness L, Melsen B, Varma H, Nair PD, et al. Bioactive nano-fibrous scaffold for vascularized craniofacial bone regeneration. J Tissue Eng Regen Med. 2018 Mar;12(3).

[39] El-Rashidy AA, Roether JA, Harhaus L, Kneser U, Boccaccini AR. Regenerating bone with bioactive glass scaffolds: A review of in vivo studies in bone defect models. Acta Biomater. 2017;62:1-28.

[40] Du X, Fu S, Zhu Y. 3D printing of ceramic-based scaffolds for bone tissue engineering: an overview. J Mater Chem B. 2018;6(27):4397-412.

[41] Meireles AB, Corrêa DK, da Silveira JVW, Millás ALG, Bittencourt E, de Brito-Melo GEA, et al. Trends in polymeric electrospun fibers and their use as oral biomaterials. Exp Biol Med. 2018;243(8):665-76.

[42] Tamay DG, Usal TD, Alagoz AS, Yucel D, Hasirci N, Hasirci V. 3D and 4D printing of polymers for tissue engineering applications. Front Bioeng Biotechnol. 2019;7(JUL).

[43] Tiffany AS, Gray DL, Woods TJ, Subedi K, Harley BAC. The inclusion of zinc into mineralized collagen scaffolds for craniofacial bone repair applications. Acta Biomater. 2019 Jul;93(217):86-96.

[44] Tomar GB, Dave JR, Mhaske ST, Mamidwar S, Makar PK. Applications of Nanomaterials in Bone Tissue Engineering. 2020;209-50.

[45] Fedore CW, Tse LYL, Nam HK, Barton KL, Hatch NE. Analysis of polycaprolactone scaffolds fabricated via precision extrusion deposition for control of craniofacial tissue mineralization. Orthod Craniofacial Res. 2017;20(March):12-7.

[46] Diaz-Gomez L, García-González CA, Wang J, Yang F, Aznar-Cervantes S, Cenis JL, et al. Biodegradable PCL/fibroin/hydroxyapatite porous scaffolds prepared by supercritical foaming for bone regeneration. Int J Pharm. 2017;527(1-2):115-25.

[47] Yadegari A, Fahimipour F, Rasoulianboroujeni M, Dashtimoghadarm E, Omidi M, Golzar H, et al. Specific considerations in scaffold design for oral tissue engineering. Biomaterials for Oral and Dental Tissue Engineering. Elsevier Ltd.; 2017. 157-183 p.

[48] Rana D, Ramasamy K, Leena M, JiménezC, CamposJ, IbarraP, etal. Surface functionalization of nanobiomaterials for application in stem cell culture, tissue engineering, and regenerative medicine. Biotechnol Prog. 2016 May;32(3):554-67.

[49] Cheng X, Wan Q, Pei X. Graphene Family Materials in Bone Tissue Regeneration: Perspectives and Challenges. Nanoscale Res Lett. 2018;13.

[50] Le Duigou A, Correa D, Ueda M, Matsuzaki R, Castro M. A review of 3D and 4D printing of natural fiber biocomposites. Mater Des. 2020;194:108911.

[51] Berton F, Porrelli D, Di Lenarda R, Turco G. A critical review on the production of electrospun nanofibres for guided bone regeneration in oral surgery. Nanomaterials. 2020;10(1).

[52] Yang Y, Wang G, Liang H, Gao C, Peng S, Shen L, et al. Additive manufacturing of bone scaffolds. Int J Bioprinting. 2019;5(1):1-25.

[53] Puwanun S, Bye FJ, Ireland MM, MacNeil S, Reilly GC, Green NH. Production and characterization of a novel, electrospun, tri-layer polycaprolactone membrane for the segregated co-culture of bone and soft tissue. Polymers (Basel). 2016;8(6):1-9.

[54] Harikrishnan P, Islam H, Sivasamy A. Biocompatibility studies of nanoengineered polycaprolactone and nanohydroxyapatite scaffold for craniomaxillofacial bone regeneration. J Craniofac Surg. 2019;30(1):265-9.

[55] Parham S, Kharazi AZ, Bakhsheshi-Rad HR, Ghayour H, Ismail AF, Nur H, et al. Electrospun Nano-fibers for biomedical and tissue engineering applications: A comprehensive review. Materials (Basel). 2020;13(9):1-25.

[56] Zafar M, Najeeb S, Khurshid Z, Vazirzadeh M, Zohaib S, Najeeb B, et al. Potential of electrospun nanofibers for biomedical and dental applications. Materials (Basel). 2016;9(2):1-21.

[57] Batool F, Strub M, Petit C, Bugueno IM, Bornert F, Clauss F, et al. Periodontal tissues, maxillary jaw bone, and tooth regeneration approaches: From animal models analyses to clinical applications. Nanomaterials. 2018;8(5).

[58] Guan L, Davies JE. Preparation and characterization of a highly macroporous biodegradable composite tissue engineering scaffold. J Biomed Mater Res. 2004 Dec;71A(3):480-7.

[59] Garagiola U, Grigolato R, Soldo R, Bacchini M, Bassi G, Roncucci R, et al. Computer-aided design/computer-aided manufacturing of hydroxyapatite scaffolds for bone reconstruction in jawbone atrophy: a systematic review and case report. Maxillofac Plast Reconstr Surg. 2016;38(1).

[60] Araneda N, Parra M, González-Arriagada WA, Del Sol M, Haidar ZS, Olate S. Morphological Analysis of the Human Maxillary Sinus Using Three-Dimensional Printing. Contemp Clin Dent. 2017;10(2):294-8.

[61] Liao W, Xu L, Wangrao K, Du Y, Xiong Q, Yao Y. Three-dimensional printing with biomaterials in craniofacial and dental tissue engineering. PeerJ. 2019;2019(7).

[62] Singh S, Prakash C, Singh R. 3D Printing in Biomedical Engineering. Singh S, Prakash C, Singh R, editors. Singapore: Springer Singapore; 2020. 346 p. (Materials Horizons: From Nature to Nanomaterials).

[63] Farré-Guasch E, Wolff J, Helder MN, Schulten EAJM, Forouzanfar T, Klein-Nulend J. Application of Additive Manufacturing

in Oral and Maxillofacial Surgery. J Oral Maxillofac Surg. 2015;73(12):2408-18.

[64] Wan Z, Zhang P, Liu Y, Lv L, Zhou Y. Four-dimensional bioprinting: Current developments and applications in bone tissue engineering. Acta Biomater. 2020;101:26-42.

[65] Haidar ZS, Di-Silvio L, Noujeim ZEF, Davies JE, Cuisinier F, Banerjee A. Engineering Solutions for Cranio-Maxillo-Facial Rehabilitation and Oro-Dental Healthcare. J Healthc Eng. 2019 Jun 18;2019:1-3.

Chapter 11

Salivary Gland Radio-Protection, Regeneration and Repair: Innovative Strategies

Ziyad S. Haidar

Abstract

Saliva has a critical role in the maintenance of oral, dental and general health and well-being. Alteration(s) in the amount/quantity and/or quality of secreted saliva may induce the development of several oro-dental variations, thereby negatively-impacting overall quality of life. Diverse factors may affect the process of saliva production and quantity/quality of secretion, including medications, systemic or local pathologies and/or reversible/irreversible damage. Indeed, chemo- and/or radio-therapy, particularly, in cases of head and neck cancer, for example, are well-documented to induce serious damage and dysfunction to the *radio-sensitive* salivary gland tissue, resulting in hypo-salivation, xerostomia (dry mouth) as well as numerous other adverse intra–/extra-oral, medical and quality-of-life issues. Although a single governing mechanism of radiation-induced salivary gland tissue damage and dysfunction has not been yet elucidated, the potential for a synergy in radio-protection (mainly, and possible -reparation) via a combinatorial approach of mechanistically distinct strategies, has been suggested and explored over the years. This is, undoubtfully, in parallel to the ongoing efforts in improving the precision, safety and efficacy of radiotherapy protocols/outcomes, as well as in developing new technological and pharmaceutical alternatives, topics covered in this chapter.

Keywords: radioprotection, salivary gland, xerostomia, head and neck cancer, oro-dental health

1. Introduction

It is well recognized that the incidence of cancer, the second leading cause of death, globally, is increasing, an ongoing major burden of disease and public health burden, World-wide. While there were 14.1 million cancer cases reported in 2012, the World Health Organization (WHO) estimated about 1 in 6 deaths is due to cancer, with 9.6 million such deaths reported in 2018. In the United States, today, cancer is the second leading, after heart disease, cause of death amongst men and women, with over 1 million new cases diagnosed, annually [1].

Despite a reduction in tobacco consumption and the significant modern advancements in medicine, the number of new cancer cases, per year, is projected to rise to 22.2 million by 2030 [1]. Cancers, often squamous cell carcinomas/neoplasms, that involve the oral cavity, nostrils, paranasal sinuses, naso–/oro–/hypo-pharynx, larynx, and the salivary glands, are commonly/collectively (despite their heterogeneity) termed head and neck cancers (HNC), which, together are responsible for nearly 200,000 deaths, a year, World-wide [2]. In the United States alone, HNC represent 4–5% of all cancers, and in Europe, HNC are the sixth most common group of cancers [3].

Besides the alarming incidence and mortality rates, HNC suffer a relatively poor prognosis, overall, whether due to delays in diagnosis, staging, treatment, particulars of the tumor site, onset, type of symptoms and/or efficacy of therapies, to mention a few. Such factors further contribute to permitting the progress and upstaging of the malignant tumor(s) which eventually result in enfeebled survival, despite the application of novel or advanced intensive therapeutic regimens. Briefly, treatment, often a multi-disciplinary case-specific approach, can employ chemo−/radio−/immune-therapy, surgery, or combinatorial strategies [4].

Herein, radiotherapy (RT), whether radical or prophylactic, remains a mainstay of HNC treatment, especially in light of modern improvements in precisely targeting and delivering the required radiation doses to the tumor, thereby allowing additional sparing of normal/healthy surrounding tissue(s), greatly reducing side or adverse effects of radiation, and consequently improving the quality of life (QoL) of patients as well as their families [5–8]. IMRT (intensity-modulated radiotherapy), VMAT (volumetric modulated arc therapy) and particle (ion-based) therapy are perhaps fine examples of modern high-precision RT [7].

RT, in general, aims to realize *localized* destruction and control of the target tumor (−cells) and halt of the reproductive potential, while minimizing toxicity onset. Specifically, high-energy radiation is deposited, causing DNA strands to break thereby damaging the cell genome either directly or indirectly (via free-radical production) and subsequently resulting in apoptosis, mitotic cell death, and tissue hypoxia, through different cascades and processes [5, 7]. Depending on the radiation dose and tissue turnover, amongst other factors, RT can almost always be expected to result in a range of side effects, of which some are reversible and others are irreversible (**Figure 1**). Indeed, HNC and oral squamous cell carcinoma (OSCC) patients receiving RT often experience pain, taste disturbances, difficulties in mastication and deglutition (swallowing) and suffer from mucositis, fungal infections, dental decay, alterations in speech, all of which are mainly due to or linked to salivary gland dysfunction which in turn results in hyposalivation and xerostomia [9–12].

Herein, xerostomia, a dry mouth sensation, is one of the main complications and complaints for HNC patients receiving RT, mainly as a sequela of the un-avoidable damage to the parotid and sub-mandibular glands (both produce over 80% of saliva) anatomically located with the radiation zone [8, 12]. Inflammation, fibrosis, atrophy and the reduced wound healing response, *i.e.* reparative and regenerative capacity of the glands, mainly due to lack of *functional* salivary gland stem/progenitor cells post-irradiation, render the *inevitable* radiotherapy-induced salivary gland damage and dysfunction, whether occurring early or late, a significant impediment to the QoL and survival of HNC and OSCC patients [10, 13, 14].

Therefore, besides modern advancements in radiation engineering technologies, ample pharmacological and pharmaceutical solutions have been explored [14]. Accumulating knowledge in understanding underlying signaling pathways, cellular and tissue responses, spatio-temporally, fuel the continuing efforts aimed to explore, develop and translate novel solutions to support in the prevention (and treatment of) radiation-induced side-effects and damage of salivary glands, a main focus of this chapter, designed to provide the *clinical* reader with a summary of relevant literature and recent innovative developments in salivary gland radioprotection and potential salivary gland repair, post-RT.

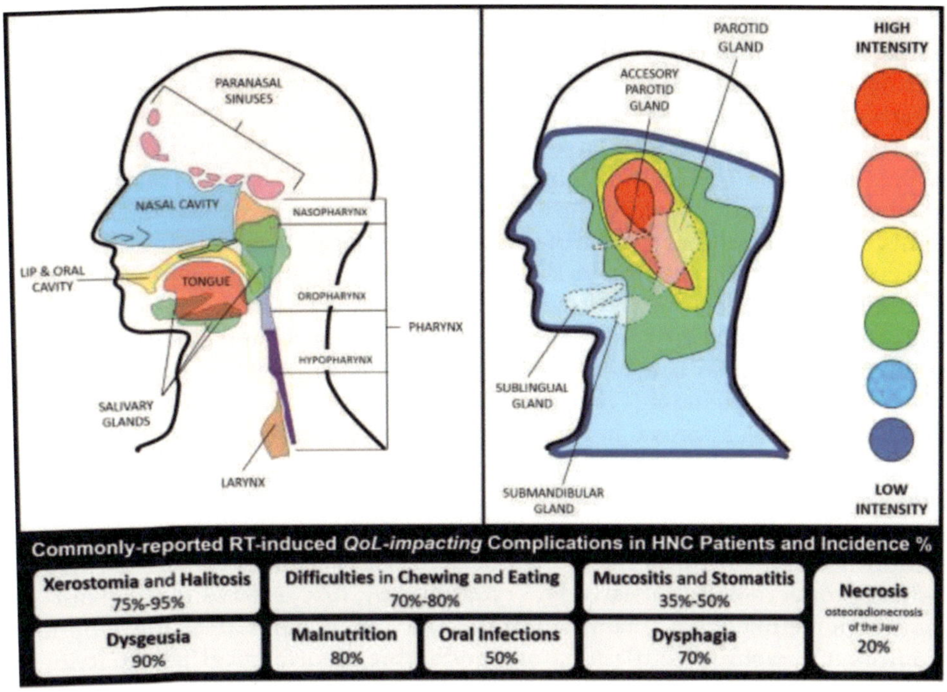

Figure 1.
Head and neck cancers regions and irradiation intensity risk during HNC radiotherapy.

2. Saliva and salivary glands: pre-, during- and post-RT

Briefly, exocrine salivary glands are classified as either major (parotid, sub-mandibular and sub-lingual) or minor (labial and buccal gland, glosso-palatine gland, and palatine and lingual) glands. Anatomically, all three major glands are highly vascularized, innervated and are architecturally similar featuring a ductal structure with a secretory/excretory (saliva-producing acini surrounded by myo-epithelial cells, myo-fibroblasts, immune cells, stromal cells, endothelial cells and nerve fibers) opening into the oral cavity/mouth [15]. The glands differ in their type of acinar cells and as a result, in the type of produced saliva. While the parotid is composed of only serous acini thereby producing watery saliva, the sub-mandibular and sub-lingual glands contain a mix of serous and mucous (glycoprotein- rich) acini, thereby producing saliva of a different composition, a seromucous secretion. Secretion of saliva is stimulated by the sympathetic (proteins) and parasympathetic (serous/ions) branches of the autonomic nervous system [15, 16].

Saliva is basically an oral lubricant fluid with multiple digestive functions critical for oro-dental health, QoL and general well-being. It is composed of a complex mixture of water (99%), electrolytes (sodium, potassium, calcium, magnesium, etc. ...), mucins, proteins, white blood cells, epithelial cells, immunoglobulins, anti-microbials/−bacterials and enzymes (1%) [16–18]. Hence, saliva is essential for moistening, chewing, swallowing and chemically-digesting foods. It also facilitates speaking, aids the tongue in taste sensing, helps protect the oral mucosa (localized immunity/mucosal resistance) and plays a role in tissue re-mineralization. A healthy adult produces/secretes a daily average of 0.5–1.5 L, at differential rates over the day, and at a near neutral (buffer) pH of 6.7 [15–17, 19–22].

Therefore, alterations in quantity (↓: hypo- or ↑: hyper-salivation) or quality of the secreted/produced saliva are associated to a variety of conditions and diseases and have been associated with some medications and therapies [23]. For instance, sialorrhea is a general term used for hyper-salivation (or drooling), often as a result of medication, systemic diseases, psychiatric disorders and/or oral pathologies, amongst others [14]. It is also often linked to conditions such as Parkinson's, epilepsy, amyotrophic lateral sclerosis or ALS, cerebral palsy, developmental disabilities, pregnancy and/or drugs including clozapine [16, 24] Common treatments for sialorrhea include surgical intervention, radiation of the salivary glands (to halt and diminish its function) and the use of oral anti-cholinergic drugs (to inhibit saliva production), however with known side or adverse effects. In recent years, numerous studies investigated the use of neuro-toxins, mainly botulinum neurotoxins or BoNTs, which basically are bacterial exotoxins that interfere and block the exocytotic release of vesicular neuro-transmitters cholinergic neuromuscular activity in the target tissue, including commercially-available RimabotulinumtoxinB (RimaBoNT-B, FDA approval in 2000) and IncobotulinumtoxinA (IncoBoNT-A, FDA approval in 2010) in patients suffering sialorrhea, with attractively promising results [24, 25].

On the other hand, salivary gland hypofunction (*progressive* loss of gland function) is commonly described or associated with the reduction of salivary flow and production, quantitatively. Frydrych [26], discussed salivary gland hypofunction etiology and classified causes into seven major areas, developmental, autoimmune/chronic inflammatory, endocrine, neurological/psychiatric, metabolic, infectious and iatrogenic [26]. In a healthy individual, un-stimulated "whole" salivary flow rate is averaged at 0.35 mL saliva per minute, with abnormalities indicated if the rate drops. For example, one of the most prevalent and studied diseases or disorders of the salivary gland is Sjögren's syndrome (SS), a chronic auto-immune inflammatory reaction characterized by lymphocytic infiltration of the exocrine glands (mostly to the salivary or lacrimal glands), which generates a significant reduction in salivary flow rate - to below 0.1 mL whole saliva per minute secreted, un-stimulated [27]. It is perhaps noteworthy herein that *whole* saliva indicates the collection of saliva (secreted from all salivary glands) present in the mouth. Other quantification techniques require direct collection from the specific gland. Moreover, often is reported in diagnosing SS that only un-stimulated whole saliva flow rates are used.

Hypo-salivation, therefore, is salivary flow rate reduction, quantified, clinically via sialometry. Xerostomia, on the other hand, is the reported perception or sensation, subjectively, of oral dryness. Hypo-salivation may or may not be accompanied by xerostomia, and vice versa. Dryness in the mouth can be a side-effect of medications or due to diseases such as HIV/AIDS, diabetes, hypertension and/or other factors including smoking, dehydration, mouth breathing, aging and/or head and neck irradiation [14, 16, 23, 28, 29]. Indeed, xerostomia is one of the most commonly reported (and expected) complications of RT (during and after RT) for HNC, and as mentioned earlier, mainly as a predictable consequence to the significant damage (and generated inflammatory immune response) caused to the salivary glands which are located and included within the RT-zone or field [30–32].

RT, besides impairing salivary gland function and salivary flow rate, impacts the quality of the secreted saliva, given the loss or atrophy of acinar and ductal cells and granules (and stem/stromal and progenitor cells) and the consequential morphological changes to salivary fluid quality (including pH and buffering capacity), thereby affecting the essential protective, functional and overall physiologic processes (**Figure 2**). Such damage [32] and impact can appear as soon as one week after the first radiation therapy session (*acute RT-induced damage is due to a disturbance in the involved signal transduction pathways on the cell membrane*). Progressive

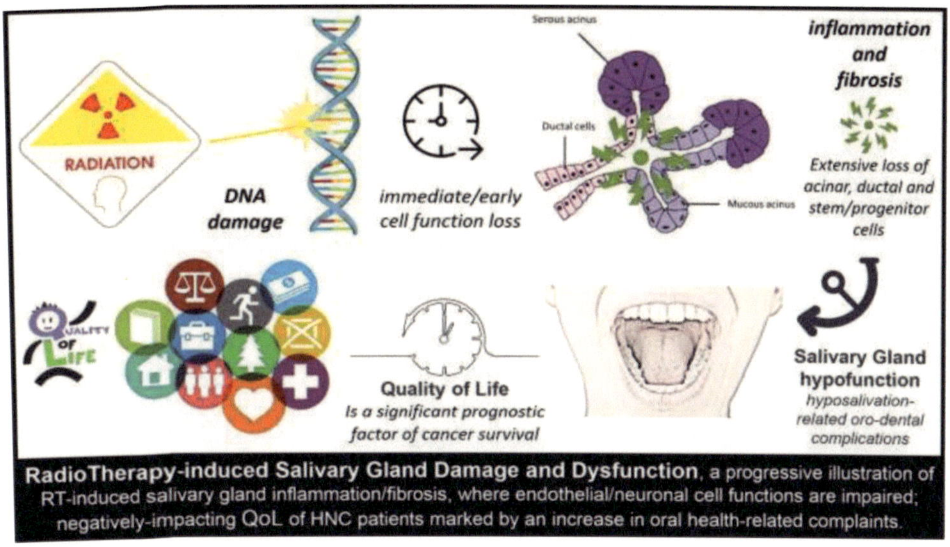

Figure 2.
Progression of RT-induced salivary gland damage and dysfunction in HNC patients.

decrease in salivary gland function is evident with more RT sessions (*delayed or late RT-induced damage is due to apoptosis-driven parenchymal cell loss, inflammation, blood vessel dilation and function loss, nerve injury and reduced parasympathetic nervous function, and fibrosis*) rendering rescue, repair and regeneration rather challenging [33–35].

As a result, the QoL of a large proportion of patients receiving RT is severely compromised [36, 37], with thicker or more viscous saliva and xerostomia leading in reported complaints [38]. Indeed, RT-related biochemical and proteomic alterations where several key glycoproteins, proteins and other molecules are affected have been identified [31, 39]. For example, Jehmlich *et al.* [40], discussed such variations post-RT, detected significant alterations in 48 proteins and highlighted the development of oral mucositis as a result of salivary gland dysfunction. Psychosocial and emotional impact on QoL of HNC patients, especially the elderly [41], where they experience and suffer from a compromised ability to and taste, chew, and swallow foods extended to their forced switching of dietary preferences to soft and carbohydrate-rich foods, thereby resulting in serious nutritional deficiencies [38, 40, 41]. Hyposalivation and sequential xerostomia also affect speaking and communication abilities, and patients experience nocturnal oral discomfort, hence, causing additional stress leading to withdrawal from everyday or day-to-day societal and emotional interactions [42–44].

Furthermore, with the prolonged oral clearance of sugars, the oral mucosa becomes painfully-dry, sticky and more susceptible to infection, the progression of dental caries (tooth decay), gingival and periodontal disease and trauma, accentuating the importance of oro-dental hygiene and care, especially in the elderly patients [41]. Other sequelae include erosion and ulceration of mucosal tissues, oral candidiasis, dysgeusia and dysphagia. Therefore, it is common for HNC patients to suffer from depression, feelings of anguish and anxiety after receipt of the RT protocol [14, 37, 45–49]. While the recovery of irradiated salivary glands at the cellular and molecular has been thus far shown to be limited, salivary recovery post-RT, from our clinical exposure and expertise, is possible, yet a lengthy (> 3 years), dire and capricious process, with underlying mechanisms not yet fully understood.

3. Radiation-induced damage prevention and potential regeneration of salivary glands

Understanding the underlying mechanisms governing cellular and molecular control of salivary gland function is highly pertinent, during- and post-RT, to aid in developing suitable and effective therapies, whether preventive or reparative. To date, it is safe to state that available therapies continue to be symptomatic and no definitive solution or approach has been shown to compensate and/or recover the impairment of salivary glands and function. Life-style modifications, synthetic saliva and/or use of salivary stimulants and sialagogues, suffer shortcomings and are not satisfactory to our patients, as they either only provide temporary (short-term) relief or might have other disquieting side-effects. Hence, global attention has been diverted to seek and develop alternative novel methods, tools and therapies, to offer to HNC patients undergoing RT, that can provide superior long-term efficacy. Herein, tissue engineering, regenerative medicine, pharmaceutics and nanotechnology may contribute.

4. Tissue engineering and reparative/regenerative medicine: current regimens and strategies

Several tissues and organs are highly sensitive to irradiation, such as the skin, esophagus and bone marrow. However, the salivary glands are intricately radiosensitive, given their highly-differentiated cell content marked with a very low or slow proliferative rate [50]. This can help explain why the salivary glands, in specific, are somewhat unique in their early- and delayed-effects post-RT, when compared to other tissues and organs. Nonetheless, salivary gland dysfunction and/or hypofunction has been shown, in some cases, to be reversible. Such treatment intervention is multi-factorial and highly-dependent on original causality, for example, in cases of alcohol abuse and dehydration or hypothyroidism. RT-induced salivary gland damage and dysfunction is a far more challenging scenario. Auto-immune/chronic inflammatory diseases, such as SS or systemic lupus erythematosus also result in irreversible damage to the salivary glands [26].

Today, as mentioned earlier, only palliative and efficacy-limited regimens are commercially-available [47]. **Tables 1–4** highlight a selection of various radio-protection strategies, at different stages of development, pre-clinically (*in vitro* and in *in vivo* testing) and clinical (human clinical trials). Briefly, database search was performed in PubMed-indexed articles using a multi-search of the following key-words: "Salivary Glands AND Radioprotection [Title/Abstract]", "Salivary Glands AND Radioprotection [MeSH]", "Salivary AND Glands AND Radioprotection [Title/Abstract]", "Salivary Gland AND Radioprotection [Title/Abstract]", "Salivary AND Gland AND Radioprotection [ALL FIELDS]", "Salivary Glands AND Radioprotection [ALL FIELDS] and "Salivary Gland AND Radioprotection [ALL FIELDS]". Eligibility and inclusion criteria included English articles reporting radio-protection data from *in vitro*, *in vivo* and/or clinical setting/trials. Articles dated back to 1978 up to the search end-date of December 31st of 2019 were analyzed. Reviews, communications or articles with preliminary results were not included in our analysis (**Figure 3**). Herein, our purpose is to screen the available literature and assess the level of development of new strategies, regimens and/or innovative solutions, to provide a usable prior-Art formatted report. Hence, not all included articles, which are tabulated for the reader, were aimed to be presented and dissected to be discussed in detail. This review attempts to provide an overview of the current understanding, status and prospect of salivary gland radioprotection

Agent	Main Findings	Ref
bFGF-PLGA microspheres	Administration of basic Fibroblast Growth Factor (bFGF) prior to and immediately after irradiation, partially protected (44%) the rat parotid gland.	[51]
pH-responsive nanoparticles for active siRNAs delivery	Introduction of siRNAs specifically targeting the Pkcδ or Bax genes significantly blocked the induction of these pro-apoptotic proteins that normally occurs post-irradiation in cultured salivary gland cells. Level of cell death from subsequent irradiation was significantly decreased.	[52]
rhHGF	Treatment of irradiated hPTS with recombinant human Hepatocyte Growth Factor (rhHGF) restored salivary marker expression and secretory function of hPTS. Changes in the phosphorylation levels of apoptosis-related proteins through HGF-MET axis inhibited irradiation-induced apoptosis.	[53]
TIGAR over-expression	*TIGAR* (a p53-inducible regulator of glycolysis and apoptosis) over-expression could diminish the radio-sensitivity of Hs 917.T cells, and decrease the autophagy level induced by ionizing irradiation.	[54]

Table 1.
Radioprotection of salivary glands, in vitro.

MICE		
Agent	**Main Findings**	**Ref**
Keratinocyte Growth Factor-1 (KGF-1)	Local delivery of keratinocyte growth factor-1 into irradiated salivary glands protected RT-induced salivary cell damage, suppressed p53-mediated apoptosis and prevented salivary hypofunction.	[55]
pH-responsive nanoparticles complexed with siRNAs	Knockdown of Pkcδ reduced the number of apoptotic cells during the acute phase of irradiation damage and also markedly improved salivary secretion at 3 months.	[52]
Dasatinib / Imatinib	Delivery of dasatinib or imatinib resulted in >75% protection/rescue of salivary gland function at 60 days end-point. Continuous dosing with dasatinib extended protection to at least 5 months and was correlated with histologic evidence of regenerated salivary gland acinar cells.	[56]
Human Adipose tissue-derived Mesenchymal Stem Cells (AdMSCs)	Local transplantation of AdMSCs improved tissue remodeling following irradiation-induced damage in salivary gland tissue. The use of a carrier enhanced the effects of AdMSC-mediated cellular protection against irradiation via paracrine secretion.	[57]
Botulinum Toxins (BTX)	Irradiated mice showed a 50% reduction in salivary flow after 3 days, whereas mice pre-injected with BTX had 25% reduction in salivary flow rate ($p < 0.05$). BTX pre-treatment ameliorates RT-induced salivary gland dysfunction.	[58]
AdMSCs secretome	Secretome modulated by hypoxic conditions to contain therapeutic factors contributed to salivary gland tissue re-modeling and demonstrated a potential to improve consequences of RT-induced salivary hypofunction.	[59]
Resveratrol (RES)	Administration of RES reversed the reduction of saliva secretion induced by irradiation and restored salivary amylase and superoxide dismutase activity. RES can protect salivary glands against the negative effects of irradiation.	[60]

MICE		
Agent	**Main Findings**	**Ref**
Amifostine	Amifostine alleviated the effects of irradiation on the bio-functions of cells, such as organelles, highly-involved in the secretory process. Amifostine can alleviate xerostomia caused by the late or delayed effects of irradiation.	[61]
Serotype 5 Adenoviral (Ad5) vector-mediated transfer of basic Fibroblast Growth Factor (AdbFGF) or Vascular Endothelial Growth Factor (AdVEGF) complementary DNAs	Single local administration of a modest dose (5×10^9 particles/gland) of a serotype 5 adenovirus (Ad5) vector encoding either bFGF or VEGF prior to irradiartion, prevents rapid micro-vessel density loss in salivary glands and reduces the loss in salivary flow rate (as measured 8 weeks post-RT).	[62]
Tempol (4-hydroxy-2,2,6,6-tetramethylpiperidine-N-oxyl)	Tempol treatment was found to protect salivary glands significantly against radiation damage (approximately 60% improvement), with no tumor protection observed.	[63]
Tempol (4-hydroxy-2,2,6,6-tetramethylpiperidine-N-oxyl)	Tempol treatment pre-irradiation significantly reduced RT-induced salivary hypofunction (approximately 50–60%). Tempol (I.V. or S.C.) administration also showed significant radio-protection. Topical use of tempol, either as a mouthwash or gel, was also reported to be radioprotective.	[64]
Isoproterenol (IPR)	IPR, stimulates adenylate cyclase/cyclic AMP (AC/cAMP) to increase the level of cAMP,25 and then increases cellular membrane ion permeability, ion active transport, and protein bio-synthesis. These events, together with the release of heavy metals, appear to reduce irradiation injury.	[65]
Tempol (4-hydroxy-2,2,6,6-tetramethylpiperidine-N-oxyl)	Irradiation resulted in a dose-dependent reduction of salivary flow rate in this mouse model.	[66]
WR-2721 WR-3689 WR779 13	Tumors examined take up less WR-3689 than the other two protectors. In RIF-1 tumor, WR-3689 is taken up most avidly, but the three drugs tend to be equally protective.	[67]
WR-2721	There is potential for protecting dose-limiting, late-responding normal tissue in the RT of human tumors with both neutrons and conventional radiotherapy.	[68]
WR-1065	Localized delivery to salivary glands markedly improved radioprotection at the cellular level. Also, mitigated the adverse side-effects associated with systemic administration.	[69]
Hypoxia pre-conditioned human Adipose tissue-derived Mesenchymal Stem Cells (hAdMSCs-HPX)	Results suggest that hAdMSCs-HPX protect salivary glands from RT-induced apoptosis, and preserve acinar structure and functions via the activation of FGFR-PI3K signaling by actions of hAdMSC-secreted factors, including FGF-10.	[70]
Entolimod	At days 8 and 15, entolimod treatment led to noticeable mitigation of damage in salivary gland tissue. Treatment 1 hr. post-RT irradiation seems more effective than 30 min pre-RT.	[71]

MICE		
Agent	**Main Findings**	**Ref**
Statins (Simvastatin)	Administration of Simvastatin could delay and reduce the extent of elevation/over-expression of TGF-β1, which in turn protects the submandibular glands from RT-induced injury.	[72]
RAT		
Agent	**Main Findings**	**Ref**
Se, Zn and Mn + *Lachesis muta* venom (O-LM)	O-LM prevented permanent submandibular gland alterations demonstrating promising results in radioprotection and recovery from RT-induced injury.	[73]
Pilocarpine, Methacholine, Reserpine and Methacholine + Reserpine	Pre-treatment with pilocarpine or methacholine improved all measured glandular functions. Pre-treatment with a combination of reserpine and methacholine showed additive protective effects on submandibular gland function, signifying cooperation of muscarinic and alpha-adrenergic receptors.	[74]
Phenylephrine Isoproterenol Methacholine or Methacholine + Phenylephrine	Pre-treatment with phenylephrine, isoproterenol and methacholine combined with phenylephrine resulted in less irradiation damage to parotid gland functions as indicated by quantified lag phase and flow rate.	[75]
WR-2721	WR-2721 provided a significant degree of protection for all glandular functional parameters including gland weight.	[76]
cAMP	The demonstrated substantial protective effect of exogenously-administered cAMP on the parotid gland supports the previously-suggested radioprotection mechanism by the beta-adrenergic agonist isoproterenol, which is known to elevate endogenous intracellular cAMP.	[77]
WR-2721 Isoproterenol	The aminothiol WR-2721 and beta-adrenergic agonist isoproterenol both conferred considerable radioprotection to the rat parotid gland. Isoproterenol acts on the beta-receptor, and its specific antagonist, propranolol, eliminated the protective effect of isoproterenol, thereby implicating the beta-receptor and cAMP in the radioprotection mechanism.	[78]
WR-2721	While non-protected glands suffered a drastic reduction in the amount of acinar tissue, ducts and blood vessels exhibited only minor morphological changes. Herein, WR-2721 protected the glands with similar signs of damage yet to a much lesser degree, in comparison.	[79]
WR-2721	WR-2721 protected against the acute phase of irradiation damage manifested during the first week post-RT. The drug also protected against chronic damage, appearing later.	[80]
Thymol	Thymol at a dose of 50 mg/Kg significantly impacted (positively) salivary gland dysfunction caused by ionizing irradiation. Short- and late- side effects of RT on the salivary glands were considered reduced by Thymol in those rats.	[81]

RAT		
Agent	**Main Findings**	**Ref**
TLK1B	After a single fraction of 16 Gy, the decline in salivary function at 8 weeks was less pronounced in TLK1B-treated animals (40%) when compared to saline-treated controls (67%).	[82]
TLK1B associated with rAAV9	AAV2/ 9-TLK1B groups showed no decline in salivary flow post-irradiation (121% increase) and salivary flow was not significantly different in irradiated and non-irradiated animals treated similarly with TLK1B.	[83]

Table 2.
Radioprotection of salivary glands, in vivo *using murine models.*

RABBIT		
Agent	**Main Findings**	**Ref**
Lidocaine HydroChloride	Pre-treatment with lidocaine improved irradiation tolerance of both, parotid and submandibular glands. Ultra-structure was largely preserved.	[84]
Lidocaine Amifostine Pilocarpin	Only animals pre-treated with lidocaine or amifostine (alone or combined with pilocarpin) showed a slight non-significant reduction in the salivary ejection fraction. Lidocaine and amifostine could largely preserve the glandular ultra-structure.	[85]
mini-PIG		
Agent	**Main Findings**	**Ref**
Orciprenaline Carbachol	Acinar cells of both glands were significantly more numerous in the pre-treatment group. Also, cells seemed better preserved. Yet, such effects were more pronounced in the parotid gland (appearing almost normal) than in the submandibular gland.	[86]
Adenoviral vector encoding FGF2 (AdLTR2EF1a-FGF2)	A single pre-administration of a hybrid serotype 5 adenoviral vector encoding FGF2 (AdLTR2EF1a-FGF2) resulted in the protection of parotid microvascular endothelial cells from irradiation damage and significantly limited the decline of parotid salivary flow.	[87]

Table 3.
Radioprotection of salivary glands, in vivo *using non-murine models.*

systems, with a look onto potential reparative and regenerative keys, where we, amongst other clinicians and researchers, do aspire for a superior, safe, efficacious and long-term innovative solution that reverses RT-induced damage to the salivary glands of our HNC patients. Moreover, we opted to avoid concluding our *overview* with calls for additional research or validation, given that vital tissue engineering strategies employing the design, characterization and optimization of novel biomaterials (and 3D printing), that can also be housing/incorporating release-controlled nanoparticles or nanocapsules that also are designed to encapsulate distinct mesenchymal stem cells, induced pluripotent stem cells (iPSCs), growth factors or cytokines and/or pharmaceutical agents or drugs, currently investigated at different levels of development are limitless in distinctions and details.

Palliative care for RT-induced salivary gland dysfunction- current and commercially-available palliative options for HNC patients undergoing RT include chewing gum (sugar-free), saliva substitutes, oral and topical lubricants, malic and ascorbic acid, saliva stimulants and sialogogue such as pilocarpine (Salagen, for

Agent	Main Findings	Ref
WR-2721	Administration of WR-2721 prior to each dose of irradiation was feasible and without significant toxicity at 100 mg/m^2. Salivary gland function improved over time after completion of RT, particularly in the parotid gland.	[88]
Botulinum Toxin A (BTX-A)	The SUVmean of the ^{225}Ac-labeled PSMA radio-ligand in the injected parotid gland (right) showed a highly significant decrease of up to 60% when compared with the left side in the 63 years old patient with advanced metastatic castration-resistant prostate cancer (suffering from sialorrhoea) receiving 80 units of BTX-A.	[89]
Amifostine	Amifostine reduces acute xerostomia and mucositis.	[90]
SMGT+IMRT	Surgical submandibular gland transfer (SMGT) was combined with intensity-modulated radiotherapy (IMRT) in a prospective phase II feasibility trial, in a single institution, including 40 HNC patients. At 12 months post-RT, the rate of absent or only mild xerostomia was 89%, and salivary flow rates were approximately 75% of pre-RT levels. Hence, patients reported decreased xerostomia and improved QoL.	[91]
Helical Tomotherapy (HT)	HT is described as an innovate, more precise and less toxic RT technique using a continuously rotating gantry to integrate 3D image guidance (a linear accelerator with computerized tomography) and deliver IMRT in a helical pattern. In 175 HNC patients, followed for up to 36 months, HT was used to deliver irradiation doses to bi-lateral parotid glands (PG-T), contra-lateral submandibular gland (cSMG), and accessory salivary glands in the oral cavity. Xerostomia was significantly decreased when the mean doses of PG-T, cSMG, and OC were kept below 29.12Gy, 29.29Gy, and 31.44Gy, respectively.	[92]

Table 4.
Radioprotection of salivary glands, clinically in human subjects.

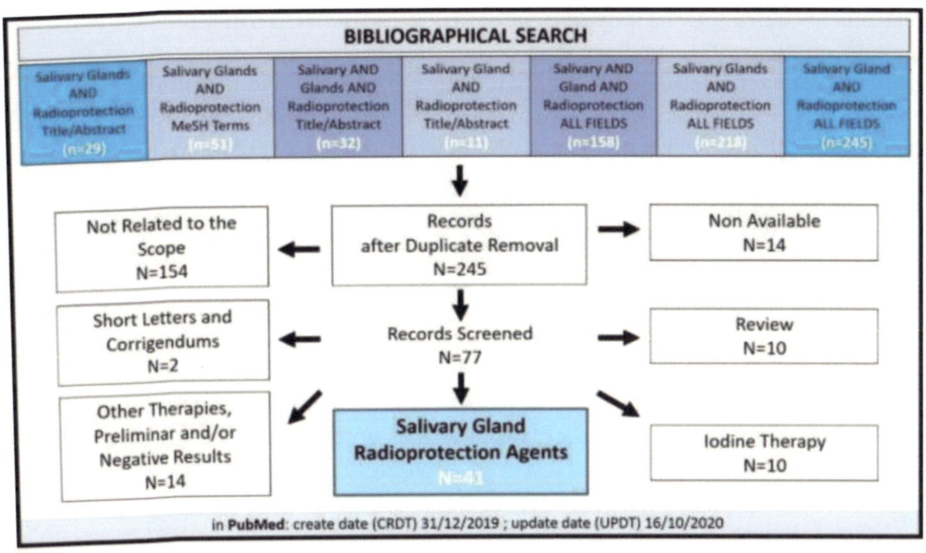

Figure 3.
PRISMA flow diagram for the bibliographic electronic search on PubMed central.

example) and cevimeline (Evoxac, for example). As mentioned above, none have proved to restore normal QoL and patient satisfaction, mainly due to their limited efficacy and effectiveness [30, 42]. On top, adverse side effects are common, and such options are often costly to patients, requiring multiple daily use over long periods of time. In parallel, patients, especially the elderly, institutionalized and frail, need to go through education and training to acquire new eating and life-style habits, learn to prevent or avoid impaired swallowing and potential choking, and improve their oral and dental hygiene practices and tools to prevent (or halt the progression of) dental and oral mucosal diseases, infections and tooth loss. Other palliative care options including acupuncture and electro-stimulation (enhancement of salivary reflexes) are currently undergoing investigation [30, 93].

The only Food and Drug Administration–approved radioprotective and anti-xerostomia drug for clinical use (adjuvant setting) is Amifostine, an organic thiophosphate, cryoprotective agent and free radical scavenger administered subcutaneously or most often intravenously upon reconstitution with normal saline prior to or simultaneously with RT to then accumulate within the salivary glands, has been extensively-studied since its development, initially under the nuclear warfare program [14, 94]. Today, while it continues to benefit some patients, prophylactically, via minimizing the effects of xerostomia and taste loss, it is often associated with severe side effects including a rapid decrease in blood pressure (hypotension), nausea and emesis or vomiting. Recent analysis of several clinical trials associated Amifostine to low-quality and mixed evidence in preventing dry mouth complaints in patients receiving RT to the head and neck region, in the short- to medium-terms (up to three months post-RT) and have questioned its potential in tumor cell protection, thereby further narrowing its clinical safety and efficacy window, especially in light of its high cost [94, 95]. Essentially, its use in radiation-induced xerostomia has already been cautioned in the year 2008 by the American Society of Clinical Oncology [96], and so, its controversial and debatable safety and use in all cancer cases lingers.

Preventive and interventional care for RT-induced salivary gland dysfunction- the main objective of any planned and/or prescribed option should be the relief of symptoms and complications associated with hypo-salivation and xerostomia in HNC patients scheduled to receive RT, in order to prevent deteriorations in their QoL thereby enhancing their battle with cancer, its treatment and consequences [97]. As discussed earlier, despite advancements in irradiation techniques and regimens including IMRT, only palliative and prophylactic options are available, all of which do suffer substantial short-comings [98, 99]. One might even consider IMPT or intensity modulated proton therapy, used to deliver a much-reduced irradiation dose and subsequently less toxic than IMRT, thereby alleviating much of the typical side effects of RT, however, IMPT is known to be more expensive and lacks accessibility and availability [43, 98, 99].

1. **Surgical Intervention alternative**- to prevent RT-induced hyposalivation, sub-mandibular gland preservation and protection from irradiation via surgical relocation to the sub-mental space, thereby away or out of irradiation zone, has been explored, with positive results. It is perhaps worth mentioning herein that sub-mandibular salivary gland supplies up to 90% of the un-stimulated saliva formation/secretion. However, such highly-invasive interventional procedures are peculiar and require exquisite surgical manipulation skills and settings. Further, surgical transfer of salivary glands is not indicated or possible for cancers of the oral cavity or patients undergoing (systemic) chemotherapy. In addition, for the gland to either retain or restore functionality, the connection of the gland to the main duct must be maintained or restored, respectively [100], altogether render it a very limit-ed/–ing option.

   In terms of innovative approaches, Rao *et al.* [101] recently described the use of a synthetic hydrogel (TraceIT, composed of water and iodinated cross-linked polyethylene glycol), injected via an 18-gauge needle, to serve as a minimally-invasive "spacer" (previously demonstrated in the treatment of prostate cancer), and displace or relocate the sub-mandibular gland in order to protect it from irradiation toxicity and be able to deliver a reduced irradiation dose, however the experimental model used comprised of four refrigerated cadaveric specimens and no further *in vivo* or clinical studies evaluated usability, malleability, safety and efficacy, amongst other factors, in clinical organ spacing.

2. **Tissue Engineering and Regenerative Medicine alternative**- clearly, better approaches need to be explored and developed, driving the search elsewhere, into the multi-disciplinary areas of tissue engineering and regenerative medicine, in order to combine with and improve current options or to innovate and translate new alternative solutions, for wound healing. This is especially true, in light of accumulating knowledge and understanding of the underlying mechanisms governing radiation-induced salivary gland damage and dysfunction [47]. Indeed, from inducing DNA damage (via: a. the generation of ROS/ reactive oxygen species or b. the breakage of the DNA double strand), to mutations to cell death (by apoptosis or necrosis, depending on cell type, injury and cellular responses), to the loss of salivary progenitors, to the accruing evidence regarding the regenerative capacity (slow yet existent) of salivary glands following RT-induced injury, more evidently upon the administration of a stimuli (exogenous delivery of stem cells and/or growth factors, for example), altogether re-emphasize the potential of such complex yet innovative approaches in finding a better clinical alternative solution.

   In a recent *clinical* study, Ho *et al.* [102] evaluated the effects of a commercially-available slowly-dissolving adhering disc/tablet formulation (OraCoat XyliMelts) on the oro-dental health, enamel remineralization, bio-film formation, saliva presence, pH and buffering in 5 patients diagnosed with xerostomia (criteria: un-stimulated whole saliva flow rate below 0.2 mL per minute and a stimulated saliva flow rate of less than 0.5 mL in 5 minutes). They also assessed patient self-reported comfort with the mint-flavored, xylitol-releasing tablets. Subjects were instructed to use the disc as often as needed for dry mouth symptoms relief. At the end, a mean of 4 + 1 discs each day and 2 discs each night, were used. Overall, desirable effects of the product on symptomatic alleviation and management of xerostomia were reported. The authors reported effective local palliation, reduced dental sensitivity, improved salivary production and buffering capacity, reduced plaque formation and alleviated xerostomia symptoms, without the need to use any systemic sialagogue medications throughout the 21 days of the study [102]. Yet, this is a pilot study, limited for involving a small of number of participants.

Biomaterials and Cell Therapy- one of the fundamental roles for the maintenance of the body of any living organism is regeneration, which enables the repair and restoration of lost or damaged tissue [47, 103]. Adult stem/stromal and progenitor cells have been identified in many tissues, and are known to have a key role in the regeneration and repair, initiated or activated either by the excessive loss of differentiated cells (pool) or via (niche) environmental cues. In the presence of functional biomaterials such as the previously-described injectable hydrogel spacer [101] and a feasible agent-delivery tablet or disc [102], *would loading, encapsulating or incorporating putative salivary progenitor or stem/stromal cells, for example, a distinct type of stimuli, yield better results?* Supplying salivary gland progenitor and stem/stromal cells, via a proper release-controlled dose-responsive carrier, might be able to re-establish the disrupted salivary stem/progenitor cell pool and niche, restore glandular tissue homeostasis, reverse hypo-salivation, and perhaps control xerostomia, a hypothesis we are currently examining in our laboratory, employing natural and synthetic polymers, liposomes, solid lipid nanoparticles and core-shell nanocapsules, and further supplementing by other pharmaceutical agents.

Modern medicine and biomedical research aim to control and enhance radio-protective as well as regenerative and reparative capabilities through the utilization of cells (cell lineages or primary cells), growing surface control using bio-scaffolds and/or manipulating growth factor/cytokine concentrations [47, 104], strategies designed to stimulate residual cells to regenerate acini and other parenchymal elements (ductal ligation) and infiltrate growth factor doses to boost salivary gland repair post-RT [105].

Growth Factor Therapy- somatomedin C is a hormone, similar to insulin in molecular structure, and actually is better known as IGF-1 or insulin-like growth factor 1 [106]. While a statement as "increased insulin-like growth factor signaling induces cell proliferation, survival and cancer progression" is true, it is traditional and partial, to a great extent. Today we understand that the issue is much more complex. For instance, IGF regulates cellular senescence which is known to halt proliferation of aged and stressed cells and do play a key role against cancer development. Actually, there is accruing evidence that, over time, IGF not only regulates but also induces pre-mature cellular senescence (tumor suppressor protein p53-dependant, in terms of acetylation, stabilization and activation) [107]. Hence, despite the *understandably-alarming, at first and for some, suggestion* to exogenously administer/supply cytokines and growth factors to sites of cancer, the recent years have indeed witnessed a note-worthy increase in the study of growth factors as cytoprotectants including their use as radioprotectors for salivary glands, and to reduce RT-induced symptoms, such as oral mucositis. To date, various growth factors have emerged as potential radioprotectors, including neurotrophic factors [108, 109], epidermal growth factor (EGF), fibroblast growth factor (FGF) [51, 110], keratinocyte growth factor (KGF) [111, 112] and the afore-mentioned insulin-like growth factor-1 or IGF-1 [55, 113, 114]. Meyer *et al.*, [113], for example, investigated and determined the radioprotectant and therapeutic effect of IGF-1, in a murine model. They found that IGF-1 is mediated by the activation and maintenance of a histone deacetylase, specifically the Sirtuin 1 (SirT-1). Pre-treatment with IGF-1 enabled the repair of double-stranded breaks in the DNA of parotid salivary gland cells within the first hours post-irradiation, thereby allowing for optimal DNA repair (*i.e.* IGF-1 promotes DNA repair in irradiated parotid salivary glands via the maintenance and activation of SirT-1) to fulfill the cell cycle checkpoints. However, hours later and as early as 8 h, RT-induced apoptotic cells were detected [113]. Such observations lead to further study the signaling cross-talk between IGF-1 and SirT-1, thereby identifying several activators, stabilizers and inhibitors, including the afore-mentioned inhibition of the p53-mediated apoptosis and the phosphoinositide 3-kinase (PI3K) – protein kinase B (Akt) pathway [107], in-depth study-worthy topics, beyond the scope of this concise review. To date, studies, collectively indicate that cytokines can be radioprotective, anti-apoptotic and suggest/promote that the exogenous and localized (via a release-controlled delivery system, preferably directly injectable) utilization of growth factors do stimulate endogenous stem cell populations/niche and will eventually contribute to the desired and/or pursued clinical solution suitable for preventing RT-induced damage, diminishing salivary hypofunction, as well as restoring salivary gland function in irradiated HNC cases.

Gene Transfer Therapy- the utilization of gene transfer, DNA transmission and cell transduction to produce high levels of transgenic protein in order to correct cellular dysfunction and/or induce a new cellular function, post-RT, is a wide area of investigation and development. Baum *et al.* [115], utilized an adenoviral technique to transfer the Aquaporin-1 (AQP1) gene into the sub-mandibular gland, reporting an increase in salivary flow when compared to control viruses into rat or mini-pig models [115, 116]. Yet, key shortcomings continue to exist for non-viral as well as viral vectors [103], rendering translation for routine clinical use difficult. Likewise, the therapeutic potential of genetic modification and application of small-interfering RNAs or siRNA for the purpose of target gene silencing are intensively investigated, progressing from pre-clinical testing in animal models to ongoing clinical trials for cancer, lung disease and liver damage in human subjects. Thus far, highly limited in salivary gland tissues and accompanied with significant safety concerns [50]. For example, AQP-1 gene transfer into the salivary glands via adeno-viral vectors to treat disorders such as SS, yielded strong immune responses, mainly due to the limited or low efficiency of intra-cellular siRNA delivery [117, 118]. Herein, similar to growth factors, cell therapy and pharmaceutical agent administration, the availability of a reproducible, scalable, safe and effective, release-controlled carrier/vehicle suitable for therapeutic siRNA delivery, directly into the salivary gland, ensuring sufficient residency/retention, is a challenge.

5. Closing remarks

5.1 Wnt/β-catenin pathway: radio-protective role and effect in RT-induced salivary gland damage

In irradiation studies and radioprotection literature, numerous cellular signaling pathways and cell-cycle alteration mechanisms have been explored. Of those, the Wnt/β-catenin signaling pathway seems to receive the utmost attention, recently, towards preventing the damage caused by irradiation [119]. Briefly, this canonical Wingless–Int (Wnt) pathway leads to the accumulation and translocation of co-activator β-catenin, a multi-functional protein involved in cell–cell adhesion, gene transcription and physiologic homeostasis (adullt), into the nucleus, via a series of molecular events initiated through the binding of specific Wnt proteins to the frizzled receptors on the cell surface. The pathway plays a critical role in cell regulating cell migration and determining cell fate, and mutations have been linked to human birth defects, cancer and other disorders and diseases [120–123].

Activating the canonical Wnt/β-catenin signaling pathway is complex. It depends on a family of glyco-proteins involved in cell-to-cell communication. To simplify, the interaction of ß-catenin with the cell adhesion molecule, e-cadherin, is involved in phenotypes: adhesion, mobility and proliferation [121, 122]. In absence of a Wnt ligand, β-catenin is degraded by the "destruction complex". Several proteins are involved within this complex whereby Axin acts as a scaffold protein facilitating the interaction of Glycogen Synthase Kinase 3β (GSK-3β), Adenomatous Polyposis Coli (APC) and Casein Kinase 1α (CK1α), for β-catenin phosphorylation [123, 124]. Then, phosphorylated β-catenin is recognized by the β-transducin-repeat-containing protein (β-TrCP) and goes through the ubiquitin-proteasome degradation pathway. When the Wnt ligand activates Wnt signaling through the plasmatic membrane receptor frizzled with other lipoprotein receptors, the cytoplasmic protein disheveled (Dvl) is recruited and thereby activated. Herein, the activation of Dvl disrupts the "destruction complex" by dissociation of the GSK-3β from the Axin and inhibits the GSK-3β. As a result, β-catenin phosphorylation is also inhibited, allowing stabilization and translocation of β-catenin into the nucleus. Nuclear β-catenin then binds to a transcription factor-T cell factor and a lymphoid-enhancing factor (Tcf/Lef) and finally activates a response, *i.e.* changes in gene expression [120, 125, 126].

The Wnt signaling pathway cross-talks with other signaling pathways, and can be modulated by several activators and inhibitors. For example, the utilization of growth factors, to activate or inhibit, has been extensively studied, further adding to the complexity given the wide range of involved genes [119]. Cross-talk between signaling pathways is possible via the common regulatory protein GSK-3β. For example, when the epidermal growth factor (EGF) is recognized by its native receptor (EGF-R), this complex activates the afore-mentioned phosphoinositide 3-kinase (PI3K) which facilitates the activation of AKT kinase regulator. Herein, the activation of AKT results in the inhibition of GSK-3β by phosphorylation [127–129] and ultimately leads to the translocation of β-catenin into the nucleus. On the other hand, the fibroblast growth factor (FGF) is also able to cross-talk with GSK-3β (common pathway with EGF) and the activation of its native receptor (FGF-R) is followed by PI3K which then results in the inhibition of GSK-3β via AKT activation [125, 130]. Herein, FGF-R activation also involves MapK activation which inhibits GSK-3β through the p90 ribosomal protein s6 kinase (p90rsk) in an AKT-independent manner [131–133]. Therefore, activating the Wnt signaling pathway (**Figure 4**) through the utilization of cytoplasmic regulatory proteins (from other signaling pathways) is potentially able to promote β-catenin stabilization, its translocation to the nucleus and the activation of survival genes [134]. Such understanding and revelations can lead to produce a plausible and innovative alternative strategy for the activation of native repair systems that may allow and promote the survival of the cells during and after RT. Possibly, can be even extended to explore plausibility for prevention.

To the best of knowledge, Hakim *et al.* [135] conducted one of the first/earliest *clinical* studies connecting signaling pathways (Wnt/β-catenin and TGF-β) with salivary gland irradiation damage. They reported an alteration in the expression pattern of Wnt1 in viable irradiated acinar cells of xerostomic patients, suggesting a possible therapeutic effect of the Wnt pathway in controlling RT-induced salivary gland damage and dysfunction [135], in accordance with previous *in vitro* studies [120]. Following this line of research, Hai *et al.* [136] carried out a study analyzing the transient activation of the Wnt/β-catenin signaling pathway to prevent

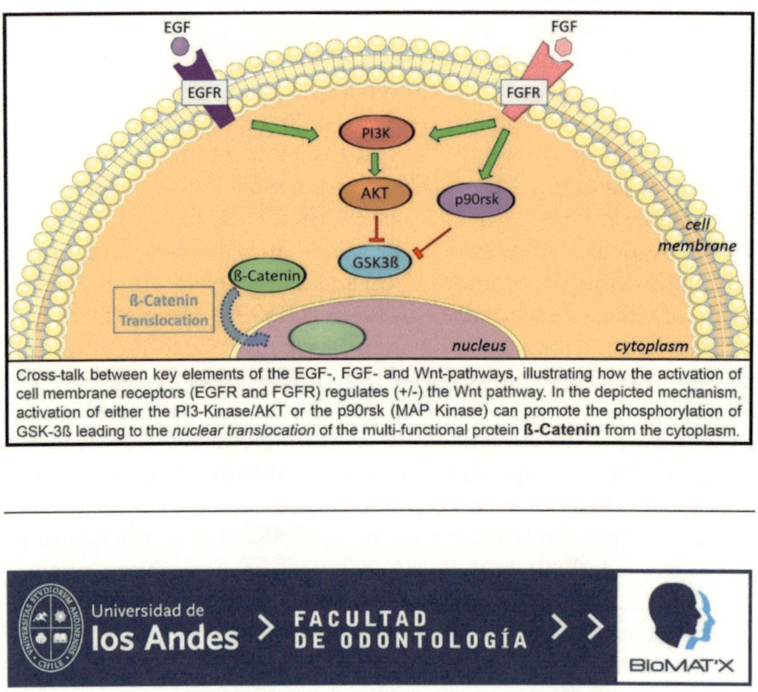

Figure 4.
EGF and FGF pathway(s) interaction with ß-catenin and canonical Wnt signaling pathway.

irradiation damage to the salivary glands. They reported, using a murine model, that activating the Wnt/β-catenin pathway through the transient activation of Wnt1 in the basal epithelium helped to prevent chronic salivary dysfunction generated by local irradiation, specifically via suppressing apoptosis and preserving or rescuing the life of salivary stem/progenitor cells. Salivation in experimental mice when compared to controls (animals receiving only RT) was increased/higher [120, 136]. However, the radioprotective effect of Wnt/β-catenin activation seems, thus far, to only occur within a limited time lapse. Activating the signaling path 3 days before or 3 days after irradiation yielded dissimilar effects on the tissues [136].

Indeed, in another approach, the activation and modulation of cell signaling pathway(s) using a cocktail (more than one) of activators has been suggested, with the Wnt signaling pathway (and its components) as therapeutic target(s). Thula *et al.* [51] evaluated the effect of EGF and bFGF (basic FGF) in salivary gland explants, reporting promising results regarding gland radioprotection [51]. Overall, taking the studied findings into account, it can be proposed that a Wnt/β-catenin signaling pathway activator might be a good candidate to be developed as a potential preventive and therapeutic strategy against the RT-induced salivary gland damage. Herein, as was and is the present scenario with cells, proteins, genes, growth factors and drugs, a suitable delivery vehicle is once more, deemed vital.

Technology Promise in Translational Tissue Engineering and NanoMedicine-the interplay between tissue engineering, regenerative medicine, biomaterials, bio-nanotechnology and nanomedicine continues to be the hallmark of current scientific research World-wide, promising to change every aspect of human life via creating revolutionary materials of biological origin for use in the diagnosis and treatment of devastating human diseases, a multi-disciplinary approach to innovative and translational solutions, suitable for scale-up, safe, efficacious and cost-effective routine clinical use [137–139]. Whether conventional small-molecule agents or emerging protein and/or peptide-based macromolecular biopharmaceutics, therapeutic effect is of vital significance. Controlled or at least predictable delivery is also substantially necessary. An intense effort is invested into engineering such complex bio-systems capable to achieve optimum cell-material interactions, while keeping intact the materials bulk properties. One of the core interests of nanobiotechnology, for example, this decade has been drug/gene/cell bio-functional delivery, driving the design and development of bio-inspired, intelligent or "smart" nano-systems [137, 138, 140]. It can be stated that a competitive and superiorly successful delivery system should offer: therapeutic outcome enhancement, patient compliance improvement and overall cost reduction of therapy. For HNC cases suffering RT-induced salivary gland damage and dysfunction, an attractive delivery system, for clinical ease-of-use, can perhaps entail a directly injectable formulation, sterilizable, capable to efficiently-hold a dose-responsive bio-load, maintain its bio-activity over time, and "predictably" control its pharmaco-kinetic release profile.

Funding and acknowledgments

This work was supported by generous funding and operating grants provided to the BioMAT'X R&D&I Group, part of CIIB (Centro de Investigación e Innovación Biomédica at UAndes), through the Faculty of Dentistry and Fondo de Ayuda a la Investigacion FAI - No. **INV-IN-2015-101** (2015–2019), Department for Research, Development and Innovation, Universidad de los Andes, Santiago de Chile. The authors wish to acknowledge supplementary funding provided under the awarded national grants from CORFO-CTecnológicos para la Innovación **#18COTE-89695** (the bioFLOSS project, 2018–2021) and CONICYT-FONDEF Chile **#ID16I10366** (the maxSALIVA project, 2016/17–2020).

Conflict of interest

The author declares that the research was conducted in the absence of any commercial or financial relationships that could be construed as a potential conflict of interest.

Author details

Ziyad S. Haidar
BioMAT'X R&D&I, Faculties of Dentistry and Medicine, Centro de Investigación e Innovación Biomédica (CiiB), Universidad de los Andes, Santiago de Chile, Chile

*Address all correspondence to: zhaidar@uandes.cl

References

[1] Cancer, Fact Sheet, World Health Organization, available from https://www.who.int/news-room/fact-sheets/detail/cancer. Accessed Oct 23, 2020.

[2] International Agency for Research on Cancer (IARC). (2019). GLOBOCAN 2018, Cancer Incidence and Mortality Worldwide. Lyon: International Agency for Research on Cancer. Avaliable from http://gco.iarc.fr/today/fact-sheets-cancers. Accessed Aug 25, 2020.

[3] Yan, K., Agrawal, N., Gooi, Z. Head and Neck Masses. Med Clin North Am **2018**, *102*,1013-1025. doi: 10.1016/j.mcna.2018.06.012.

[4] Cognetti, D. M., Weber, R. S., Lai, S. Y. Head and neck cancer: an evolving treatment paradigm. Cancer **2008**, *113*, 1911-1932, doi:10.1002/cncr.23654.

[5] Jaffray, D. A., Gospodarowicz, M. K. *Radiation Therapy for* Cancer, 2015, ISBN 9781464803499.

[6] Shetty, A. V, Wong, D. J. Systemic Treatment for Squamous Cell Carcinoma of the Head and Neck. Otolaryngol. Clin. North Am. **2017**, *50*, 775-782, doi:10.1016/j.otc.2017.03.013.

[7] Barazzuol, L., Coppes, R. P., van Luijk, P. Prevention and treatment of radiotherapy-induced side effects. Molecular oncology. **2020**, 14, 1538-1554. https://doi.org/10.1002/1878-0261.12750

[8] Gil, Z., Fliss, D. M. Contemporary management of head and neck cancers. Isr. Med. Assoc. J. **2009**, *11*, 296-300.

[9] Deloch, L., Derer, A., Hartmann, J., Frey, B., Fietkau, R., Gaipl, U. S. Modern Radiotherapy Concepts and the Impact of Radiation on Immune Activation. Front. Oncol. **2016**, *6*, 141, doi:10.3389/fonc.2016.00141.

[10] Baskar, R., Dai, J., Wenlong, N., Yeo, R., Yeoh, K.W. Biological response of cancer cells to radiation treatment. Front Mol Biosci **2014**,*1*,24. doi:10.3389/fmolb.2014.00024.

[11] Manukian, G., Bar-Ad, V., Lu, B., Argiris, A., Johnson, J.M. Combining Radiation and Immune Checkpoint Blockade in the Treatment of Head and Neck Squamous Cell Carcinoma. Front Oncol **2019**. doi:10.3389/fonc.2019.00122.

[12] Jensen, SB., Vissink, A., Limesand, K.H., Reyland, M.E. Salivary Gland Hypofunction and Xerostomia in Head and Neck Radiation Patients. J Natl Cancer Inst Monogr **2019**, 53. doi:10.1093/jncimonographs/lgz016.

[13] Wu, V. W. C., Leung, K. Y. A Review on the Assessment of Radiation Induced Salivary Gland Damage After Radiotherapy. Front Oncol **2019**. doi:10.3389/fonc.2019.01090.

[14] Miranda-Rius, J., Brunet-Llobet, L., Lahor-Soler, E., Farré, M. Salivary Secretory Disorders, Inducing Drugs, and Clinical Management. Int. J. Med. Sci. **2015**, *12*, 811-824, doi:10.7150/ijms.12912.

[15] Ghannam, M. G., Singh, P. Anatomy, Head and Neck, Salivary Glands. *StatPearls* **2019** Available from https://www.ncbi.nlm.nih.gov/books/NBK538325/. Accessed Jan 29, 2020.

[16] Punj, A. Secretions of Human Salivary Gland. Secretions of Human Salivary Gland, Salivary Glands - New Approaches in Diagnostics and Treatment, Işıl Adadan Güvenç, IntechOpen. **2018**. doi: 10.5772/intechopen.75538. Available from: https://www.intechopen.com/books/salivary-glands-new-approaches-in-diagnostics-and-treatment/secretions-of-human-salivary-gland.

[17] Benn, A. M., Thomson, W. M. Saliva: an overview. N. Z. Dent. J. **2014**, *110*, 92-96.

[18] Tiwari, M. Science Behind Human Saliva. J Nat Sci Biol Med **2011**, 2, 53-58. doi: 10.4103/0976-9668.82322.

[19] Proctor, G. B. The physiology of salivary secretion. Periodontol. *2000* **2016**, *70*, 11-25, doi:10.1111/prd.12116.

[20] Qin, R., Steel, A., Fazel, N. Oral mucosa biology and salivary biomarkers. Clin. Dermatol. **2017**, *35*, 477-483, doi:10.1016/j.clindermatol.2017.06.005.

[21] Farnaud, S. J. C., Kosti, O., Getting, S. J., Renshaw, D. Saliva: physiology and diagnostic potential in health and disease. ScientificWorldJournal. **2010**, *10*, 434-456, doi:10.1100/tsw.2010.38.

[22] Fábián, T. K., Beck, A., Fejérdy, P., Hermann, P., Fábián, G. Molecular mechanisms of taste recognition: considerations about the role of saliva. Int. J. Mol. Sci. **2015**, *16*, 5945-5974, doi:10.3390/ijms16035945.

[23] von Bültzingslöwen, I., Sollecito, T. P., Fox, P. C., Daniels, T., Jonsson, R., Lockhart, P. B., Wray, D., Brennan, M. T., Carrozzo, M., Gandera, B., Fujibayashi, T., Navazesh, M., Rhodus, N. L., Schiødt, M. Salivary dysfunction associated with systemic diseases: systematic review and clinical management recommendations. *Oral Surg. Oral Med. Oral Pathol. Oral Radiol. Endod.* **2007**, *103 Suppl*, S57.e1-15, doi:10.1016/j.tripleo.2006.11.010.

[24] Dashtipour, K., Bhidayasiri, R., Chen, J. J., Jabbari, B., Lew, M., Torres-Russotto, D. RimabotulinumtoxinB in sialorrhea: systematic review of clinical trials. J. Clin. Mov. Disord. **2017**, *4*, 9, doi:10.1186/s40734-017-0055-1.

[25] Jost, W.H., Friedman, A., Michel, O., Oehlwein, C., Slawek, J., Bogucki, A., Ochudlo, S., Banach, M., Pagan, F., Flatau-Baqué, B., Dorsch, U., Csikós, J., Blitzer, A. Long-term incobotulinumtoxinA treatment for chronic sialorrhea: Efficacy and safety over 64 weeks. Parkinsonism Relat Disord **2020**, *70*, 23-30. doi: 10.1016/j.parkreldis.2019.11.024.

[26] Frydrych, A. M. Dry mouth: Xerostomia and salivary gland hypofunction. Aust. Fam. Physician **2016**, *45*, 488-492.

[27] Azuma, N., Katada, Y., Kitano, S., Sekiguchi, M., Kitano, M., Nishioka, A., Hashimoto, N., Matsui, K., Iwasaki, T., Sano, H. Correlation between salivary epidermal growth factor levels and refractory intraoral manifestations in patients with Sjögren's syndrome. Mod. Rheumatol. **2014**, *24*, 626-632, doi:10.3109/14397595.2013.850766.

[28] Millsop, J. W., Wang, E. A., Fazel, N. Etiology, evaluation, and management of xerostomia. Clin. Dermatol. **2017**, *35*, 468-476, doi:10.1016/j.clindermatol.2017.06.010.

[29] Tan, E. C. K., Lexomboon, D., Sandborgh-Englund, G., Haasum, Y., Johnell, K. Medications That Cause Dry Mouth As an Adverse Effect in Older People: A Systematic Review and Metaanalysis. J. Am. Geriatr. Soc. **2018**, *66*, 76-84, doi:10.1111/jgs.15151.

[30] Vissink, A., Mitchell, J. B., Baum, B. J., Limesand, K. H., Jensen, S. B., Fox, P. C., Elting, L. S., Langendijk, J. A., Coppes, R. P., Reyland, M. E. Clinical management of salivary gland hypofunction and xerostomia in head-and-neck cancer patients: successes and barriers. Int. J. Radiat. Oncol. Biol. Phys. **2010**, *78*, 983-991, doi:10.1016/j.ijrobp.2010.06.052.

[31] Schaue, D., Kachikwu, E. L., McBride, W. H. Cytokines in radiobiological responses: a review.

Radiat. Res. **2012**, *178*, 505-523, doi:10.1667/RR3031.1.

[32] Williams, J. P., McBride, W. H. After the bomb drops: a new look at radiation-induced multiple organ dysfunction syndrome (MODS). Int. J. Radiat. Biol. **2011**, *87*, 851-868, doi:10.3109/09553002.2011.560996.

[33] Mohammadi, N., Seyyednejhad, F., Oskoee, P.A., Oskoee, S.S., Mofidi, N. Evaluation of Radiation-induced Xerostomia in Patients with Nasopharyngeal Carcinomas. J Dent Res Dent Clin Dent Prospects **2007**, 1, 65-70. doi: 10.5681/joddd.2007.011

[34] Strojan, P., Hutcheson, K. A., Eisbruch, A., Beitler, J. J., Langendijk, J. A., Lee, A. W. M., Corry, J., Mendenhall, W. M., Smee, R., Rinaldo, A., Ferlito, A. Treatment of late sequelae after radiotherapy for head and neck cancer. Cancer Treat. Rev. **2017**, *59*, 79-92, doi:10.1016/j.ctrv.2017.07.003.

[35] Franzén, L., Funegård, U., Ericson, T., Henriksson, R. Parotid gland function during and following radiotherapy of malignancies in the head and neck. A consecutive study of salivary flow and patient discomfort. *Eur. J. Cancer* **1992**, *28*, 457-462.

[36] Siddiqui, F., Movsas, B. Management of Radiation Toxicity in Head and Neck Cancers. Semin. Radiat. Oncol. **2017**, *27*, 340-349, doi:10.1016/j.semradonc.2017.04.008.

[37] Berk, L. B., Shivnani, A. T., Small, W. Jr. Pathophysiology and management of radiation-induced xerostomia. J. Support. Oncol. **2005**, *3*, 191-200.

[38] Hammerlid, E., Silander, E., Hörnestam, L., Sullivan, M. Health-related quality of life three years after diagnosis of head and neck cancer--a longitudinal study. Head Neck **2001**, *23*, 113-125.

[39] Hall, S. C., Hassis, M. E., Williams, K. E., Albertolle, M. E., Prakobphol, A., Dykstra, A. B., Laurance, M., Ona, K., Niles, R. K., Prasad, N., Gormley, M., Shiboski, C., Criswell, L. A., Witkowska, H. E., Fisher, S. J. Alterations in the Salivary Proteome and N-Glycome of Sjögren's Syndrome Patients. J. Proteome Res. **2017**, *16*, 1693-1705, doi:10.1021/acs.jproteome.6b01051.

[40] Jehmlich, N., Stegmaier, P., Golatowski, C., Salazar, M. G., Rischke, C., Henke, M., Völker, U. Differences in the whole saliva baseline proteome profile associated with development of oral mucositis in head and neck cancer patients undergoing radiotherapy. J. Proteomics **2015**, *125*, 98-103, doi:10.1016/j.jprot.2015.04.030.

[41] Thomson, W. M. Dry mouth and older people. *Aust. Dent. J.* **2015**, *60 Suppl 1*, 54-63, doi:10.1111/adj.12284.

[42] Cereda, E., Cappello, S., Colombo, S., Klersy, C., Imarisio, I., Turri, A., Caraccia, M., Borioli, V., Monaco, T., Benazzo, M., Pedrazzoli, P., Corbella, F., Caccialanza, R. Nutritional counseling with or without systematic use of oral nutritional supplements in head and neck cancer patients undergoing radiotherapy. Radiother. Oncol. **2018**, *126*, 81-88, doi:10.1016/j.radonc.2017.10.015.

[43] Li, Y., Taylor, J. M. G., Ten Haken, R. K., Eisbruch, A. The impact of dose on parotid salivary recovery in head and neck cancer patients treated with radiation therapy. Int. J. Radiat. Oncol. Biol. Phys. **2007**, *67*, 660-669, doi:10.1016/j.ijrobp.2006.09.021.

[44] Jiang, N., Zhao, Y., Jansson, H., Chen, X., Mårtensson, J. Experiences of xerostomia after radiotherapy in patients with head and neck cancer: A qualitative study. J. Clin. Nurs. **2018**, *27*, e100–e108, doi:10.1111/jocn.13879.

[45] Wang, W., Xiong, W., Wan, J., Sun, X., Xu, H., Yang, X. The decrease of PAMAM dendrimer-induced cytotoxicity by PEGylation via attenuation of oxidative stress. Nanotechnology **2009**, *20*, 105103, doi:10.1088/0957-4484/20/10/105103.

[46] Nadig, S. D., Ashwathappa, D. T., Manjunath, M., Krishna, S., Annaji, A. G., Shivaprakash, P. K. A relationship between salivary flow rates and Candida counts in patients with xerostomia. J. Oral Maxillofac. Pathol. **2017**, *21*, 316, doi:10.4103/jomfp.JOMFP_231_16.

[47] Kagami, H., Wang, S., Hai, B. Restoring the function of salivary glands. Oral Dis. **2008**, *14*, 15-24, doi:10.1111/j.1601-0825.2006.01339.x.

[48] Villa, A., Abati, S. Risk factors and symptoms associated with xerostomia: a cross-sectional study. Aust. Dent. J. **2011**, *56*, 290-295, doi:10.1111/j.1834-7819.2011.01347.x.

[49] Bressan, V., Bagnasco, A., Aleo, G., Catania, G., Zanini, M. P., Timmins, F., Sasso, L. The life experience of nutrition impact symptoms during treatment for head and neck cancer patients: a systematic review and meta-synthesis. Support. Care Cancer **2017**, *25*, 1699-1712, doi:10.1007/s00520-017-3618-7.

[50] Grundmann, O., Mitchell, G. C., Limesand, K. H. Sensitivity of salivary glands to radiation: from animal models to therapies. J. Dent. Res. **2009**, *88*, 894-903, doi:10.1177/0022034509343143.

[51] Thula, T. T., Schultz, G., Tran-Son-Tay, R., Batich, C. Effects of EGF and bFGF on irradiated parotid glands. Ann. Biomed. Eng. **2005**, *33*, 685-695.

[52] Arany, S., Xu, Q., Hernady, E., Benoit, D. S. W., Dewhurst, S., Ovitt, C. E. Pro-apoptotic gene knockdown mediated by nanocomplexed siRNA reduces radiation damage in primary salivary gland cultures. J. Cell. Biochem. **2012**, *113*, 1955-1965, doi:10.1002/jcb.24064.

[53] Yoon, YJ., Shin, HS., Lim, JY. A hepatocyte growth factor/MET-induced antiapoptotic pathway protects against radiation-induced salivary gland dysfunction. Radiother Oncol. **2019**, 138, 9-16. doi: 10.1016/j.radonc.2019.05.012.

[54] Tai, G., Zhang, H., Du, J., Chen, G., Huang, J., Yu, J., Cai, J., Liu, F. TIGAR overexpression diminishes radiosensitivity of parotid gland fibroblast cells and inhibits IR-induced cell autophagy. Int J Clin Exp Pathol. **2015**, 8, 4823-4829.

[55] Choi, J.S., Shin, H.S., An, H.Y., Kim, Y.M., Lim, J.Y. Radioprotective effects of Keratinocyte Growth Factor-1 against irradiation-induced salivary gland hypofunction. Oncotarget **2017**, *8*, 13496-13508, doi:10.18632/oncotarget.14583.

[56] Wie, S. M., Wellberg, E., Karam, S. D., Reyland, M. E. Tyrosine Kinase Inhibitors Protect the Salivary Gland from Radiation Damage by Inhibiting Activation of Protein Kinase C-δ. Mol. Cancer Ther. **2017**, *16*, 1989-1998, doi:10.1158/1535-7163.MCT-17-0267.

[57] Choi, J.S., An, H.Y., Shin, H.S., Kim, Y.M., Lim, J.Y. Enhanced tissue remodelling efficacy of adipose-derived mesenchymal stem cells using injectable matrices in radiation-damaged salivary gland model. J. Tissue Eng. Regen. Med. **2018**, *12*, e695–e706, doi:10.1002/term.2352.

[58] Zeidan, Y. H., Xiao, N., Cao, H., Kong, C., Le, Q.T., Sirjani, D. Botulinum Toxin Confers Radioprotection in Murine Salivary Glands. Int. J. Radiat. Oncol. Biol. Phys. **2016**, *94*, 1190-1197, doi:10.1016/j.ijrobp.2015.12.371.

[59] An, H.Y., Shin, H.S., Choi, J.S., Kim, H. J., Lim, J.Y., Kim, Y.M. Adipose

Mesenchymal Stem Cell Secretome Modulated in Hypoxia for Remodeling of Radiation-Induced Salivary Gland Damage. PLoS One **2015**, *10*, e0141862, doi:10.1371/journal.pone.0141862.

[60] Xu, L., Yang, X., Cai, J., Ma, J., Cheng, H., Zhao, K., Yang, L., Cao, Y., Qin, Q., Zhang, C., Zhang, Q., Sun, X. Resveratrol attenuates radiation-induced salivary gland dysfunction in mice. Laryngoscope **2013**, *123*, E23–E29, doi:10.1002/lary.24276.

[61] Okumura, H., Nasu, M., Yosue, T. Effects of amifostine administration prior to irradiation to the submandibular gland in mice: autoradiographic study using 3H-leucine. Okajimas Folia Anat. Jpn. **2009**, *85*, 151-160.

[62] Cotrim, A. P., Sowers, A., Mitchell, J. B., Baum, B. J. Prevention of irradiation-induced salivary hypofunction by microvessel protection in mouse salivary glands. Mol. Ther. **2007**, *15*, 2101-2106, doi:10.1038/sj.mt.6300296.

[63] Cotrim, A. P., Hyodo, F., Matsumoto, K., Sowers, A. L., Cook, J. A., Baum, B. J., Krishna, M. C., Mitchell, J. B. Differential radiation protection of salivary glands versus tumor by Tempol with accompanying tissue assessment of Tempol by magnetic resonance imaging. Clin. Cancer Res. **2007**, *13*, 4928-4933, doi:10.1158/1078-0432.CCR-07-0662.

[64] Cotrim, A. P., Sowers, A. L., Lodde, B. M., Vitolo, J. M., Kingman, A., Russo, A., Mitchell, J. B., Baum, B. J. Kinetics of tempol for prevention of xerostomia following head and neck irradiation in a mouse model. Clin. Cancer Res. **2005**, *11*, 7564-7568, doi:10.1158/1078-0432.CCR-05-0958.

[65] Aonuma, M., Nasu, M., Iwata, H., Yosue, T. Radioprotection of the murine submandibular gland by isoproterenol: autoradiography study with 3H-leucine. Odontology **2004**, *92*, 14-21, doi:10.1007/s10266-004-0032-7.

[66] Vitolo, J. M., Cotrim, A. P., Sowers, A. L., Russo, A., Wellner, R. B., Pillemer, S. R., Mitchell, J. B., Baum, B. J. The stable nitroxide tempol facilitates salivary gland protection during head and neck irradiation in a mouse model. Clin. Cancer Res. **2004**, *10*, 1807-1812.

[67] Rasey, J. S., Krohn, K. A., Menard, T. W., Spence, A. M. Comparative biodistribution and radioprotection studies with three radioprotective drugs in mouse tumors. Int. J. Radiat. Oncol. Biol. Phys. **1986**, *12*, 1487-1490.

[68] Rasey, J. S., Nelson, N. J., Mahler, P., Anderson, K., Krohn, K. A., Menard, T. Radioprotection of normal tissues against gamma rays and cyclotron neutrons with WR-2721: LD50 studies and 35S-WR-2721 biodistribution. Radiat. Res. **1984**, *97*, 598-607.

[69] Varghese J.J., Schmale I.L., MickelsenD.,HansenM.E.,NewlandsS.D., Benoit D.S.W., Korshunov V.A., Ovitt C.E. Localized Delivery of Amifostine Enhances Salivary Gland Radioprotection. J Dent Res. **2018,** doi: 10.1177/0022034518767408.

[70] Shin H.S., Lee S., Kim Y.M., Lim J.Y. Hypoxia-Activated Adipose Mesenchymal Stem Cells Prevents Irradiation-Induced Salivary Hypofunction by Enhanced Paracrine Effect Through Fibroblast Growth Factor 10. Stem Cells. **2018**, doi: 10.1002/stem.2818.

[71] Toshkova, IA., Gleibermana, SA., Metta, VL., Hutsonb, AS., Singhc, AK., Gudkovde, AV., Burdelyad, LG. Mitigation of Radiation-Induced Epithelial Damage by the TLR5 Agonist Entolimod in a Mouse Model of Fractionated Head and Neck Irradiation. Radiat. Res. **2017**, 187, 570-580.

[72] Xu, L., Yang, X., Chen, J., Ge, X., Qin, Q., Zhu, H., Zhang, C., Sun, X.

Simvastatin attenuates radiation-induced salivary gland dysfunction in mice. Drug Des Devel Ther. **2016**, 10, 2271-2278.

[73] Crescenti, E. J., Medina, V. A., Croci, M., Sambuco, L. A., Prestifilippo, J. P., Elverdin, J. C., Bergoc, R. M., Rivera, E. S. Radioprotection of sensitive rat tissues by oligoelements Se, Zn, Mn plus Lachesis muta venom. J. Radiat. Res. **2011**, *52*, 557-567.

[74] Coppes, R. P., Vissink, A., Zeilstra, L. J., Konings, A. W. Muscarinic receptor stimulation increases tolerance of rat salivary gland function to radiation damage. Int. J. Radiat. Biol. **1997**, *72*, 615-625.

[75] Coppes, R. P., Zeilstra, L. J., Vissink, A., Konings, A. W. Sialogogue-related radioprotection of salivary gland function: the degranulation concept revisited. Radiat. Res. **1997**, *148*, 240-247.

[76] Menard, T. W., Izutsu, K. T., Ensign, W. Y., Keller, P. J., Morton, T. H., Truelove, E. L. Radioprotection by WR-2721 of gamma-irradiated rat parotid gland: effect on gland weight and secretion at 8-10 days post irradiation. Int. J. Radiat. Oncol. Biol. Phys. **1984**, *10*, 1555-1559.

[77] Sodicoff, M., Conger, A. D. Radioprotection of the rat parotid gland by cAMP. Radiat. Res. **1983**, *96*, 90-94.

[78] Sodicoff, M., Conger, A. D. Radioprotection of the rat parotid gland by WR-2721 and isoproterenol and its modification by propranolol. Radiat. Res. **1983**, *94*, 97-104.

[79] Pratt, N. E., Sodicoff, M., Liss, J., Davis, M., Sinesi, M. Radioprotection of the rat parotid gland by WR-2721: morphology at 60 days post-irradiation. Int. J. Radiat. Oncol. Biol. Phys. **1980**, *6*, 431-435.

[80] Sodicoff, M., Conger, A. D., Pratt, N. E., Trepper, P. Radioprotection by WR-2721 against long-term chronic damage to the rat parotid gland. Radiat. Res. **1978**, *76*, 172-179.

[81] Abedi, SM., Yarmand, F., Motallebnejad, M., Seyedmajidi, M., Moslemie, D., Bijanif, A., Hosseinimehrg, SJ. Radioprotective Effect of Thymol Against Salivary Glands Dysfunction Induced by Ionizing Radiation in Rats. Iran J Pharm Res. 2016, 15, 861-866.

[82] Palaniyandi, S., Odaka, Y., Green, W., Abreo, F., Caldito, G., De Benedetti, A., Sunavala-Dossabhoy, G. Adenoviral delivery of Tousled kinase for the protection of salivary glands against ionizing radiation damage. Gene Ther. **2011**, 18, 275-282.

[83] Shanmugam, PST., Dayton, RD., Palaniyandi, S., Abreo, F., Caldito, G., Klein, RL., Sunavala-Dossabhoy. Recombinant AAV9-TLK1B Administration Ameliorates Fractionated Radiation-Induced Xerostomia. Hum Gene Ther. 2013, 24, 604-612.

[84] Hakim, S.G., Benedek, G. A., Su, Y.X., Jacobsen, H.C., Klinger, M., Dendorfer, A., Hemmelmann, C., Meller, B., Nadrowitz, R., Rades, D., Sieg, P. Radioprotective effect of lidocaine on function and ultrastructure of salivary glands receiving fractionated radiation. Int. J. Radiat. Oncol. Biol. Phys. **2012**, *82*, e623–e630, doi:10.1016/j.ijrobp.2011.09.017.

[85] Hakim, S. G., Kosmehl, H., Lauer, I., Nadrowitz, R., Wedel, T., Sieg, P. A comparative study on the protection profile of lidocaine, amifostine, and pilocarpin on the parotid gland during radiotherapy. Cancer Res **2005**, 65, 10486-10493, doi:10.1158/0008-5472.CAN-05-0023.

[86] Lotz, S., Caselitz, J., Tschakert, H., Rehpenning, W., Seifert, G. Radioprotection of minipig salivary glands by orciprenaline-carbachol. An ultrastructural and semiquantitative light microscopic study. Virchows Arch. A. Pathol. Anat. Histopathol. **1990**, *417*, 119-128.

[87] Guo, L., Gao, R., Xu, J., Jin, L., Cotrim, AP., Yan, X., Zheng, C., Goldsmith, CM., Shan, Z., Hai, B., Zhou, J., Zhang, C., Baum, BJ., Wang, S. AdLTR2EF1α-FGF2-mediated prevention of fractionated irradiation-induced salivary hypofunction in swine. Gene Ther. **2014**, 21, 866-873.

[88] McDonald, S., Meyerowitz, C., Smudzin, T., Rubin, P. Preliminary results of a pilot study using WR-2721 before fractionated irradiation of the head and neck to reduce salivary gland dysfunction. Int. J. Radiat. Oncol. Biol. Phys. **1994**, *29*, 747-754.

[89] Baum, R. P., Langbein, T., Singh, A., Shahinfar, M., Schuchardt, C., Volk, G. F., Kulkarni, H. Injection of Botulinum Toxin for Preventing Salivary Gland Toxicity after PSMA Radioligand Therapy: an Empirical Proof of a Promising Concept. Nucl. Med. Mol. Imaging **2018**, *52*, 80-81, doi:10.1007/s13139-017-0508-3.

[90] Vacha, P., Fehlauer, F., Mahlmann, B., Marx, M., Hinke, A., Sommer, K., Richter, E., Feyerabend, T. Randomized phase III trial of postoperative radiochemotherapy +/− amifostine in head and neck cancer. Is there evidence for radioprotection? Strahlenther. Onko. **2003**, *179*, 385-389, doi:10.1007/s00066-003-1016-1.

[91] Scrimger, R.A., Seikaly, H., Vos, L.J., Harris, J., O'Connell, D., Ghosh, S., Debenham, B., Jha, N. Combination of submandibular salivary gland transfer and intensity-modulated radiotherapy to reduce dryness of mouth (xerostomia) in patients with head and neck cancer. Head Neck **2018**, 40:2353-2361. doi: 10.1002/hed.25339.

[92] Teng, F., Fan, W., Luo, Y., Ju, Z., Gong, H., Ge, R., Tong, F., Zhang, X., Ma, L. Reducing Xerostomia by Comprehensive Protection of Salivary Glands in Intensity-Modulated Radiation Therapy with Helical Tomotherapy Technique for Head-and-Neck Cancer Patients: A Prospective Observational Study. *Biomed Res Int* **2019**, 14, 2019:2401743. doi: 10.1155/2019/2401743.

[93] de Castro, G. Jr, Guindalini, R. S. Supportive care in head and neck oncology. Curr. Opin. Oncol. **2010**, *22*, 221-225, doi:10.1097/CCO.0b013e32833818ff.

[94] Gu, J., Zhu, S., Li, X., Wu, H., Li, Y., Hua, F. Effect of amifostine in head and neck cancer patients treated with radiotherapy: a systematic review and meta-analysis based on randomized controlled trials. PLoS One **2014**, *9*, e95968, doi:10.1371/journal.pone.0095968.

[95] Riley, P., Glenny, A.M., Hua, F., Worthington, H.V. Pharmacological interventions for preventing dry mouth and salivary gland dysfunction following radiotherapy. Cochrane database Syst. Rev. **2017**, *7*, CD012744, doi:10.1002/14651858.CD012744.

[96] The American Society of Clinical Oncology. Clinical Practice Guideline Update: Use of Chemotherapy and Radiation Therapy Protectants. *J Oncol Pract* **2008**, *4*, 277-279. Written by: Hensley, M.L., Hagerty, K.L., Kewalramani, T., Green, D.M., Meropol, N. J., Wasserman, T.H., Cohen, G.I., Emami, B., Gradishar, W.J., Mitchell, R.B., Thigpen, J.T., Trotti, A., von Hoff, D., Schuchter, L. M. doi: 10.1200/JOP.0868502

[97] Vissink, A., Jansma, J., Spijkervet, F. K., Burlage, F. R., Coppes, R. P. Oral sequelae of head and neck radiotherapy. Crit. Rev. Oral Biol. Med. **2003**, *14*, 199-212.

[98] Braam, P. M., Terhaard, C. H., Roesink, J. M., Raaijmakers, C. P. Intensity-modulated radiotherapy significantly reduces xerostomia compared with conventional radiotherapy. Int. J. Radiat. Oncol. Biol. Phys. **2006**, *66*, 975-980, doi:10.1016/j.ijrobp.2006.06.045.

[99] Teng, F., Fan, W., Luo, Y., Ju, Z., Gong, H., Ge, R., Tong, F., Zhang, X., Ma, L. Reducing Xerostomia by Comprehensive Protection of Salivary Glands in Intensity-Modulated Radiation Therapy with Helical Tomotherapy Technique for Head-and-Neck Cancer Patients: A Prospective Observational Study. Biomed Res Int **2019**. doi: https://doi.org/10.1155/2019/2401743.

[100] Marzouki, H. Z., Elkhalidy, Y., Jha, N., Scrimger, R., Debenham, B. J., Harris, J. R., O'Connell, D. A., Seikaly, H. Modification of the submandibular gland transfer procedure. Laryngoscope **2016**, *126*, 2492-2496, doi:10.1002/lary.26029.

[101] Rao, A. D., Coquia, S., De Jong, R., Gourin, C., Page, B., Latronico, D., Dah, S., Su, L., Clarke, S., Schultz, J., Rosati, L. M., Fakhry, C., Wong, J., DeWeese, T. L., Quon, H., Ding, K., Kiess, A. Effects of biodegradable hydrogel spacer injection on contralateral submandibular gland sparing in radiotherapy for head and neck cancers. Radiother. Oncol. **2018**, *126*, 96-99, doi:10.1016/j.radonc.2017.09.017.

[102] Ho, J., Firmalino, M. V., Anbarani, A. G., Takesh, T., Epstein, J., Wilder-Smith, P. Effects of A Novel Disc Formulation on Dry Mouth Symptoms and Enamel Remineralization in Patients With Hyposalivation: An *In Vivo* Study. *Dent. (Sunnyvale, Calif.)* **2017**, *7*, doi:10.4172/2161-1122.1000411.

[103] Ogawa, M., Oshima, M., Imamura, A., Sekine, Y., Ishida, K., Yamashita, K., Nakajima, K., Hirayama, M., Tachikawa, T., Tsuji, T. Functional salivary gland regeneration by transplantation of a bioengineered organ germ. Nat. Commun. **2013**, *4*, 2498, doi:10.1038/ncomms3498.

[104] Zhang, N.N., Huang, G.L., Han, Q.B., Hu, X., Yi, J., Yao, L., He, Y. Functional regeneration of irradiated salivary glands with human amniotic epithelial cells transplantation. Int. J. Clin. Exp. Pathol. **2013**, *6*, 2039-2047.

[105] Okazaki, Y., Kagami, H., Hattori, T., Hishida, S., Shigetomi, T., Ueda, M. Acceleration of rat salivary gland tissue repair by basic fibroblast growth factor. Arch. Oral Biol. **2000**, *45*, 911-919.

[106] Michalopoulou, F., Petraki, C., Philippou, A., Analitis, A., Msaouel, P., Koutsilieris, M. Expression of IGF-IEc Isoform in Renal Cell Carcinoma Tissues. Anticancer Res **2020**, 40, :6213-6219. doi: 10.21873/anticanres.14641.

[107] Tran, D., Bergholz, J., Zhang, H., He, H., Wang, Y., Zhang, Y., Li, Q., Kirkland, J. L., Xiao, Z. X. Insulin-like growth factor-1 regulates the SIRT1-p53 pathway in cellular senescence. Aging cell **2014**, 13, 669-678. https://doi.org/10.1111/acel.12219.

[108] Xiao, N., Lin, Y., Cao, H., Sirjani, D., Giaccia, A. J., Koong, A. C., Kong, C. S., Diehn, M., Le, Q.T. Neurotrophic factor GDNF promotes survival of salivary stem cells. J. Clin. Invest. **2014**, *124*, 3364-3377, doi:10.1172/JCI74096.

[109] Swick, A., Kimple, R. J. Wetting the whistle: neurotropic factor improves salivary function. J. Clin. Invest. **2014**, *124*, 3282-3284, doi:10.1172/JCI77194.

[110] Kojima, T., Kanemaru, S., Hirano, S., Tateya, I., Suehiro, A., Kitani, Y., Kishimoto, Y., Ohno, S., Nakamura, T., Ito, J. The protective efficacy of basic fibroblast growth factor in radiation-induced salivary gland dysfunction in mice. Laryngoscope **2011**, *121*, 1870-1875, doi:10.1002/lary.21873.

[111] Borges, L., Rex, K. L., Chen, J. N., Wei, P., Kaufman, S., Scully, S., Pretorius, J. K., Farrell, C. L. A protective role for keratinocyte growth factor in a murine model of chemotherapy and radiotherapy-induced mucositis. Int. J. Radiat. Oncol. Biol. Phys. **2006**, *66*, 254-262, doi:10.1016/j.ijrobp.2006.05.025.

[112] Lombaert, I. M., Brunsting, J. F., Wierenga, P. K., Kampinga, H. H., de Haan, G., Coppes, R. P. Keratinocyte growth factor prevents radiation damage to salivary glands by expansion of the stem/progenitor pool. Stem Cells **2008**, *26*, 2595-2601, doi:10.1634/stemcells.2007-1034.

[113] Meyer, S., Chibly, A. M., Burd, R., Limesand, K. H. Insulin-Like Growth Factor-1-Mediated DNA Repair in Irradiated Salivary Glands Is Sirtuin-1 Dependent. J. Dent. Res. **2017**, *96*, 225-232, doi:10.1177/0022034516677529.

[114] Grundmann, O., Fillinger, J. L., Victory, K. R., Burd, R., Limesand, K. H. Restoration of radiation therapy-induced salivary gland dysfunction in mice by post therapy IGF-1 administration. BMC Cancer **2010**, *10*, 417, doi:10.1186/1471-2407-10-417.

[115] Baum, B. J., Zheng, C., Cotrim, A. P., Goldsmith, C. M., Atkinson, J. C., Brahim, J. S., Chiorini, J. A., Voutetakis, A., Leakan, R. A., Van Waes, C., Mitchell, J. B., Delporte, C., Wang, S., Kaminsky, S. M., Illei, G. G. Transfer of the AQP1 cDNA for the correction of radiation-induced salivary hypofunction. Biochim. Biophys. Acta **2006**, *1758*, 1071-1077, doi:10.1016/j.bbamem.2005.11.006.

[116] Redman, R. S. On approaches to the functional restoration of salivary glands damaged by radiation therapy for head and neck cancer, with a review of related aspects of salivary gland morphology and development. Biotech. Histochem. **2008**, *83*, 103-130, doi:10.1080/10520290802374683.

[117] Cotrim, A. P., Sowers, A., Mitchell, J. B., Baum, B. J. Prevention of irradiation-induced salivary hypofunction by microvessel protection in mouse salivary glands. Mol. Ther. **2007**, *15*, 2101-2106, doi:10.1038/sj.mt.6300296.

[118] Guo, L., Gao, R., Xu, J., Jin, L., Cotrim, AP., Yan, X., Zheng, C., Goldsmith, CM., Shan, Z., Hai, B., Zhou, J., Zhang, C., Baum, BJ., Wang, S. AdLTR2EF1α-FGF2-mediated prevention of fractionated irradiation-induced salivary hypofunction in swine. Gene Ther. **2014**, 21, 866-873.

[119] Song, G., Ouyang, G., Bao, S. The activation of Akt/PKB signaling pathway and cell survival. J. Cell. Mol. Med. **2005**, *9*, 59-71.

[120] Wang, J.F., Liu, C., Zhang, Q., Huang, G.H. Research progress in the radioprotective effect of the canonical Wnt pathway. Cancer Biol. Med. **2013**, *10*, 61-71, doi:10.7497/j.issn.2095-3941.2013.02.001.

[121] Vidya Priyadarsini, R., Senthil Murugan, R., Nagini, S. Aberrant activation of Wnt/β-catenin signaling pathway contributes to the sequential progression of DMBA-induced HBP carcinomas. Oral Oncol. **2012**, *48*, 33-39, doi:10.1016/j.oraloncology.2011.08.008.

[122] Huang, J.;Qu, Q., Guo, Y., Xiang, Y., Feng, D. Tankyrases/β-catenin Signaling Pathway as an

Anti-proliferation and Anti-metastatic Target in Hepatocarcinoma Cell Lines. J Cancer **2020**, *11*, 432-440. doi: 10.7150/jca.30976.

[123] Orme, M. H., Giannini, A. L., Vivanco, M. D., Kypta, R. M. Glycogen synthase kinase-3 and Axin function in a beta-catenin-independent pathway that regulates neurite outgrowth in neuroblastoma cells. Mol. Cell. Neurosci. **2003**, *24*, 673-686.

[124] Garan, A., Akyüz, S., Oztürk, L. K., Yarat, A. Salivary parameters and caries indices in children with black tooth stains. J. Clin. Pediatr. Dent. **2012**, *36*, 285-288.

[125] Nusse, R., Clevers, H. Wnt/β-Catenin Signaling, Disease, and Emerging Therapeutic Modalities. Cell **2017**, *169*, 985-999, doi:10.1016/j.cell.2017.05.016.

[126] Huang, H., He, X. Wnt/beta-catenin signaling: new (and old) players and new insights. Curr. Opin. Cell Biol. **2008**, *20*, 119-125, doi:10.1016/j.ceb.2008.01.009.

[127] Doble, B. W., Woodgett, J. R. GSK-3: tricks of the trade for a multi-tasking kinase. J. Cell Sci. **2003**, *116*, 1175-1186.

[128] Cross, D. A., Alessi, D. R., Cohen, P., Andjelkovich, M., Hemmings, B. A. Inhibition of glycogen synthase kinase-3 by insulin mediated by protein kinase B. Nature **1995,** *378*, 785-789, doi:10.1038/378785a0.

[129] Krasilnikov, M. A. Phosphatidylinositol-3 kinase dependent pathways: the role in control of cell growth, survival, and malignant transformation. Biochemistry. (Mosc). **2000**, *65*, 59-67.

[130] Huang, L., Fu, L. Mechanisms of resistance to EGFR tyrosine kinase inhibitors. Acta Pharm. Sin. B **2015**, *5*, 390-401, doi:10.1016/j.apsb.2015.07.001.

[131] Torres, M. A., Eldar-Finkelman, H., Krebs, E. G., Moon, R. T. Regulation of ribosomal S6 protein kinase-p90(rsk), glycogen synthase kinase 3, and beta-catenin in early Xenopus development. Mol. Cell. Biol. **1999**, *19*, 1427-1437.

[132] Dailey, L., Ambrosetti, D., Mansukhani, A., Basilico, C. Mechanisms underlying differential responses to FGF signaling. Cytokine Growth Factor Rev. **2005**, *16*, 233-247, doi:10.1016/j.cytogfr.2005.01.007.

[133] Alcaraz, E., Vilardell , J., Borgo, C., Sarró, E., Plana, M., Marin, O., Pinna, L.A., Bayascas, J.R., Meseguer, A., Salvi, M., Itarte, E., Ruzzene, F. Effects of CK2β subunit down-regulation on Akt signalling in HK-2 renal cells. PLoS One **2020**. doi: https://doi.org/10.1371/journal.pone.0227340.

[134] Kennedy, S. G., Wagner, A. J., Conzen, S. D., Jordán, J., Bellacosa, A., Tsichlis, P. N., Hay, N. The PI 3-kinase/Akt signaling pathway delivers an anti-apoptotic signal. Genes Dev. **1997**, *11*, 701-713.

[135] Hakim, S. G., Ribbat, J., Berndt, A., Richter, P., Kosmehl, H., Benedek, G. A., Jacobsen, H. C., Trenkle, T., Sieg, P., Rades, D. Expression of Wnt-1, TGF-β and related cell-cell adhesion components following radiotherapy in salivary glands of patients with manifested radiogenic xerostomia. Radiother. Oncol. **2011**, *101*, 93-99, doi:10.1016/j.radonc.2011.07.032.

[136] Hai, B., Yang, Z., Shangguan, L., Zhao, Y., Boyer, A., Liu, F. Concurrent transient activation of Wnt/β-catenin pathway prevents radiation damage to salivary glands. Int. J. Radiat. Oncol. Biol. Phys. **2012**, *83*, e109–e116, doi:10.1016/j.ijrobp.2011.11.062.

[137] Haidar, Z.S. Bio-Inspired/-Functional Colloidal Core-Shell Polymeric-Based NanoSystems: Technology Promise in Tissue Engineering, Bioimaging and NanoMedicine. Polymers 2010, 2, 323-352. https://doi.org/10.3390/polym2030323.

[138] Riley, P., Glenny, A.M., Hua, F., Worthington, H.V. Pharmacological interventions for preventing dry mouth and salivary gland dysfunction following radiotherapy. Cochrane Database of Systematic Reviews **2017**, *7*. doi: 10.1002/14651858.CD012744.

[139] Ocampo, J., Vásquez, B., Sandoval, C., Navarrete, J., Haidar, Z.S., Olate, S. Características Morfocuantitativas de la Glándula Submandibular de Ratón (Mus musculus)/ Morphocuantitative Characteristics of the Mouse (Mus musculus) Submandibular Gland. International Journal of Morphology **2020**, 38, 570-577. https://dx.doi.org/10.4067/S0717-95022020000300570.

[140] Ocampo, J., Olate, S., Haidar, Z.S., Vásquez, B. Hiposialia y Xerostomía Post Irradiación: Terapias Innovadoras en el Campo Biomolecular/ Hyposialia and Xerostomy Post Irradiation: Innovative Therapies in the Biomolecular Field. International Journal of Morphology **2019**, 37, 1564-1571. https://dx.doi.org/10.4067/S0717-95022019000401564.